More information about this series at http://www.springer.com/series/1114

Vimla L. Patel • Thomas G. Kannampallil
David R. Kaufman

Editors

Cognitive Informatics for Biomedicine

Human Computer Interaction in Healthcare

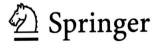 Springer

Editors
Vimla L. Patel
Center for Cognitive Studies
  in Medicine and Public Health
The New York Academy of Medicine
New York, NY, USA

Columbia University
Weill Cornell College of Medicine
New York, NY, USA

Arizona State University
Scottsdale, AZ, USA

David R. Kaufman
Arizona State University
Scottsdale, AZ, USA

Thomas G. Kannampallil
University of Illinois at Chicago
Chicago, IL, USA

The New York Academy of Medicine
New York, NY, USA

ISSN 1431-1917   ISSN 2197-3741 (electronic)
Health Informatics
ISBN 978-3-319-17271-2   ISBN 978-3-319-17272-9 (eBook)
DOI 10.1007/978-3-319-17272-9

Library of Congress Control Number: 2015947140

Springer Cham Heidelberg New York Dordrecht London

Springer International Publishing AG Switzerland is part of Springer Science+Business Media (www.springer.com)

To John T Bruer

For his 30-year commitment to research on medical cognition and for the resulting impact of his vision and support

Foreword

When I was first introduced to computing (in university, not on my parents' laps the way it happens today), the notion of interface design was pretty much irrelevant. Initially (1966) I wrote my programs on paper and then translated them onto punch cards that were run through mainframe computers in batch mode. A direct interface with the computer did not actually occur. Within a few years, I was able to type code into minicomputers using teletype machines—all upper case, noisy, and certainly not mobile. The results of a program then came back as text on the same teletype. And, a few years after that, we had moved on to the use of video display terminals, although the screens still displayed only ascii characters and efforts to draw pictures were achieved solely by using keyboard characters aligned above or adjacent to others to suggest an image of some sort.

I moved in the early 1970s to what would soon become known as Silicon Valley, and there (as a Stanford medical student and computer science graduate student) I was exposed to remarkably inventive activities at Stanford Research Institute (now known simply as SRI International). Developed in their Artificial Intelligence Center, "Shakey the robot" was demonstrating whole new ways to interact with computing devices (this computer-on-wheels had "sensory" inputs, could solve problems, and then would perform their solution by moving in a room with a platform and pushing objects up or down ramps as required).[1] A few years earlier, SRI scientist Doug Engelbart had developed a new way to interact with characters and activities on a display screen utilizing a manual device that rolled on a desktop and used a button to make selections—a creation that he wistfully called a "mouse" because of the wire "tail" that emerged from it to connect to the display device.[2] But most of us were still using keyboards for all our work, depending on paper printouts to review our programs and their results (initially produced on large line printers, next on portable thermal paper devices, and then on early laser printers).

---

[1] http://en.wikipedia.org/wiki/Shakey_the_robot (Accessed November 29, 2014).

[2] http://www.dougengelbart.org/firsts/mouse.html (Accessed November 29, 2014).

Nearby SRI was Xerox's Palo Alto Research Center, known simply as Xerox PARC, and we at Stanford had close interactions with many of the creative developers there. By 1973 we had been exposed to their work on the Xerox Alto, the first computer to use a desktop metaphor and incorporating a mouse pointing device of the sort that Engelbart had invented at SRI.[3] And, by the end of that decade, two other key innovations were unveiled: (1) the introduction of commercial microcomputers (notably the Apple II, first presented to the public in April 1977,[4] and the first IBM PC, which did not appear until four years later[5]) and (2) the introduction of local networking in the form of Ethernet technology, developed by Bob Metcalfe at Xerox PARC and then spun off into a company called 3Com in 1979.[6]

But even at the end of that decade, most of us were still using character-based devices without graphical capabilities, and our access to networks was limited to the wide-area technology of the ARPANET.[7] I do not remember any discussions of interface design or human-computer interaction during the 1970s, although pertinent notions were beginning to develop, mostly at Xerox PARC in light of their Alto experience. Everything changed in the following decade. Xerox did introduce commercial products based on its Alto work (an office document management system known as the Star[8] and a set of machines that were designed to support work coded in the Lisp programming language[9]), but their innovations had led to expensive special-purpose machines and failed to succeed in the marketplace (Smith 1999). The 1983 introduction of the Apple Lisa[10] (a personal computer with a graphical user interface, icons, and mouse pointing device), followed a year later by a less expensive and commercially successful successor, the Apple Macintosh,[11] changed computing (and human-computer interaction) in key ways. Before long the notion of a computer "desktop" became standard, with icons, files, folders, and images. It was in this context that it became clear that programmers needed to understand their intended users and to design systems that would be intuitive, usable, and well matched with the user's needs and assumptions.

I have summarized this history here because I fear that we too often forget that our remarkable advances in computing and communications happened gradually, with key early insights and inventions that led incrementally to the interconnected world of ubiquitous computing that we expect and accept today. The same is true of our knowledge of human-computer interaction, which began as a subject of study

---

[3] http://en.wikipedia.org/wiki/Xerox_Alto (Accessed November 29, 2014).

[4] http://en.wikipedia.org/wiki/History_of_Apple_Inc.#Apple_II (Accessed November 29, 2014).

[5] http://www-03.ibm.com/ibm/history/exhibits/pc25/pc25_birth.html (Accessed November 29, 2014).

[6] http://standards.ieee.org/events/ethernet/history.html (Accessed November 29, 2014).

[7] http://en.wikipedia.org/wiki/ARPANET (Accessed November 29, 2014).

[8] http://en.wikipedia.org/wiki/Xerox_Star (Accessed November 29, 2014).

[9] http://en.wikipedia.org/wiki/Lisp_machine (Accessed November 29, 2014).

[10] http://oldcomputers.net/lisa.html (Accessed November 29, 2014).

[11] http://apple-history.com/128k (Accessed November 29, 2014).

(as I have stressed) decades after we first began to work with early computing devices. Most of us began with highly intuitive notions of how a computer should interact with its users, and there were no courses or books to guide us. It was largely with the introduction of graphical user interfaces that notions of right and wrong ways to build interfaces began to emerge.

I was accordingly impressed, in 1980, when I encountered the first of Ben Shneiderman's books on psychological issues and human factors in the design of computer systems (Shneiderman 1980). This initial volume focused more on programming styles, team organization, and personality factors, but I was intrigued and impressed by the psychological emphasis and the notion that cognition was a crucial consideration in the design and construction of computing systems. It was his landmark book on user interface design, which appeared in its first edition in 1986, that ultimately persuaded me that there was an important set of scientific issues to be explored and that building the interface to a computer system should be based on theory and established principles rather than intuition. Now in its fifth edition, that book continues to be a classic volume for those interested in how to achieve effective human-computer interaction through principled interface design (Shneiderman et al. 2009).

As a physician and computer scientist who has watched biomedical informatics evolve from an exploratory discipline to a more mature field that feeds into a vibrant health information technology industry, I can identify poor human engineering as a key barrier to the successful fielding of computer systems for healthcare and biomedicine. Physicians and other health professionals, who too often despise or reject the systems they are asked to use, will almost always focus on problems with the interface design and performance: "confusing," "inefficient," "slow," "difficult to learn," "annoying," "condescending," "unusable," and many more similar characterizations. I accordingly applaud the effort to focus on human-computer interaction and usability in the design and implementation of clinical systems.

The best of intentions, and great cleverness in information and knowledge management, will come to naught if the systems that provide clinical functionalities are constructed without deep insight into the cognitive issues that affect the intended users. The growing field of cognitive informatics, with its focus on health and biomedicine as demonstrated in the current volume, is accordingly a crucial element in the evolution and success of the informatics field (Shortliffe 2013). As this book makes clear, there are core principles and theories that need to be understood, and a set of methods for exploring the cognitive processes of both users and system developers, that will determine the utility and success of the systems that are built for use in healthcare settings. Their importance cannot be overstated, and it will be crucially important for students of biomedical informatics to learn these skills and insights and to bring them to bear in future work. I applaud the efforts of Drs. Patel, Kannampallil, and Kaufman, and all the chapter authors, and commend this volume to all those who want to assure that the systems they build, and the interactive environments that they promote, will reflect the rigor and dedication to human-computer interaction principles that will ultimately enhance both the user's experience and the quality and safety of the care that we offer to patients.

Arizona State University   Edward H. Shortliffe, MD, PhD
Phoenix, Arizona
November 2014

References

Shneiderman, B. (1980). *Software psychology: Human factors in computer and information systems*. Winthrop Publishers. ISBN-13:978-0876268162.

Shneiderman, B., Plaisant, C., Cohen, M., & Jacobs, S. (2009). *Designing the user interface: Strategies for effective human-computer interaction*. Prentice Hall. ISBN-13:978-0321537355.

Shortliffe, E. H. (2013). Chapter 23: Reflections on the role of cognitive science in biomedical informatics. In V. L. Patel, D. Kaufman, & T. Cohen (Eds.), *Cognitive informatics in health and biomedicine: Case studies on critical care, complexity and errors* (pp. 467-475). London: Springer.

Smith, D. K., & Alexander, R. C. (1999). *Fumbling the future: How xerox invented, then ignored, the first personal computer*. iUniverse. ISBN-13:978–1583482667.

Preface

One might ask how it is that cognitive scientists have prepared a book that deals with a topic—human-computer interaction (HCI)—that has largely been the purview of computer scientists. Computer science is well represented in this volume, but the orientation of the discussion is distinctly from a cognitive perspective. Some background may be helpful in explaining how this cognitive focus on the medical realities of human-computer interaction evolved.

As I embarked on my investigations into the nature of cognitive complexity and error in medicine, I was aware of the pervasive role of computers and technology in high intensity settings such as emergency departments and intensive care units. However, my primary focus was on the role of cognition, and I did not initially appreciate the central role that technology would play in our discussions and, in turn, in our studies. Our six-year journey into these multi-site, team-based investigations showed us that technology could sometimes overwhelm or be taken for granted by clinical teams, occasionally exacerbating errors or leading to new ones. However, it also became clear that technology could play a major role in error mitigation, if human cognition and its interaction with the socio-cultural environment were seriously considered in the context of system design and use. Furthermore, it was evident that advances in technology could support data collection and analyses, as well as the modeling of human behavior, to help us make better predictions regarding the use and impact of patient-oriented decision tools, and thus the outcomes of care. In addition, new sensor-based techniques allowed us to track healthcare providers in naturalistic practice settings, observing unobtrusively how they worked in the context of clinical workflow. We leveraged these methods to capture real-world data in a more precise way (at one- or two-second intervals), and then used visualization methods to display and support the analysis in our laboratory, studying the subjects' 2-dimensional movement patterns within the clinical units.

During this time, we also saw a dramatic change in patient behavior, wherein patients increasingly came to the emergency room, or to see their personal physicians bringing pieces of paper with information that they had gathered from the

Internet. Similarly, an increase in the use of social media to seek and share health information became very apparent. We accordingly asked whether health information technology could help to mitigate errors by providing cognitive support to health care providers and patients, in part by facilitating the delivery of information and computer-supported care even in their homes, without generating unintended negative consequences. These are other questions about the effect of technology in shaping human behavior, especially in terms of how information is organized, retrieved and used safely, occupied our thoughts throughout the process.

Then, during the last few years, I became actively involved in teaching a course on *Human-Computer Interaction and Human Factors in Health Care*, offered to both biomedical informatics and computer science graduate students. We soon found that there were no books that covered this field in a coherent, systematic way, especially ones that offered a cognitive perspective that resonated with our view of the field. Most books failed to also offer no special insights or examples drawn from the healthcare environment. I have co-taught the class with my colleague David Kaufman, an educational and cognitive psychologist with an interest both in HCI and in medical applications. We were forced to use papers from various journals and books, covering HCI from the perspective of biomedical informatics, psychology, computer science, and engineering, as well as cognitive anthropology. I viewed HCI as a cognitive topic as much as a technical one and reached out to my colleague, Thomas Kannampallil, who has a background in computer science and cognition, as a logical person to work with me on a new HCI textbook that would take a cognitive perspective. We then extended our invitation to David Kaufman, who agreed to join us as a third co-editor. The next step was to outline the key topics to be included in the volume, after which we invited as chapter authors several well-known and respected people who offered pertinent expertise. Then, as we edited the contributed chapters, we continued to focus on cognitive themes, and particularly asked what these technologies and methods do to the human mind as well as how they facilitate effective completion of the tasks by users.

We were delighted that the chapter authors enthusiastically agreed to participate in this project. In fact, they embraced the idea, seeing the need for such a volume. The resulting book highlights the state of the art in HCI in health care and offers subject reviews, drawing from the current research in HCI and providing a graduate level textbook that is suitable for use in an introductory HCI course for biomedical informatics, cognitive science, computer science and social science students. Since many of the examples are drawn from medicine and health, the volume is particularly pertinent for biomedical informatics students, but our classroom experience has shown us that medical examples can be concrete motivating examples for students in computer science or other fields who may not have a long-term professional interest in working in the healthcare arena.

This work would not have been possible without dedicated support and collegial brainstorming with my colleagues and co-editors, Thomas and David. We spent many hours communicating and providing timely input to the authors. All chapters were reviewed by one of the editors and one additional reviewer. Cindy Guan, from the *Center for Cognitive Studies in Medicine and Public Health* at The New York Academy of Medicine, provided much needed support in editing and keeping track of the chapter processing efforts. We are also grateful to the Center's advisory board members (Bill Clancey, Alan Lesgold, Randy Miller, Michael Shabot, and Ted Shortliffe), who shaped our thoughts about the book while offering advice and guidance regarding the role of technology in mitigating errors as well as in providing cognitive support. I offer my very special thanks to John Bruer, President of the James S. McDonnell Foundation, who supported the work of our Center, and much of our work to put together this volume. Without his vision and commitment regarding the importance of cognition and education in biomedicine and health, much of the work we have done, including this and our previous books on cognitive complexity and error in critical care and ER, and on cognitive science in medicine: biomedical modeling, would not have been possible. I am indebted to him for his support, and for facilitating this wonderful and fruitful journey that I have enjoyed with my colleagues for more than a decade.

New York, NY, USA   Vimla L. Patel, PhD, DSc
Scottsdale, AZ, USA
April 2015

Contents

Editors and Contributors

Editors

Vimla L. Patel Center for Cognitive Studies in Medicine and Public Health, The New York Academy of Medicine, New York, NY, USA

Columbia University, Weill Cornell Medical College, New York, NY, USA

Arizona State University, Scottsdale, AZ, USA

Thomas G. Kannampallil University of Illinois at Chicago, Chicago, IL, USA

The New York Academy of Medicine, New York, NY, USA

David R. Kaufman Arizona State University, Scottsdale, AZ, USA

Contributors

Joanna Abraham Department of Biomedical and Health Information Sciences, College of Applied Health Sciences, University of Illinois at Chicago, Chicago, IL, USA

Zia Agha Department of Medicine, School of Medicine, University of California, San Diego, La Jolla, CA, USA

West Health Institute, La Jolla, CA, USA

Suresh K. Bhavnani Institute for Translational Sciences, University of Texas Medical Branch, Galveston, TX, USA

Elizabeth Borycki School of Health Information Science, University of Victoria, Victoria, BC, Canada

Yunan Chen Department of Informatics, University of California, Irvine, Irvine, CA, USA

J. Franck Diaz-Garelli School of Biomedical Informatics, University of Texas Health Science Center at Houston, Houston, TX, USA

Karen Dunn Lopez Department of Health Systems Science, College of Nursing, University of Illinois at Chicago, Chicago, IL, USA

Amy Franklin School of Biomedical Informatics, University of Texas Health Science Center at Houston, Houston, TX, USA

Paul N. Gorman Department of Medical Informatics and Clinical Epidemiology, Oregon Health & Science University, Portland, OR, USA

David A. Hanauer Department of Pediatrics, University of Michigan Medical School, Ann Arbor, MI, USA

School of Information, University of Michigan, Ann Arbor, MI, USA

Holly B. Jimison College of Computer and Information Science and College of Health Sciences, Northeastern University, Boston, MA, USA

Todd R. Johnson School of Biomedical Informatics, University of Texas Health Science Center at Houston, Houston, TX, USA

Elsbeth Kalenderian Department of Oral Health Policy and Epidemiology, Harvard School of Dental Medicine, Boston, MA, USA

Joseph Kannry Icahn School of Medicine at Mount Sinai, New York, NY, USA

Peter Killoran School of Biomedical Informatics, University of Texas Health Science Center at Houston, Houston, TX, USA

Andre Kushniruk School of Health Information Science, University of Victoria, Victoria, BC, Canada

Albert M. Lai Department of Biomedical Informatics, The Ohio State University, Columbus, OH, USA

Kristin Mainello College of Computer and Information Science and College of Health Sciences, Northeastern University, Boston, MA, USA

Helen Monkman School of Health Information Science, University of Victoria, Victoria, BC, Canada

Daniel G. Morrow Department of Educational Psychology, University of Illinois at Urbana-Champaign, Champaign, IL, USA

Andrea Parker College of Computer and Information Science and College of Health Sciences, Northeastern University, Boston, MA, USA

Misha Pavel College of Computer and Information Science and College of Health Sciences, Northeastern University, Boston, MA, USA

Rachel Ramoni Oral Health Policy and Epidemiology, Harvard School of Dental Medicine, Boston, MA, USA

Center for Biomedical Informatics, Harvard Medical School, Boston, MA, USA

Katie A. Siek School of Informatics and Computing, Indiana University, Bloomington, IN, USA

Hardeep Singh Houston VA HSR&D Center for Innovations in Quality, Effectiveness and Safety (IQuESt), The Michael E. Debakey Veterans Affairs Medical Center and the Section of Health Services Research, Department of Medicine, Baylor College of Medicine, Houston, TX, USA

Dean F. Sittig The UT-Memorial Hermann Center for Healthcare Quality & Safety, University of Texas School of Biomedical Informatics at Houston, Houston, TX, USA

Charlotte Tang Department of Computer Science, Engineering and Physics, University of Michigan-Flint, Flint, MI, USA

Harold Thimbleby Department of Computer Science, Swansea University, Swansea, Wales, UK

Muhammad Walji Department of Diagnostic and Biomedical Sciences, School of Dentistry, University of Texas Health Science Center at Houston, Houston, TX, USA

Nadir Weibel Department of Computer Science and Engineering, Jacobs School of Engineering, University of California, San Diego, La Jolla, CA, USA

Veteran Affairs Medical Research Foundation, HSRD VA San Diego Healthcare System, San Diego, CA, USA

Yan Xiao Human Factors & Patient Safety Science, Baylor Scott & White Health, Dallas, TX, USA

Kai Zheng Department of Health Management and Policy, School of Public Health, University of Michigan, Ann Arbor, MI, USA

School of Information, University of Michigan, Ann Arbor, MI, USA

Chapter 1
A Multi-disciplinary Science of Human Computer Interaction in Biomedical Informatics

Vimla L. Patel, Thomas G. Kannampallil, and David R. Kaufman

1.1 Human Computer Interaction in Healthcare

Modern healthcare relies on a connected, integrated and sophisticated backbone of health information technology (HIT). Clinicians rely on HIT (e.g., electronic health records, EHRs) to deliver safe patient care. As has been extensively documented in recent research literature, HIT use is fraught with numerous challenges, some of which compromise patient safety (Koppel et al. 2005; Horsky et al. 2005; IOM 2011). Usability and more specifically, workflow, data integration and data presentation are among the principal pain points identified by clinicians in a recent HIMSS survey (2010). These issues are the subject of a growing body of applied research in human-computer interaction (HCI) and allied disciplines.

HCI is an interdisciplinary science at the intersection of social and behavioral sciences, and computer and information technology. Drawing from the fields of psychology, computer and social sciences, HCI is concerned with understanding

V.L. Patel (✉)
Center for Cognitive Studies in Medicine and Public Health, The New York Academy of Medicine, 1216 Fifth Avenue, New York, NY 10029, USA

Columbia University, Weill Cornell College of Medicine, New York, NY, USA

Arizona State University, Scottsdale, AZ, USA
e-mail: vpatel@nyam.org

T.G. Kannampallil
University of Illinois at Chicago, Chicago, IL, USA

The New York Academy of Medicine, New York, NY, USA
e-mail: tgk2@uic.edu

D.R. Kaufman
Arizona State University, Scottsdale, AZ, USA
e-mail: David.Kaufman.1@asu.edu

© Springer International Publishing Switzerland 2015
V.L. Patel et al. (eds.), *Cognitive Informatics for Biomedicine*, Health Informatics,
DOI 10.1007/978-3-319-17272-9_1

1

how people interact with devices and systems, and how to make these interactions more useful and usable (Carroll 2003).

HCI research was originally spurred by the advent of personal computers in the early 1980s. HCI developed as an applied science, drawing heavily on software psychology, to enhance the design and evaluation of human-computer interfaces (Shneiderman 1992). With early work rooted in modeling human performance and efficiency of using interfaces (Card et al. 1983), HCI has been transformed by developments in technology and software. HCI also became both a focal area of inquiry and application for cognitive science, and a fertile test bed for evaluating cognitive theories.

With advances in computing and technology, HCI research has greatly expanded, spawning several research genres: computer supported cooperative work (CSCW), mobile and ubiquitous computing (UbiComp), and intelligent user interfaces (IUI). While early work on HCI drew heavily on theories and empirical research in cognitive psychology (e.g., research on memory, perception and motor skills), and human factors to explain and improve human interactions with machines, the advent of personal computers transformed the field. Grudin (2012) provides a comprehensive history and development of HCI. The transformation and development of HCI as a field had a profound impact in healthcare as it did in other professional sectors. An extended history is beyond the scope of this chapter. However, we provide a brief synopsis as an entry-point to discuss HCI in the context of healthcare.

HCI research in healthcare has paralleled the theoretical and methodological developments in the field beginning with cognitive evaluations of electronic medical records in the mid-1990s (Kushniruk et al. 1996), extending to a focus on distributed health information systems (Horsky et al. 2003; Hazlehurst et al. 2007) and analysis of unintended sociotechnical consequences of computerized provider order entry systems (Koppel et al. 2005). HCI work in biomedicine extends across clinical and consumer health informatics, addressing a range of user populations including providers, biomedical scientists and patients. While the implications of HCI principles for the design of HIT are acknowledged, the adoption of the tools and techniques among clinicians, informatics researchers and developers of HIT are limited. There is a general consensus that HIT has not realized its potential as a tool that facilitates clinical decision-making, coordination of care, and improvement of patient safety (Middleton et al. 2013; IOM 2011; Schumacher and Lowry 2010). For interested readers, a recent chapter by Patel and Kaufman (2014) provides a detailed discussion on the relationship between HCI and biomedical informatics.

Theories and methods in HCI continue to evolve to better meet the needs of evaluating systems. For example, classical cognitive or symbolic information processing theory viewed mental representations as mediating all activity (Card et al. 1983). Although methods and theories emerging from the classical cognitive approach continue to be useful and productive, they are limited in their characterization of interactivity or of team/group activities. In more contemporary theories of HCI, such as distributed cognition, cognition is viewed as the process of coordinating internal (mental states) and external representations. The scope has broadened to include external mediators of cognition including artifacts and is also seen as stretched across social agents (e.g., a clinical care team). The socio-technical approach has further expanded the focus of HCI research to include a range of social and organizational factors that influence the productive use and acceptance of technology (Berg 1999).

The scope of HCI in biomedicine and healthcare is currently very broad encompassing thousands of journal articles across medical disciplines and con-sumer health domains. Although the 14 chapters in this volume cover considerable terrain, it would not be possible to cover the full range of research and application of HCI in biomedicine and healthcare. In general, there is a strong focus in this volume on issues in clinical informatics. The chapters by Jimison and colleagues on consumer health informatics (Chap. 12), and by Lai and Siek (Chap. 13) on mobile health are notable exceptions.

Human factors and HCI are sister disciplines and share many of the same methods and foci. Although they remain distinct disciplines, the boundaries of research have become increasingly blurred, often using similar theories and methods (Patel and Kannampallil 2014). In addition, patient safety and clinical workflow are focal topics in applied human factors in healthcare. However, we elected not to specifically cover human factors research because of its immense scope. The handbook edited by Carayon and colleagues (2012) provides excellent coverage (in the 50+ chapters) of this important field. Pervasive computing in healthcare is a burgeoning cutting-edge field of growing importance (Orwat et al. 2008), but is only briefly addressed in a couple of chapters. Similarly, HCI and global health informatics is an important emerging field of research (Chan and Kaufman 2010), but is not dealt with in this volume. Finally, our focus is predom-inantly on evaluation of HIT in the modern healthcare environment rather than the design (or design approaches) for HIT. Although the chapters in this volume embrace a range of theoretical perspectives, it should be noted that this is part of the Cognitive Informatics series and the frameworks are somewhat skewed toward the cognitive rather than the social perspectives. The omissions in this text leave room for future volumes that will encompass some of these other fields.

1.2 Scope and Purpose of the Book

The objective of this book is to provide a pedagogical description of HCI within the context of healthcare settings and HIT. Although there is a growing awareness of the importance of HCI in biomedical informatics, there is limited training at the graduate level in HCI for biomedical informatics (BMI) students. An informal review of the curriculum of graduate programs led us to the conclusion that fewer than 25 % of the US-based BMI programs had any course in HCI or related topics. Part of the reason for this, we believe, is the relative inaccessibility of advanced level graduate materials for students. While there are considerable original mate-rials in the form of journal and conference articles, these are idiosyncratic in their coverage of issues and demand greater understanding of cognitive and informatics-related issues. Our purpose with this book is to provide an aggregated source of a collection of HCI topics that are relevant to BMI students and researchers. The role of HCI in the biomedical informatics curriculum is reflected in the presence of HCI-related courses in some academic graduate programs and in the growing number of research programs. Most courses are taught with a combination of research papers, general HCI textbooks with minimal focus on HIT, and instructor prepared material. Within this scope, we have identified a set of topics – both from a classical HCI perspective and others from an applied HCI in BMI focus. These chapters, as we acknowledged above, do not provide comprehensive coverage of all HCI topics. However, the selected topics represent a mix of topics that coalesces the past with the future of HCI.

1.3   Organization of Chapters

The book is organized in the following manner: the early Chaps. (2, 3, 4, 5, and 6) focus on the theoretical and methodological basis of HCI. The major themes covered include cognition, communication, socio-technical considerations, and evaluation methods for research. Chapters 7, 8, 9, 10, and 11 describe the application of HCI methods and theories to address several key issues including usability and user-centered design, team activities, and unintended consequences of technology use. The last three Chaps. (12, 13, and 14) describe recent trends in consumer health informatics, mobile computing in health, and visualization approaches. The themes that are addressed in the various chapters have been selected with the purpose of addressing specific biomedical informatics challenges related to HIT (and consumer health tools) evaluation. As a result, key topics that are often covered in HCI books, such as motor and visual/perceptual theories, have not been discussed. We have also followed a specific structure: each chapter includes a description of the key HCI problem and its relevance to biomedical informatics, detailed examples where applicable (in some chapters, explicit case studies), a set of discussion questions and additional follow up readings for interested readers. A brief overview of each of the chapters is provided below.

As previously described, HCI has its original roots in psychology, and more specifically in cognitive science. In Chap. 2, Kaufman, Kannampallil and Patel describe these cognitive foundations within the context of biomedicine and healthcare. Cognitive theories relevant to HCI including human information processing, interactive environments, mental models, role of external representation in HCI, and distributed cognition are described. In Chap. 3, Morrow and Dunn-Lopez describe the information processing and interactive approaches to communication, focusing on how these can be used to improve communication effectiveness, leading to more efficient work activities, collaboration and patient safety. In the following chapter, Sittig and Singh describe a socio-technical model for HIT evaluation. They describe an 8-dimensional socio-technical model and illustrate its application for HIT development and implementation.

In Chap. 5, Kannampallil and Abraham discuss the various methods for evaluating HIT. Methods of evaluation that encompass issues of HCI and those from a more contextual and situated perspectives are described, including the appropriateness of each method in various evaluation contexts. In contrast to the traditional methods described in Chap. 5, Zheng and colleagues discuss in Chap. 6 a new family of HCI methods called "computational ethnography." Computational ethnography relies on digital trace data available in healthcare environments to characterize human-computer interactions. Examples of such data include audit logs, motion capture, and Radio Frequency Identification (RFID). Examples from various clinical situations are used to illustrate how these methods have been applied in healthcare to study end users' interactions with technological interventions.

In Chap. 7, Kushniruk and colleagues discuss the importance of user-centered design (UCD) in improving the usability of clinical systems. A range of approaches including the use of laboratory style usability testing to the use of clinical simulations conducted in real-world clinical settings are described. The authors also introduce new approaches to low-cost rapid usability engineering methods that can be applied throughout the design and implementation cycle of clinical information systems. Johnson and colleagues in Chap. 8 provide an alternative perspective on the interaction challenges with medical devices—an almost ubiquitous component of clinical environments. They discuss the challenges of developing medical device interfaces as a function of the interplay between the complexities of the clinical environment, users of medical devices and device constraints. Regulatory considerations and their impact on medical devices interactions are also described.

In Chap. 9, Kalenderian, Walji and Ramoni provide an example of the application of HCI evaluation methods in the re-design of a dental EHR interface. In addition to showing how these principles can be applied for the design of dental EHRs, they describe the importance of participatory design process for the design and development of usable HIT. The case study example provides further context for the methods described in Chap. 5. Tang and colleagues (Chap. 10) characterize the role of team activities and teamwork in modern healthcare practice. They discuss how team composition and interactions create significant challenges for maintaining seamless team activities in clinical settings. They draw on socio-technical systems theory to illustrate how team activities are situated within the context of HIT use. Case studies from the field are used to further exemplify the nuances of team activities and interactions in complex clinical settings.

In Chap. 11, Franklin provides an overview of the nature and types of unintended consequences of the use of HIT in clinical environments—both its positive serendipitous results, as well as negative, unintended, and potentially harmful consequences of technology. A review of different classification systems for studying the unanticipated effects of HIT, especially EHR and CPOE use, is considered with several examples from research.

In Chap. 12, Jimison and colleagues illustrate the challenges of designing healthcare solutions for consumers. They detail the issues of varying cultural backgrounds, levels of literacy and access that cause considerable challenges in design. The authors review these issues and describe the role of participatory user-centered design for developing safe and usable consumer health tools.

Recent advances have spurred the widespread adoption and use of mobile devices in healthcare settings. In Chap. 13, Lai and Siek examine the use of mobile devices in healthcare both among consumers (e.g., patients) and clinicians, including design considerations, requirements and challenges of its use. Modern wearable devices, such as smart watches and Google Glass, and their potential applications within healthcare settings are also considered. Finally, in Chap. 14, Bhavnani introduces the relatively new domain of biomedical visualization, specifically focusing on how visualization approaches can amplify our ability to analyze large and complex data. Using examples from network analysis, the significant power of visualization for data analysis and interpretation is demonstrated, from a scientific and translational perspective. Opportunities for visualization in biomedical informatics, available tools, and the challenges of biomedical visualization are also described.

1.4 Future Directions for HCI in Healthcare

The range of users of HIT including clinicians, biomedical researchers, health consumers and patients continue to expand, as does the range of functions supported by HIT. The challenges of supporting these populations are well known. HCI methods of evaluation and iterative design will play an increasingly pivotal role (Kushniruk et al., Chap. 7). The approaches encompass tried and tested methods that continue to yield valuable insight into system usability, and related matters such as learning, adoption and training. The approaches also include cutting-edge methodologies including computational ethnography (Zheng et al., Chap. 6), which continue to broaden the scope of applied HCI, and to ask questions about workflow and related matters that were not previously possible. There is no doubt that the fields of mHealth (mobile Health) and pervasive computing will continue to push the envelope on creating new worlds in HIT. HCI methods will have to continue to advance to play a productive role and meet the new demands realized by these developments.

We see future research as having a greater focus on the role of HIT and safe design of the healthcare workplace, including its involvement in patient safety. Although it has been shown that HIT has significant potential to improve safety, it must be acknowledged that it can also cause harm. One of our future challenges will be to ensure that we include both the private and public sectors in our efforts to understand the risks associated with HIT, including development of standards and criteria for safe design and implementation. The role of HCI in engendering such a change in HIT design and development cannot be overstated.

References

Berg, M. (1999). Patient care information systems and health care work: A sociotechnical approach. *International Journal of Medical Informatics, 55*(2), 87–101.

Carayon, P., Alyousef, B., & Xie, A. (2012). Human factors and ergonomics in health care. In G. Salvendy (Ed.), *Handbook of human factors and ergonomics* (4th ed., pp. 1574–1595). Hoboken: Wiley.

Card, S. K., Newell, A., & Moran, T. P. (1983). *The psychology of human-computer interaction.* Hillsdale: Erlbaum Associates.

Carroll, J. M. (Ed.). (2003). *HCI models, theories, and frameworks: Toward a multidisciplinary science.* San Francisco: Morgan Kaufmann.

Chan, C. V., & Kaufman, D. R. (2010). A technology selection framework for supporting delivery of patient-oriented health interventions in developing countries. *Journal of Biomedical Informatics, 43*(2), 300–306.

Grudin, J. (2012). A moving target: The evolution of human-computer interaction. In J.A. Jacko (Ed.), *The human-computer interaction handbook–fundamentals, evolving technologies, and emerging applications* (2nd ed., pp. 1–24). CRC Press.

Horsky, J., Kaufman, D. R., Oppenheim, M. I., & Patel, V. L. (2003). A framework for analyzing the cognitive complexity of computer-assisted clinical ordering. *Journal of Biomedical Informatics, 36*(1), 4–22.

Hazlehurst, B., McMullen, C. K., & Gorman, P. N. (2007). Distributed cognition in the heart room: How situation awareness arises from coordinated communications during cardiac surgery. *Journal of Biomedical Informatics, 40*(5), 539–551.

HIMMS EHR Usability Task Force – User Pain Points Group. (2010). *EHR usability pain points survey Q4-2009.* Available online at: http://www.himss.org/files/HIMSSorg/content/files/Usability_Pain_PointsHIMSS10.pdf

Horsky, J., Kuperman, G. J., & Patel, V. L. (2005). Comprehensive analysis of a medication dosing error related to CPOE. *Journal of the American Medical Informatics Association, 12*(4), 377–382.

Institute of Medicine (IOM). (2011). *Health IT and patient safety: Building safer systems for better care.* Washington, DC: Institute of Medicine.

Koppel, R., et al. (2005). Role of computerized physician order entry systems in facilitating medication errors. *JAMA, 293*(10), 1197–1203.

Kushniruk, A. W., et al. (1996). Assessment of a computerized patient record system: A cognitive approach to evaluating medical technology. *MD Computing, 13*(5), 406–415.

Middleton, B., et al. (2013). Enhancing patient safety and quality of care by improving the usability of electronic health record systems: Recommendations from AMIA. *Journal of the American Medical Informatics Association, 20*(e1), e2–e8.

Orwat, C., Graefe, A., & Faulwasser, T. (2008). Towards pervasive computing in health care – A literature review. *BMC Medical Informatics and Decision Making, 8*(1), 26.

Patel, V. L., & Kannampallil, T. G. (2014). Human factors in health information technology: Current challenges and future directions. *Yearbook of Medical Informatics, 9*(1), 58–66.

Patel, V. L., & Kaufman, D. R. (2014). Cognitive science and biomedical informatics. In E. H. Shortliffe & J. J. Cimino (Eds.), *Biomedical informatics: Computer applications in health care and biomedicine* (4th ed., pp. 133–185). New York: Springer.

Schumacher, R. M., & Lowry, S. Z. (2010). *NIST guide to the processes approach for improving the usability of electronic health records.* National Institute of Standards and Technology.

Shneiderman, B. (1992). *Designing the user interface: Strategies for effective human-computer interaction* (Vol. 2). Reading: Addison-Wesley.

Chapter 2
Cognition and Human Computer Interaction in Health and Biomedicine

David R. Kaufman, Thomas G. Kannampallil, and Vimla L. Patel

2.1 Introduction

Do we really need a theory of cognition? What advantages are conferred by a cognitive theory or a collection of theories? How can cognitive theory advance our knowledge as it pertains to the design and use of health information technology? The past 30 years have produced a cumulative body of experiential and practical knowledge about user experience, system design and implementation that provide insights to guide further work. This practical knowledge embodies the need for sensible and intuitive user interfaces, an understanding of workflow, and the ways in which systems impact individual and team performance (Patel and Kaufman 2014). Human-computer interaction (HCI) in health care and other domains are at least partly an empirical science where the growing knowledge base can be leveraged as needed. However, practical or empirical knowledge, for example, in the form of case studies is inadequate for producing robust generalizations, or sound design and implementation principles.

D.R. Kaufman (✉)
Arizona State University, Scottsdale, AZ, USA
e-mail: David.Kaufman.1@asu.edu

T.G. Kannampallil
University of Illinois at Chicago, Chicago, IL, USA

The New York Academy of Medicine, New York, NY, USA
e-mail: tgk2@uic.edu

V.L. Patel
Center for Cognitive Studies in Medicine and Public Health, The New York Academy of Medicine, 1216 Fifth Avenue, New York, NY 10029, USA

Columbia University, Weill Cornell College of Medicine, New York, NY, USA

Arizona State University, Scottsdale, AZ, USA
e-mail: vpatel@nyam.org

© Springer International Publishing Switzerland 2015
V.L. Patel et al. (eds.), *Cognitive Informatics for Biomedicine*, Health Informatics,
DOI 10.1007/978-3-319-17272-9_2

We argue that there is a need for a theoretical foundation. Of course, theory is a core part of any basic or applied science and is necessary to advance knowledge, to test hypotheses and to discern robust generalizations from the increasingly idiosyncratic field of endeavor.

Cognitive theory has been a central part of HCI since its inception. However, HCI has expanded greatly since its beginning as a discipline focused on a small subset of interactive tasks such as text editing, information retrieval and software programming (Grudin 2008). It is currently a flourishing area of inquiry that covers all manners of interactions with technology from smart phones to ticketing kiosks. Similarly, in health care, HCI research has focused on an enormous range of health information technologies from electronic health record (EHR) systems to consumer fitness devices such as the Fitbit™. In addition, technology is no longer the realm of the solo agent; rather, it is increasingly a team game. This has led to the adaptation of cognitive theories to HCI that stress the importance of the social and/or distributed nature of computing (Rogers 2004).

Rogers (2004, 2012) critiques the rapid pace of theory change. She argues "the paint has barely dried for one theory before a new coat is applied. It makes it difficult for anything to become established and widely used." Although we perceive this to be a legitimate criticism, we must acknowledge the extraordinary diversity in HCI subjects of inquiry. In addition, cognitive theories have endured; however, they have also evolved in response to new sets of circumstances such as the emphasis on real-world research in complex messy settings, on the role of artifacts as mediators of performance and on team cognition.

What role can theory play in HCI research and application? Bederson and Shneiderman (2003) categorize five types of theories that can inform HCI practice:

- Descriptive – providing concepts, terminology, methods and focusing further inquiry;
- Explanatory – elucidating relationships and processes (e.g., explaining why user performance on a given system is suboptimal);
- Predictive – enabling predictions to be made about user performance or of a given system (e.g., predicting increased accuracy or efficiency as a result of a new design);
- Prescriptive – providing guidance for design from high level principles to specific design solutions;
- Generative – seeding novel ideas for design including prototype development and new paradigms of interaction.

Cognitive theories have played an instrumental role in all five categories, although predicting performance across a spectrum of users (e.g., from novice to expert) remains a challenge. In addition, generative theories have begun to play a more central role in HCI design. Although theoretical frameworks such as ethnomethodology, activity theory and ecological psychology, to name a few, have made substantive contributions to the field, this chapter is focused primarily on cognitive theories including classical human information processing, external cognition and distributed cognition.

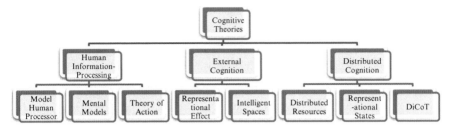

Fig. 2.1 Partial space of frameworks and cognitive theories

In this chapter, we take a historical approach in documenting the evolution of cognitive theories beginning with the early application of information-processing theories and exploring external as well as distributed cognition. Each of these constitutes a family of theories or a framework that embraces core principles, but differs in important respects. A framework is a general pool of constructs for understanding a domain, but it is not sufficiently cohesive or fully realized to constitute a theory (Anderson 1983). The field of HCI as applied to healthcare is remarkably broad in scope and the domain of medicine is characterized by immense complexity and diversity in both tasks and activities (Kannampallil et al. 2011). Specific HCI theories are often limited in scope especially as applied to a rich and complex knowledge domain. Patel and Groen (1992) make an analogous argument for the use of cognitive theories as applied to medical education. Frameworks can provide a theoretical rationale for innovative design concepts and serve to motivate HCI experiments. They can become further differentiated into theories that cover or emphasize a particular facet of interaction (e.g., analyzing teamwork) in the context of a broader framework (e.g., distributed cognition).

We provide a survey of these different theories and illustrate their application with case studies and examples, focusing mostly on issues pertaining to health technology, but also drawing on other domains. This chapter is not intended to be comprehensive or a critical look at the state of the art on HCI in health and biomedicine. Rather, it is written for a diverse audience including those who are new to cognitive science and cognitive psychology. The scope of this chapter is limited with a primary focus on cognitive theories, as they have been applied in healthcare contexts.

A partial space of cognitive theories, as reflected in the chapter, is illustrated in Fig. 2.1. As described, it isn't intended to be exhaustive. It's illustrative of how to conceptualize the theoretical frameworks. It should also be noted that the boundaries between frameworks are somewhat permeable. For example, external and distribute cognition frameworks are co-extensive. However, it serves the purpose of emphasizing the evolution of cognitive theories and highlight specific facets such as the effect of representations on cognition or the social coordination of computer-mediated work. Although the theories within a framework may differ on key issues, the primary difference is in their points of emphasis. In other words, they privilege some aspect as it pertains to cognition and interaction.

2.2 Human Information Processing

A computational theory of mind provides the fundamental underpinning for most contemporary cognitive theories. The basic premise is that much of human cognition can be characterized as a series of operations which reflect computations on mental representations. Early theories and models of human performance were often described in terms of the perceptual and motor activities and assumptions by their structural components (e.g., limits of short-term memory). These were primarily derived from the stimulus-response paradigm, and considered the human as an "information processor." In other words, within this paradigm the human was an information controller, perceiving and responding to activities (Anderson 2005). This approach led to the development of several commonly used models such as Fitts Law (Mackenzie 1992) and the theory of bimanual control (Mackenzie 2003) – that predict performance of human activities in a variety of tasks (e.g., task acquisition, flight controls, and air traffic control). Detailed descriptions of the use of these theories can be found in Chap. 5 of this volume.

With the advent of computers, and more recently significantly interactive environments, there was a need for more integrated information-processing models that accounted for the human-computer interaction (HCI). There were two important requirements: first, the models needed to account for the sequential and integrated actions that evolve during human-computer interactions; second, in addition to the layout and format of the interface, the models also needed to account for the content that was presented on the interfaces (John 2003). In its most general form, the human information processor consists of input, processing and output components (see Fig. 2.2). The input to the processor involves perception of stimuli from the external world; the input/stimuli would be processed by a processor and involves a series of processing stages. Typically, these stages include encoding of the

Fig. 2.2 Input-output model of human information processing. STM refers to short-term memory and LTM is an abbreviation for long-term memory

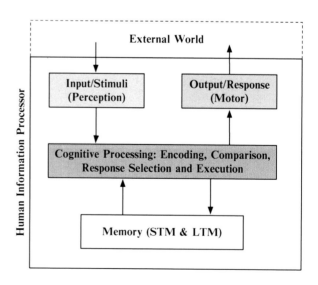

perceived stimuli, comparing and matching it to known mental representations in memory, and selection and execution of an appropriate response. The response is realized through motor actions. For example, consider a clinician's interaction with an EHR interface, where he/she has to select a medication from a dropdown menu. The input component would perceive the dropdown menu from the interface, which would be matched in memory and a click action response would be triggered. This click action would be relayed to the motor components (output), which executes the action by clicking the dropdown menu item. This cycle repeats till the entire task of selecting the medication is completed. In the next sections, we consider core constructs associated with this approach including the model human processor, Norman's theory of action, and mental models.

2.2.1 Model Human Processor

One of the earliest and most commonly described instantiations of a theoretical human information processing system is the Model Human Processor (MHP). MHP can be described as a set of processors, memories and their interactions that operate based on a set of principles (Card et al. 1983). As per MHP, the human mind consists of three interacting processors: perceptual, cognitive and motor. These processors can operate in serial (e.g., pressing a key) or in parallel (e.g., driving a car and listening to radio). Information processing of MHP occurs in cycles. First, the perceptual processor retrieves sensory (visual or audio) information from the external world and is transmitted to the working memory (WM). Once the information is in the WM, information is processed using a *recognize-act* cycle of cognitive processor. During each cycle, contents of WM are connected to actions that are linked to them (from long term memory). These actions, in turn, modify the contents of the WM resulting in a new cycle of actions. MHP can be used to develop an integrated description regarding the psychological effects of human computer interaction performance. While it is considered a significant oversimplification for general users (see applications of the MHP using the GOMS model in Chap. 5), it provided a preliminary mechanism on which much of the human performance modeling research was developed. MHP is useful to predict and compare different interface designs, task performance and learnability of user interfaces. It can be used to develop guidelines for interface design such as spatial layout, response rates and recall. It also provides a significant advantage, as these human performance measures can be determined even without a functional prototype or actual users.

Although the use of MHP approach has not commonly been applied in healthcare contexts, there have been a few noteworthy studies. For example, Saitwal et al. (2010) used the keystroke level model (KLM, an instantiation of the GOMS approach) to compute the time taken, and the number of steps required to complete a set of 14 EHR-based tasks. Using this approach, they characterized the challenges of the user interface and identified opportunities for improvement.

Detailed description of this study and the use of the GOMS approach can be found in Chap. 5.

2.2.2 Norman's Theory of Action

In the mid 1980s, cognitive science was beginning to flourish as a discipline and HCI was viewed as both a test bed for these theories and as a domain of practice. The MHP work was indicative of those efforts. At the same time, microcomputers were becoming increasingly common in homes, work and school. As a result, computers were transitioning from being a tool that was used by experts (i.e., computer scientists and those with high degrees of technical expertise) exclusively to one that was used broadly by individuals in all walks of life. Systems at that point in time were particularly unwieldy and often, extremely difficult to learn. In a seminal paper on cognitive engineering (Norman 1986), Norman sought to craft a theory "to understand the fundamental principles behind human action and performance that are relevant for the development of engineering principles of design" (p 32). A second objective was to devise systems that are "pleasant to use."

A critical insight of the theory is the discrepancy between psychologically expressed goals, and the physical controls and variables of a system. For example, a goal may be to scroll down towards the bottom of a document, and a scroll bar embodies the physical controls to realize such a goal. Shneiderman presented a similar analysis in his theory of direct manipulation (Shneiderman 1982). The key question is how an individual's goals and intentions get expressed as a set of physical actions that transform a virtual system and result in the desired change of state (e.g., reaching the intended section of the document). The Norman model draws on many of the same basic cognitive concepts as the MHP model, but embodies it in a seven stage model of action (Norman 1986), illustrated in Fig. 2.3.

The action cycle begins with a *goal*, for example, retrieving a patient's surgical history. The goal is a generic one independent of any system. In this context, let us presuppose that the clinician has access to paper record as well as those in an EHR. The second stage involves the formation of an *intention*, which in this case might be to retrieve the patient record in an EHR. The intention leads to the *specification of an action* sequence, which may include signing on to the system (which in itself may necessitate several actions), engaging a component system or simply a field that can be used to locate a patient in the database, and entering the patient's identifying information (e.g., last name or medical record number, if it is known). The specification results in *executing an action*, which may necessitate several actions. The system responds in some way or in the case of a failed attempt, may not respond at all. A change in system state may or may not provide a clear indication of the new state or a failure to provide feedback as to why the desired state has not appeared (e.g., system provides no indicators of a wait state or why no response is forthcoming). The perceived system response must then be *interpreted* and *evaluated* to determine whether the goal has been achieved. If the response provided by

Fig. 2.3 Norman's action
cycle

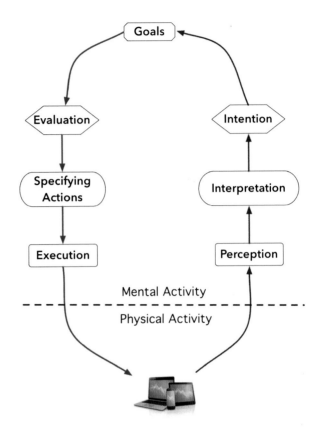

the system is "record not found," that could mean a number of things including that a name was mistyped or the number was incorrectly listed. On the basis of this determination, a next action will be chosen.

Any task of moderate complexity will involve substantial nesting of sub-goals, requiring a series of actions. To an experienced user, the action cycle may appear as a completely transparent and seamless process. However to a less experienced user, the process may breakdown at any of the seven stages. Norman (1986) describes two primary means in which the action cycle can break down. The *gulf of execution* reflects the difference between the goals and intentions of the user and the kinds of actions enabled by the system. For example, a user may not know the appropriate action sequence or the interface may not provide discernible clues to make such sequences transparent. For instance, a transaction may appear to be complete, but further action is needed to execute the selection process (e.g., pressing enter to accept a transaction).

The *gulf of evaluation* reflects the degree to which the user can make sense of the state of a system and determine how well their expectations have been met. For example, it is sometimes difficult to interpret a state transition and to know whether one has arrived at the correct state or whether the user has chosen an incorrect path.

Goals that necessitate multiple state or screen transitions are more likely to present difficulties for users, especially as they learn the system. Bridging gulfs involves both bringing about changes to the system design and training users to become better attuned to the affordances offered by a system resources. Gulfs can be partially explained by differences in the designer's models and the users' mental models, as discussed in the next section. The designer's model is the conceptual model to be built, based on analysis of the task, requirements, and an understanding of the users' capabilities (Norman 1986). The users' mental models of system behavior are developed through interacting with similar systems and gaining an understanding of how actions (e.g., selecting an item from a menu) will produce predictable and desired outcomes. Graphical user interfaces that involve direct manipulation of screen objects and widgets represent an attempt to reduce the distance between a designer's and user's model (Shneiderman 1982). Obviously, the distance is likely to be more difficult to bridge in a system like an EHR that incorporates a wide range of functions and components that may provide different layouts and forms of interaction.

Norman's theory of action has given rise, or in some cases, reinforced the need for sound design principles. For example, the state of a system should be plainly visible to the user and feedback should be transparent. In illustration, dialog boxes or alert messages can trigger the intention of reminding users to what is possible or needed to complete the task. There is a need to provide good mappings between the actions (e.g., clicking on a tab) and the results of the action as reflected in the state of the system (e.g., providing access to the expected display).

Norman's theory of action informed a great deal of research and design across domains. The seven-stage action theory was used to good effect by Zhang and colleagues in their development of a taxonomy of errors (Zhang et al. 2004). The theory also draws on Reason's categorization of errors as either slips or mistakes (Reason 1992). Slips result from the incorrect execution of a correct action sequence and mistakes are the product of the correct completion of an incorrect action sequence. Slips and mistakes are further categorized into execution errors and evaluation errors. They are further categorized into each of the descriptors that correspond to the Norman's seven stages (e.g., goals, intentions). Zhang et al. (2004) provide the following example of an intention slip: "A nurse intended to enter the rate of infusion using the up–down arrow keys, because this is the technique on the pump she most frequently uses; however, on this pump the arrow keys move the selection region instead of changing the selected number" (p 98). An example of an evaluation/intention slips is that a nurse interprets a yellow flashing light on a device analogically (based on prior knowledge of yellow as a warning) and interprets it as noncritical when it is in fact signaling a critical event. Norman's seven-stage action theory proved to be a useful model for characterizing a wide range of medical error types.

Although theory of action has been very influential in the world of design and research, it also has shortcomings (Sharp et al. 2007). The theory proposes that stages are followed sequentially. However, users do not necessarily proceed in such a sequential manner, especially in a domain such as medicine, which is constituted by numerous and complex nonlinear tasks. Contemporary GUIs, for example, web-based or app-based systems provide users greater flexibility in achieving the desired state or access the needed information. As discussed in subsequent sections, external representations (e.g., as expressed in text displays or visualizations) offer guidance to the user or even structure their interactions in such a way that a planned action sequence may not be necessary.

2.2.3 *Mental Models*

Mental models are an important construct in cognitive science and have been widely used in HCI research (Van der Veer and Melguizo 2003). Mental models are an analog-based construct for describing how individuals form internal models of systems. They are employed to answer questions such as "how does it work?" or "what will happen if I make the following move?" "Analog" suggests that the representation explicitly shares some aspect of the structure of the world it represents. For example, one can envision in the mind's eye a set of connected visual images of the succession of ATM screens one has to negotiate to get $200 out of one's checking account or buildings one passes on the way home from a local grocery store. This is in contrast to an abstraction-based form such as propositions or schemas in which the mental structure consists of either the gist, or a summary representation, for example, the procedures needed to complete an ATM transaction. Like other forms of mental representation, mental models are invariably incomplete, imperfect and subject to the processing limitations of the cognitive system (Norman 1983). Mental models can be derived from perception, language or from one's imagination (Payne 2003). Running a model corresponds to a process of mental simulation to generate possible future states of a system from observed or hypothetical state.

The constructs discussed in the prior sections emphasize how the general limits of the human-information processing system (e.g., limits in perception, attention and retrieval from memory) influence performance on a given task in a particular context (Payne 2003). On the other hand, mental models emphasize mental content, namely, knowledge and beliefs. An individual's mental model provides predictive and explanatory capabilities regarding the functions of a particular system. The construct has been used to characterize differences in expertise in a range of knowledge domains such as physics (Payne 2003). Experts have richer and more robust models of a range of phenomena, whereas novices are more prone to imprecision and errors. Mental models has been used to characterize models that have a spatial and temporal context, as is the case in reasoning about the behavior of electrical circuits (White and Frederiksen 1990). The model can be used to simulate a process (e.g., predict the effects of network interruptions on downloading a movie from www.amazon.com).

Kaufman et al. (1996) characterized clinician's mental model of the human cardiovascular system (specifically, cardiac output). The study characterized progressions in understanding of the system as a function of expertise. The research also documented various conceptual flaws in subjects' mental models and how these flaws impacted subjects' predictions and explanations of physiological manifestations (e.g., changes in blood flow in the venous system). In general, mental models are a useful explanatory construct for characterizing errors that are due to problems in understanding and not ones associated with flawed execution of procedures.

Mental models are a particularly useful explanatory device in understanding human-computer interaction (Staggers and Norcio 1993). The premise is that by exploring what users can understand and how they reason about the systems, it is possible to design them in a way that support the acquisition of the appropriate mental model and to reduce errors while performing with them. It is also useful to distinguish between a designer's conceptual model of a given system and a user's mental model (Staggers and Norcio 1993). The wider the gap, the more difficulties individuals will experience in using the system. For example, Kaufman and colleagues (2003) evaluated the usability of a home-based telemedicine system targeting older adults with diabetes. The study documented a substantial gulf between patients' mental models of the system and the designer's intent of how the system should be used. Although most of the participants had a shallow understanding of how such systems worked, there were some who possessed more elaborate mental models, and were better able to negotiate the system to perform a range of tasks including uploading blood glucose values and monitoring one's condition over time.

It is believed that novice users of a system can benefit from instructions that imparts a conceptual model or supports a mental simulation process (i.e., helping the users mentally step through problem states) (Payne 2003). Diagrammatic models of the device or system are often used to support such a learning process. For example, Halasz and Moran (1983) found that such a model was particularly beneficial to students learning to use a programmable calculator. Kieras and Bovair (1984) demonstrated a similar benefit for students learning to master a simple control panel device. They conducted a series of studies contrasting two groups learning to use a device. One group was trained to operate the device through learning the procedures by rote. The second group was trained using a model of how the device works. The model group learned the procedures faster, executed them more rapidly and improvised when necessary, e.g., replacing inefficient procedures with simpler ones. The study provides an illustration of how having a more robust mental model of a system can impact performance. A more advanced model can enable a user to discover alternative ways to achieve the same goal and overcome obstacles.

The construct of mental models fell into disuse in the last couple of decades as theories that emphasized interaction and externalization of representations flourished. However, the construct has resurfaced in recent years as a means to characterize how individuals' conceptualizations differ from representations in systems. For example, Smith and Koppel (2014) take the approach a step further in that they conceptualize three models: the patient's reality, that reality as represented in an EHR and as reflected in a clinician's understanding or mental model of the problem. Drawing on data from a wide range of sources (e.g., observations and log files) and findings, they constructed "scenarios of misalignment" or misrepresentation including categories such as "IT data too broadly focused" (i.e., lacking precise descriptions). For example, medical problem lists that do not permit sufficient qualification or classification illustrate an example of IT as being too broad or coarse. For instance, clinicians were not able to specify that a stroke resulted from a left-sided cerebrovascular accident. The typology provides a useful basis for IT designers to potentially reduce the gaps, better support users and diminish the potential for unintended consequences.

Shared mental models (SMM) represent an extension of the concept of mental models. The construct is rooted in research on teamwork in areas such as aviation (Orasanu 1990). Clinical care is recognized as a highly collaborative practice and there is a need to develop shared understanding about the processes involved in patient care as well as the evolving conditions of patients that are currently under their care. Breaks in communication among team members are known to be significant contributors to medical errors (Coiera 2000). There are only a few studies that demonstrate a relationship between SMM and clinical performance (Custer et al. 2012). Mamykina and colleagues (2014) investigated the development of SMM in an intensive care unit. The data included observations, audio recorded transcripts of patient handoff (i.e., transfer of patient during shift change) and rounds. In a recent paper, the analysis focused on a single care team including an attending physician, residents, nurses, medical students and physician assistants. The results indicated that the team initially had rather divergent perspectives on how well patients were doing, and the relative success of the treatment. Rounds served as an important coordinating event and the team endeavored to construct shared mental models (i.e., achieving a shared understanding) through an iterative process of resolving discrepancies. There was substantial evidence of change in SMM and in the coordination of patient care over a 3 day period. Whereas conversations on the first day focused on creating basic alignment and making immediate modifications to the care, discussions on the third day focused on understanding of underlying reasons for the situation, and developing a long-term plan more consistent with this collective causal understanding (Mamykina et al. 2014).

As mentioned previously, the concept of mental models has diminished as a construct employed by HCI researchers. One of the reasons is that mental models are not observable and can only be inferred indirectly. However, we believe that it has enduring value as an explanatory device for characterizing how individuals understand a system. The construct is too often used as a synonym for understanding, or for generic mental representation (i.e., with no commitment to the form of the representation). We favor the more specific instantiation of it as a model that can be used to simulate a process and project forward to predict events or outcomes or to explain why a particular outcome occurred. This enables us to develop theories or models for a given domain and then be able to predict and explain variation in performance. This should apply to a wide range of contexts whether the goal is to teach patients with diabetes to understand the basic physiology of their disease or for clinicians to use a newly implemented EHR. There is also evidence that a model-centric approach to teaching, in which an effort is made to foster an understanding of how a system works, confers some advantages over rote learning approaches to acquire the procedures needed to complete a task (Payne 2003; Gott and Lesgold 2000).

2.3   External Cognition

Internal representations reflect mental states that correspond to the external world. The term external representation refers to any object in the external world that has the potential to be internalized or to be used to augment cognitive processes (without internalizing). External representations such as images, graphs, icons, audible sounds, texts with symbols (e.g., letter and numbers), shapes and textures are vital sources of knowledge, means of communication and cultural transmission. The classical model of information-processing cognition viewed external representations as mere inputs to the mind that were processed and then internalized (Zhang 1997). The landscape began to change in the early 1990s when new cognitive theories focused on interactivity rather than solely modeling what was assumed to happen inside the head. Rogers (2012) cites Larkin and Simon's (1987) classic paper on "why a diagram may be worth a thousand words" as seminal to researchers in HCI. It offered the first alternative empirical account that focused on how people interact with external representations. The core idea was that cognition can be viewed as the interplay between internal and external representations, rather than only about modeling an individual's mental state and processes. Similar ideas had been put forth by others (Hutchins et al. 1985), but Larkin and Simon provided an explicit computational account that inspired the HCI community (Rogers 2012). Larkin and Simon (1987) made an important distinction between two kinds of external representation: diagrammatic and sentential representations. Although they are informationally equivalent, they are considered to be computationally different. That is, they contain the same information about the problem but the amount of cognitive effort required to come to the solution differs. For example, effective displays facilitate problem solving by allowing users to substitute perceptual operations (i.e., recognition) for effortful cognitive operations (e.g., memory retrieval and computationally-intensive reasoning) and effective displays can reduce the amount of time spent searching for critical information (Patel and Kaufman 2014). On the other hand, cluttered or poorly organized displays may increase the burden.

In the next two sections, we consider two extensions of external cognition, namely, the representational effect and the theory of intelligent spaces.

2.3.1 Representational Effect

The representational effect can be construed as a generalization of Larkin and Simon's (1987) conceptualization of the cognitive impact of external representations (Zhang and Norman 1994). It is well-known that different representations of a common abstract structure can have a significant impact on cognition (Zhang and Norman 1994; Kahneman 2011). For example, different forms of displaying patients' lab values can be more or less efficient for tasks. A display may be oriented to support a quick readout of discrete values or alternatively, one that allows clinicians to discern trends over a period of time. A simple illustration of the effect is that Arabic numerals are more efficient for arithmetic calculations (e.g., 26×92) than Roman numerals (XXVI × XCII) even though the representations are identical in meaning. Similarly, a digital clock provides a quick readout for precisely determining the time at a glance (Norman 1993). On the other hand, an analog clock enables one to more easily determine time intervals (e.g., elapsed or remaining time) without recourse to mental calculations. Norman (1993) proposed that external representations play a critical role in enhancing cognition and intelligent behavior. These durable representations (at least those that are visible) persist in the external world and are continuously available to augment memory, reasoning, and computation. Imagine the cognitive burden of having to do multi-digit multiplication without the use of external aids. Even a pencil and paper will allow you to hold partial results (interim calculations) externally. Calculations can be extremely computationally intensive without recourse to external representations (or memory aids).

Zhang and colleagues (Zhang 1997; Zhang et al.; Zhang and Patel 2006) summarized the following properties of external representations:

- Provide memory aids that can reduce cognitive load
- Provide information that can be directly perceived and used such that minimal processing is needed to explicitly interpret the information
- Support perception so that one can recognize features easily and make inferences directly
- Structure cognitive behavior without cognitive awareness
- Change the nature of a task by generating more efficient action sequences

Several researchers have described the mediating role of information technology on clinical reasoning. For example, Kushniruk et al. (1996) studied how clinicians learned to use an EHR over multiple sessions. They found that as users familiarized themselves with the system, their sequential information-gathering and reasoning strategies were driven by the organization of information on the user interface. In other words, the users followed a "screen-driven" strategy when taking a medical history from a patient. This had both positive consequences in that it promoted a more thorough consideration of the patient history, as well as negative consequences in that the clinician failed to search for findings not available on the display or inconsistent with their operative diagnostic hypothesis. In general, a screen-driven strategy can enhance performance by reducing the cognitive load imposed by information-gathering goals and enable the physician to allocate more cognitive resources toward patient evaluation (Patel and Kaufman 2014). On the other hand, this strategy can induce a certain sense of complacency or excessive reliance on the display to guide the process.

Similar results were reported by Patel et al. (2000) in a study contrasting the use of EHRs with paper records in a diabetic clinic setting. Physicians entered significantly more information about the patient's chief complaint using the EHR similarly following a screen-driven strategy. Likewise, the structure of the paper records document was such that physicians represented more information about the history of present illness and review of systems using paper-based records. The introduction of an EHR changed information-gathering and documentation strategies, thereby changing the information representation and meaning. The effects of the EHR persisted even after the re-introduction of paper records.

External representations can mediate cognition in a number of ways with both positive and negative impact. The following real-world example was drawn from a study related to a comprehensive causal analysis of a medication dosing error, in which an overdose of Potassium Chloride (KCl) was administered through a commercial computer order entry system (CPOE) in an ICU (Horsky et al. 2005). The authors' detailed analysis included the use of inspection of system logs, interviews with clinicians and a cognitive evaluation of the order-entry system involved. For the purpose of this paper, we highlight one element of the error to illustrate the interplay between technology and user interaction for clinical decision-making. In this case, the system provided screen order-entry forms for medication with intravenous drip and IV bolus orders that were superficially similar, yet required different calculations to estimate the dose. In this case, orders for IV bolus were specified by dose. In contrast, orders for other intravenous drip administration were indicated by duration, rather than by volume of administered fluid as suggested by the order-entry field "Total Volume." The latter referred to the size of the IV bag rather than the total amount of fluid to be delivered, which may exceed the volume indicated. In addition, intravenous fluid orders were not displayed on the medication review screen, further complicating the task of calculating an appropriate KCl bolus for a patient receiving intravenous medications. Calculating the correct infusion dosage was a vitally important task. However, not only did the interface not provide tools to facilitate this process, it also proved to be an obstacle.

It is well documented that IV medication errors commonly result in potentially harmful events (Taxis and Barber 2003; Husch et al. 2005). The configuration of external resources or representations, for example on a visual display, can have a significant impact on how the system facilitates (or alternatively, hinders) cognition. Critical care settings are immensely complex environments and medical error can be the product of a host of factors including workflow and communication (Patel et al. 2014). As discussed in subsequent sections, the organization of displays are just one of several facets that mediate interaction.

2.3.2 Intelligent Use of Space

Theories of external cognition tend to emphasize the computational offloading that eases the cognitive burden of a user. However, external representations can also be manipulated by individuals in a variety of ways to facilitate creative thinking as well (Rogers 2012; Zhang and Norman 1994; Kirsh 2005). According to Kirsh, "cognitive processes flow to wherever it is cheaper to perform them. The human 'cognitive operating system' extends to states, structures, and processes outside the mind and body" (Kirsh 2010) (p. 172). For example, one may choose to create a diagram to help interpret a complex sentence and that will alleviate some of the cognitive burden of sense-making. Kirsch draws on a range of examples, in illustration, how people follow a cooking recipe by arranging and re-arranging items (e.g., utensils and ingredients) to coordinate their activities. The central premise is that people interact and create external structure (or representations) because through these interactions, it is easier to process more efficiently and more effectively than by working inside the head alone. In essence, individuals are able to improve their thinking and comprehension by creating and using external representations (Kirsh 2010).

Kirsh (1995) studied how individuals restructured their environments when performing a range of tasks. He found that they constantly rearrange items to track the task state, support memory, predict effects of actions, and so forth. Restructuring often can reduce the cost of visual search, make it easier to notice, identify and remember items, and simplify task representation (Senathirajah et al. 2014a). The theory of intelligent spaces is an extension of this idea. Kirsh classified intelligent uses of space into three categories: (1) arrangements that simplify choice, (2) arrangements that simplify perception (e.g., calling attention to a group of items), and (3) spatial dynamics that simplify mental computation. The theory of intelligent spaces suggests that the idiosyncratic arrangements of individuals including clinicians may serve to simplify inferences or computations. The theory is potentially extensible across a range of domains including health information technology (HIT).

Although EHRs are very elaborate complex systems that support a wide range of functions, they often fail to support the varied needs of healthcare practitioners. Systems often fail to take into consideration the significant variability of medical information needs, which differ according to setting, specialty, role, individual patient and institution (Senathirajah et al. 2014b). In addition, they are not responsive to the highly collaborative nature of the work. In response to these challenges, Senathirajah and colleagues (2014a, b) developed a new model for health information systems, embodied in MedWISE, a widget-based highly configurable EHR platform. MedWISE supports drag/drop user configurations and the sharing of user-created elements such as custom laboratory result panels and user-created interface tabs. It was hypothesized that such a system could afford the clinician greater flexibility and better fit to the tasks they were required to perform. The intelligent spaces theoretical framework informed the design of MedWISE.

In an experiment conducted by Senathirajah et al. (2014b), 13 clinicians used the MedWISE system to review four patient cases. The data included video recordings of clinicians' interactions with the system and the screen layouts they created via the drag/drop capabilities. The focus here was on the creation of spatial layouts. The study documented three strategies which were labeled "opportunistic selection" (rapidly gathering items on the screen and reviewing), structured (organizing the layout categorically) and "dynamic stage" approach. The latter approach involved the user interacting with small groups of widgets at a time, using the space as a staging area to examine a specific concern and then shift to the next. An example of dynamic stage approach was that the clinician kept the index note (initial note) open at the bottom of column 2 (middle column) and stacked the unexamined labs and reports, closed, in column 1 (leftmost column), opened them in column 2 to compare them with the index note, and closed and moved them to column 3. This interaction pattern could reflect examination of specific diagnostic concerns (e.g., ruling out a diagnostic hypothesis). An example of the structured approach is indicated in Fig. 2.4. The clinician has stated that he is keeping the right side as a free space for thinking space, for studies, and for to-do items. A to-do list is at upper

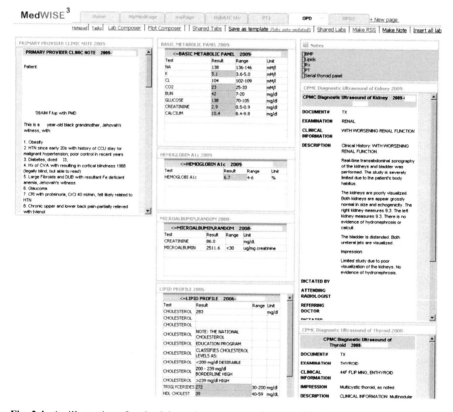

Fig. 2.4 An illustration of a physician using a structured approach in MedWISE

right (in the yellow sticky note), while orienting items including the primary provider clinic note is at left, with lab data down the middle. This reflects a common pattern found of going from left to right with orienting material, data, and then action items. The clinician has grouped labs according to related diagnostic facets, for example, the HbA1c and micro albumin (diabetes-related) are together, and then thyroid-related results (TSH, T3 and T4) are grouped at the bottom of the center column.

The clinicians employed spatial arrangement in ways consistent with theory and research on workplace spatial arrangement (Senathirajah et al. 2014b). This includes assignment of screen regions for particular purposes, juxtaposition of elements to facilitate calculation (e.g., ratios), and grouping elements with common meanings or relevance to the diagnostic facets of the case (e.g., thyroid findings). Clinicians also made deliberate use of the space following a common pattern of left-to-right progression of orienting materials, data, and action items or reflection space. Widget selection was based on an assessment of what information was useful or relevant immediately or likely to be in the near future (as more information is gathered). The study demonstrated how a user-composable EHR in which users have substantial control over how a display is populated and arranged can embody the advantages predicted by the intelligent use of space theory.

The external cognition framework has introduced a set of concepts that has enabled researchers and designers to characterize designs in ways not previously accessible to them (Rogers 2012). As evidenced in the work on MedWISE, it provided a language that framed how people manipulate representations, interact with objects, and organize their space. This provides a basis for designing tools that facilitate different kinds of interaction. It also suggests that there are more and less optimal ways to configure a display for particular tasks and that the impact of such configurations are measurable.

2.4 Distributed Cognition

The external cognition framework seeded important design concepts. It also provides a means to engage in a more rigorous approach to evaluation. The distributed cognition (DCog) approach takes the argument further beyond the internal-external representation divide (Rogers 2012). DCog re-conceptualizes cognitive phenomena in terms of individuals, artifacts, and internal and external representations and their interactions (Rogers 2012). It provides a more extensive account than external cognition. The core approach entails describing a "cognitive system," which involves interactions among people, artifacts they employ, and the environment they are situated in. Hutchins and colleagues proposed a new paradigm for fundamentally rethinking our assumptions about cognition (Hutchins 1995).

DCog represents a shift in the study of cognition from an exclusive focus on the mind of the individual to being "stretched" across groups, material artifacts and cultures (Hutchins 1995; Suchman 1986). This paradigm has gained substantial currency in HCI research. In the distributed approach, cognition is viewed as a process of coordinating distributed internal (i.e., what's in the mind) and external representations (e.g., visual displays, post-it notes, paper records). Distributed cognition has two focal points of inquiry, one that emphasizes the inherently social and collaborative nature of cognition (e.g., attending physicians, residents, nurses and respiratory therapists in cardiothoracic intensive care unit jointly contributing to a decision process), and one that characterizes the mediating effects of technology (e.g., EHRs, mobile devices apps) or other artifacts on cognition.

Hollan et al. (2000) emphasize that distributed cognition is more than the social distribution of cognitive processes; rather it is a broader conceptualization that includes emergent phenomena in social interactions as well as interactions between people and the structure of their environment. According to Hollan et al., the perspective "highlights three fundamental questions about social interactions: (1) how are the cognitive processes we normally associate with an individual mind implemented in a group of individuals, (2) how do the cognitive properties of groups differ from the cognitive properties of the people who act in those groups, and (3) how are the cognitive properties of individual minds affected by participation in group activities?" (Hollan et al. 2000) (p 177).

DCog is concerned with representational states and the informational flows around the media carrying these representations (Perry 2003). The framework enables researchers to consider all factors relevant to a task, coalescing individuals, the problem and the tools into a single unit of analysis. This makes it a productive means to develop an understanding of how representations act as intermediaries in the dynamically changing and coordinated processes of work activities (Perry 2003).

Hutchins' (1995) seminal analysis of ship navigation of a U.S. navy vessel provided a compelling account of how crews took the ships bearing and how this information was interpreted processed, and transformed across representational states (embodied in media and technology such as ship navigation instruments like the ship's compass and communication among interdependent actors that constitute the ship's crew). The succession of states resulted in the determination of a ships location, progress and how they could be aligned with intended trajectories. The entities operating within the functional system are not viewed from the perspective of the individual, but as a collective (Perry 2003). Both people and artifacts are considered as representational components of the system. As should be clear at this point, external representations are not mere inputs or stimuli to the mind, but play a more instrumental role in cognition.

In the next sections, we review two extensions of DCog including the distributed resource model and the propagation of representational states.

2.4.1 Distributed Resources Model

One of the strengths of the DCog, as applied to HCI, is that it can be used to understand how properties of objects on the screen (e.g., links, menus) can serve as external representations and reduce cognitive load. Wright et al. (2000) proposed a distributed resources model to address the question of the information needed to carry out a task and where it should be located: as an interface object or as knowledge that a user brings to the task. The relative difference in the distribution of representations is pivotal in determining the efficacy of a system designed to support a complex task such as computer provider entry (Horsky et al. 2003). The distributed resources model includes two primary components. The first is a characterization of information structures (i.e., resource types), pertaining to the control of action and the second is a process-oriented description of how these information structures can be used for action (interaction strategies) to complete a task. The information structures can be embodied in any artifact (e.g., paper charts or an EHR). Wright et al. enumerated several of these information structures including plans, goals, history and state. Plans include possible sequence of actions, events, and anticipated states. Goals refer to the desired states the user wants to accomplish. They may be generated internally or emerge from the interaction with the system. History refers to the part of a plan that has already been accomplished. The history of past actions may be maintained in a web browser, for example, as a list of previously visited pages that can be accessed via a drop-down list. State is the current configuration of resources, for example, as represented in the display screen at a given point in time. These are all considered to be resources for action rather than static structures. They can be externalized, manipulated and subjected to evaluation (Wright et al. 2000).

Horsky et al. (2003) employed the distributed resource model to investigate the usability of a CPOE system. The goal was to analyze order-entry tasks and to identify areas of complexity that may impede performance. The research consisted of two component analyses: a cognitive walkthrough evaluation that was modified based on the distributed resource model and an experiment involving a simulated clinical ordering task performed by seven physicians who were experienced users of the CPOE. The walkthrough analysis revealed that the configuration of resources (e.g., very long menus and complexly configured screens) placed an unnecessarily heavy cognitive load on the user. In addition, successful interaction was too often dependent on the recall of system-related knowledge. The resources model was also used to explain patterns of errors produced by clinicians including, selecting an inappropriate order set, omissions and redundant entries. The authors concluded that the reconfiguration of resources may yield guiding principles and design solutions in the development of complex interactive systems (Horsky et al. 2003). In addition, system design that better reflects the constraints of the task (e.g., hospital admission) and domain (e.g., internal medicine) may minimize the need for more robust mental models or extensive system knowledge.

2.4.2 Propagation of Representational States

Horsky et al. conducted a DCog analysis that emphasized the technology-mediating effects of a CPOE interface on clinical performance. Hazlehurst and colleagues (2007) emphasize both the socially-distributed nature and mediating impact of artifacts on communication during cardiac surgery. Towards that end, they employed a cognitive ethnography method to understand how system resources are configured and used for cardiac surgery and to prevent adverse events. DCog focuses on the activity system as the unit of analysis and seeks to understand how properties of this system determine performance (Hutchins 1995; Horsky et al. 2003; Hazlehurst et al. 2007).

Following Hutchins (1995), Hazlehurt views the 'propagation of representational states' through activity systems as explanatory of cognitive behavior and sought to investigate the organizing features of this propagation as an explanation of system and human performance (Hazlehurst et al. 2007). Accordingly, "a representational state is a particular configuration of an information-bearing structure, such as a monitor display, a verbal utterance, or a printed label, that plays some functional role in a process within the system (Hazlehurst et al. 2007) (p 540)". They identified six patterns of communication between surgeon and perfusionist that relate to the functional properties of the activity system. For example, *direction* is a pattern that seeks to transition the activity system to a new state (e.g., administering medications that affect blood coagulation). *Goal sharing* involves creating an expectation of a desired future, but not specifically the action sequence necessary to achieve the target state. These patterns of communication serve to enhance situation awareness, for example, by making the current situation clear and mutually understood.

The distributed cognition approach has been widely used in HCI to examine existing practices and workflow (Rogers 2012). It has also been used to inform the iterative design process by characterizing how the quality and configuration of resources and representations might be transformed and how this change may impact work practices. It is an approach that is inherently well suited to a complex, media-rich and collaborative domain such as medicine. However, a distributed cognitive analysis can be extremely difficult to conduct (requiring substantial specialized knowledge of the analytic approach as well as the knowledge domain), rather complex and very time consuming. In the next section, we describe an approach which endeavors to make the DCog approach more tractable and bring it closer to the design process (Blandford and Furniss 2006).

2.4.3 Distributed Cognition of Teamwork (DiCoT)

DCog's has developed a rather comprehensive and penetrating approach to understanding the different dimensions of human-computer interaction. However, there is no 'off-the-shelf' methodology for using it in research or as a practitioner (Furniss et al. 2014). According to Rogers, the application of DCog theory and methods are complicated by the fact that there are no set of features to attend to and no checklist or prescribed method to follow (Rogers 2012). In addition, the analysis and abstraction requires a very high level of skill. However, there have been various structured approaches to gathering and analyzing data including the Distributed Resources (DR) Model (Wright et al. 2000) described in a previous section. DiCoT (Distributed Cognition for Teamwork) was developed to provide a structured approach to analyze work systems and teamwork (Furniss et al. 2014; Furniss and Blandford 2006). The approach is informed by theoretical principles from the DCog literature.

The DiCoT framework focuses on developing five interdependent models with different foci: artifacts, physical, information flow, social and evolutionary (Furniss et al. 2014). Each of the models is informed by a set of principles. For example, the artifacts model includes the premise that mediating artifacts are brought into coordination (e.g., paper and electronic health records) in the completion of a task. A second principle is reflected in the fact that we use our environment continuously by "creating scaffolding" to simplify cognitive tasks (Hollan et al. 2000). The physical model refers to the physical organization of work. It is guided by principles such as space and cognition, which states how humans manipulate space towards the facilitation of decision making or problem solving (e.g., grouping objects into categories). This is similar to the intelligent uses of space (Kirsh 1995). Information transformation is one of the principles of information flow. It suggests that transformation occurs when the representation of information changes. As described previously, more effective representations provide better support for reasoning.

DiCoT has been used to analyze complex systems in a range of healthcare contexts including ambulance control room dispatch (Furniss and Blandford 2006) and infusion pump use in intensive care (Rajkomar and Blandford 2012). Emergency medical dispatch is constituted by a team that coordinates the delivery of services (e.g., dispatching an ambulance) to respond to a call for medical assistance. Furniss and Blandford (2006) conducted a study of an EMD team using the DiCoT approach. The focus was on describing the work system, identifying sources of weakness and projecting the likely consequences of a redesign (e.g., what is likely to happen when a centrally available shared display is visible or accessible to each member of the team). On the basis of characterizing systemic weaknesses, they suggested changes to the physical layout that could enhance "cross-boundary working". Their observations revealed a discontinuity between the central ambulance control and the crews in the field. In response, Furniss and Blandford (2006) proposed the use of more flexible communication channels so the crew could be contacted whether they are at a station or are mobile. The multifaceted model enables the researchers to envision a set of consequences to the redesign scheme along a range of dimensions (e.g., information flow). Clinical practitioners and other stakeholders review and comment on the concrete redesign solutions.

The DCog framework, which incorporates a number of interrelated theories, offers the most comprehensive and in our view, the most compelling theoretical approach to explain the technology-mediated and social/collaborative nature of clinical work. Each theory within this framework privileges different aspects of interactions.

2.5   Conclusions

It is reasonable to conclude that we need a theory (or theories) of cognition in the context of HCI and health care. Although we have learned much from empirical studies and applied work, a theoretical framework is needed to account for the broad scope of the field and the complexity that is inherent in the domain of medicine. Without a sound theoretical framework, generalizations would be limited, and principled approaches to design would be largely illusory. In this chapter, we traced the evolution of cognitive theory from the classical information-processing approach to external cognition through distributed cognition. The information-processing approach drew extensively on concepts from cognitive psychology and embraced a computational approach to the study of interaction. The MHP theory (Card et al. 1983) provides insight into cognitive processes and provides a predictive model of behavior, albeit one that is limited in scope. Norman's theory of action (Norman 1986) offers an explanatory account of the challenges involved in using systems. It also offers general prescriptions, for example, emphasizing the importance of quality feedback to the user. The theory of mental models as applied to HCI builds on the idea of gulfs to further explicate the kinds of knowledge needed to productively use a system. It also broadly prescribes how to narrow the divide between designer models and users' mental models. Although these theories are inherently incomplete in their focus on the solitary individual, they continue to be productive as explanatory theories of HCI.

Theories of external cognition expanded the scope of analysis to include a focus on external representations. Several studies have demonstrated how representations mediate cognition and how differential mediation (as reflected in display configurations) can contribute to medical errors. The theory of intelligent spaces (Kirsh 1995) is a generative theory, which seeded concepts that were realized in the design of the MedWISE system. DCog theories are the most encompassing in their focus on both technology-mediated and socially distributed cognition. The theories offer rich descriptive and explanatory accounts of technology use in the medical workplace. Distributed resource theory (Wright et al. 2000) works both as a descriptive theory characterizing the state of affairs and a prescriptive theory that can be used to reconfigure interfaces to alleviate some of the cognitive burden on users. Significant challenges remain in the domain of health information technology. Although cognitive theory cannot provide all of the answers, it remains a powerful tool for advancing knowledge and furthering the scientific enterprise.

Discussion Questions

1. What role can cognitive theory play in HCI research and application? Describe the different kinds of theories that can inform HCI in practice situations.
2. Explain the gulfs of execution and evaluation and how they can be used to inform HCI design.
3. Mental models are an analog-based construct for describing how individuals form internal models of systems. Explain what is meant by analog. How can mental models inform our understanding of the user experience?
4. Describe the meaning and significance of the representational effect. How can it influence the design of visual displays to represent lab results?
5. What implications can one draw from the theory of intelligent spaces? How can it be used to seed design concepts in health care?
6. What are the essential differences between theories of external representation and theories of distributed cognition?

Additional Readings

Carroll, J. M. (2003). *HCI models, theories, and frameworks: Toward a multidisciplinary science*. San Francisco: Morgan Kaufmann.
Patel, V. L., & Kaufman, D. R. (2014). Cognitive science and biomedical informatics. In E. H. Shortliffe & J. J. Cimino (Eds.), *Biomedical informatics: Computer applications in health care and biomedicine* (pp. 133–185). New York: Springer.
Rogers, Y. (2012). HCI theory: Classical, modern, and contemporary. *Synthesis Lectures on Human-Centered Informatics, 5*(2), 1–129.

References

Anderson, J. R. (1983). *The architecture of cognition*. Cambridge, MA: Cambridge University Press.
Anderson, J. R. (2005). *Cognitive psychology and its implications*. New York: Macmillan.
Bederson, B. B., & Shneiderman, B. (2003). *The craft of information visualization: Readings and reflections*. San Francisco, CA: Morgan Kaufmann.
Blandford, D., & Furniss, D. (2006). DiCoT: A methodology for applying distributed cognition to the design of teamworking systems. In S. W. Gilroy & M. D. Harrison (Eds.), *Interactive systems: Design, specification, and verification* (pp. 26–38). Berlin: Springer.
Card, S. K., Newell, A., & Moran, T. P. (1983). *The psychology of human-computer interaction*. New York: Erlbaum Associates.
Coiera, E. (2000). When conversation is better than computation. *Journal of the American Medical Informatics Association, 7*(3), 277–286.
Custer, J. W., et al. (2012). A qualitative study of expert and team cognition on complex patients in the pediatric intensive care unit. *Pediatric Critical Care Medicine, 13*(3), 278–284.
Furniss, D., & Blandford, A. (2006). Understanding emergency medical dispatch in terms of distributed cognition: A case study. *Ergonomics, 49*(12–13), 1174–1203.

Furniss, D., et al. (2014). Exploring medical device design and use through layers of distributed cognition: How a glucometer is coupled with its context. *Journal of Biomedical Informatics, 53*, 330–341.

Gott, S. P., & Lesgold, A. M. (2000). Competence in the workplace: How cognitive performance models and situated instruction can accelerate skill acquisition. In R. Glaser (Ed.), *Advances in instructional psychology: Educational design and cognitive science* (pp. 239–327). Mahwah: Erlbaum Associates.

Grudin, J. (2008). A moving target: The evolution of human-computer interaction. In *The human-computer interaction handbook–fundamentals, evolving technologies, and emerging applications* (pp. 1–24). Mahwah: Erlbaum Associates.

Halasz, F. G., & Moran, T. P. (1983). Mental models and problem solving in using a calculator. In *Proceedings of the SIGCHI conference on human factors in computing systems* (pp. 212–216). New York: ACM.

Hazlehurst, B., McMullen, C. K., & Gorman, P. N. (2007). Distributed cognition in the heart room: How situation awareness arises from coordinated communications during cardiac surgery. *Journal of Biomedical Informatics, 40*(5), 539–551.

Hollan, J., Hutchins, E., & Kirsh, D. (2000). Distributed cognition: Toward a new foundation for human-computer interaction research. *ACM Transactions on Computer-Human Interaction (TOCHI), 7*(2), 174–196.

Horsky, J., et al. (2003). A framework for analyzing the cognitive complexity of computer-assisted clinical ordering. *Journal of Biomedical Informatics, 36*(1), 4–22.

Horsky, J., Kuperman, G. J., & Patel, V. L. (2005). Comprehensive analysis of a medication dosing error related to CPOE. *Journal of the American Medical Informatics Association: JAMIA, 12*(4), 377–382.

Husch, M., et al. (2005). Insights from the sharp end of intravenous medication errors: Implications for infusion pump technology. *Quality & Safety in Health Care, 14*(2), 80–86.

Hutchins, E. (1995). *Cognition in the wild*. Cambridge, MA: MIT Press.

Hutchins, E. L., Hollan, J. D., & Norman, D. A. (1985). Direct manipulation interfaces. *Human-Computer Interaction, 1*(4), 311–338.

John, B. E. (2003). Information processing and skilled behavior. In J. M. Carroll (Ed.), *HCI models, theories and frameworks: Towards a multidisciplinary science* (pp. 55–102). San Francisco: Morgan Kaufmann.

Kahneman, D. (2011). *Thinking, fast and slow*. New York: McMillan Farrar, Straus and Giroux.

Kannampallil, T. G., et al. (2011). Considering complexity in healthcare systems. *Journal of Biomedical Informatics, 44*(6), 943–947.

Kaufman, D. R., Patel, V. L., & Magder, S. A. (1996). The explanatory role of spontaneously generated analogies in reasoning about physiological concepts. *International Journal of Science Education, 18*(3), 369–386.

Kaufman, D. R., et al. (2003). Usability in the real world: Assessing medical information technologies in patients' homes. *Journal of Biomedical Informatics, 36*(1), 45–60.

Kieras, D. E., & Bovair, S. (1984). The role of a mental model in learning to operate a device. *Cognitive Science, 8*(3), 255–273.

Kirsh, D. (1995). The intelligent use of space. *Artificial Intelligence, 73*(1), 31–68.

Kirsh, D. (2005). Metacognition, distributed cognition and visual design. In P. Gardenfors & P. Johansson (Eds.), *Cognition, education, and communication technology* (pp. 147–180). London: Routledge.

Kirsh, D. (2010). Thinking with external representations. *AI and Society, 25*, 441–454.

Kushniruk, A. W., et al. (1996). Assessment of a computerized patient record system: A cognitive approach to evaluating medical technology. *MD Computing, 13*(5), 406–415.

Larkin, J. H., & Simon, H. A. (1987). Why a diagram is (sometimes) worth ten thousand words. *Cognitive Science, 11*(1), 65–100.

Mackenzie, I. S. (1992). Fitts' law as a research and design tool in human-computer interaction. *Human-Computer Interaction, 7*(1), 91–139.

Mackenzie, I. S. (2003). Motor behavior models for human-computer interaction. In J. M. Carroll (Ed.), *HCI models, theories, and frameworks: Toward a multidisciplinary science*. San Francisco: Morgan Kaufmann.

Mamykina, L., Hum, R. S., & Kaufman, D. R. (2014). Investigating shared mental models in critical care. In V. L. Patel, D. R. Kaufman, & T. Cohen (Eds.), *Cognitive informatics in health and biomedicine* (pp. 291–315). London: Springer.

Norman, D. A. (1983). Some observations on mental models. In D. Gentner & A. L. Stevens (Eds.), *Mental models* (pp. 7–14). Hillsdale: Erlbaum Associates.

Norman, D. A. (1986). Cognitive engineering. In D. A. Norman & S. W. Draper (Eds.), *User centered system design* (pp. 31–61). Hillsdale: Erlbaum Associates.

Norman, D. A. (1993). Cognition in the head and in the world: An introduction to the special issue on situated action. *Cognitive Science, 17*(1), 1–6.

Orasanu, J. M. (1990). *Shared mental models and crew decision making* (CSL technical report no. 46). Princeton: Princeton University, Cognitive Sciences Laboratory.

Patel, V. L., & Groen, G. J. (1992). Cognitive framework for clinical reasoning: Application for training and practice. In D. A. Evans & V. L. Patel (Eds.), *Advanced models of cognition for medical training and practice* (pp. 193–212). Heidelberg: Springer-Verlag GmbH & Co. Kg.

Patel, V. L., & Kaufman, D. R. (2014). Cognitive science and biomedical informatics. In E. H. Shortliffe & J. J. Cimino (Eds.), *Biomedical informatics: Computer applications in health care and biomedicine* (pp. 133–185). New York: Springer.

Patel, V. L., et al. (2000). Impact of a computer-based patient record system on data collection, knowledge organization, and reasoning. *Journal of the American Medical Informatics Association: JAMIA, 7*(6), 569–585.

Patel, V. L., Kaufman, D. R., & Cohen, T. (Eds.). (2014). *Cognitive informatics in health and biomedicine: Case studies on critical care, complexity and errors*. London: Springer.

Payne, S. J. (2003). Users' mental models: The very ideas. In J. M. Carroll (Ed.), *HCI models, theories, and frameworks: Toward a multidisciplinary science* (pp. 135–156). San Francisco: Morgan Kaufmann.

Perry, M. (2003). Distributed cognition. In J. M. Carroll (Ed.), *HCI, models, theories, and frameworks: Toward a multidisciplinary science* (pp. 193–223). San Francisco: Morgan Kaufmann.

Rajkomar, A., & Blandford, A. (2012). Understanding infusion administration in the ICU through distributed cognition. *Journal of Biomedical Informatics, 45*(3), 580–590.

Reason, J. (1992). *Human error*. Cambridge: Cambridge University Press.

Rogers, Y. (2004). New theoretical approaches for human-computer interaction. *Annual Review of Information Science and Technology, 38*(1), 87–143.

Rogers, Y. (2012). HCI theory: Classical, modern, and contemporary. *Synthesis Lectures on Human-Centered Informatics, 5*(2), 1–129.

Saitwal, H., et al. (2010). Assessing performance of an electronic health record (EHR) using cognitive task analysis. *International Journal of Medical Informatics, 79*(7), 501–506.

Senathirajah, Y., Bakken, S., & Kaufman, D. (2014a). The clinician in the driver's seat: Part 1 – A drag/drop user-composable electronic health record platform. *Journal of Biomedical Informatics, 52*, 165–176.

Senathirajah, Y., Kaufman, D., & Bakken, S. (2014b). The clinician in the driver's seat: Part 2 – Intelligent uses of space in a drag/drop user-composable electronic health record. *Journal of Biomedical Informatics, 52*, 177–188.

Sharp, H., Rogers, Y., & Preece, J. (2007). *Interaction design: Beyond human-computer interaction*. New York: Wiley.

Shneiderman, B. (1982). The future of interactive systems and the emergence of direct manipulation. *Behaviour & Information Technology, 1*(3), 237–256.

Smith, S. W., & Koppel, R. (2014). Healthcare information technology's relativity problems: A typology of how patients' physical reality, clinicians' mental models, and healthcare information technology differ. *Journal of the American Medical Informatics Association: JAMIA, 21*(1), 117–131.

Staggers, N., & Norcio, A. F. (1993). Mental models: Concepts for human-computer interaction research. *International Journal of Man-Machine Studies, 38*(4), 587–605.

Suchman, L. (1986). *Plans and situated actions: The problem of human machine interaction.* Cambridge, MA: Cambridge University Press.

Taxis, K., & Barber, N. (2003). Causes of intravenous medication errors: An ethnographic study. *Quality & Safety in Health Care, 12*(5), 343–347.

Van der Veer, G. C., & Melguizo, P. (2003). Mental models. In A. Sears & J. A. Jacko (Eds.), *The human-computer interaction handbook: Fundamentals, evolving technologies, and emerging applications* (pp. 58–80). Mahwah: Erlbaum Associates.

White, B. Y., & Frederiksen, J. R. (1990). Causal model progressions as a foundation for intelligent learning environments. *Artificial Intelligence, 42*(1), 99–157.

Wright, P. C., Fields, R. E., & Harrison, M. D. (2000). Analyzing human-computer interaction as distributed cognition: The resources model. *Human-Computer Interaction, 15*(1), 1–41.

Zhang, J. (1997). The nature of external representations in problem solving. *Cognitive Science, 21*(2), 179–217.

Zhang, J., & Norman, D. A. (1994). Representations in distributed cognitive tasks. *Cognitive Science, 18*(1), 87–122.

Zhang, J., & Patel, V. L. (2006). Distributed cognition, representation, and affordance. *Pragmatics & Cognition, 14*(2), 333–341.

Zhang, J., et al. (2004). A cognitive taxonomy of medical error. *Journal of Biomedical Informatics, 37*(3), 193–204.

Zhang, J., Johnson, K. A., Malin, J., & Smith, J. W. (2002). Human-centered information visualization. Paper presented at *International workshop on dynamic visualization and learning*, Tubingen, Germany, July 18–19, 2002.

Chapter 3
Theoretical Foundations for Health Communication Research and Practice

Daniel G. Morrow and Karen Dunn Lopez

3.1 Introduction

At first glance, communication among clinicians may seem to be the least complicated component of the health care domain, which involves providing care for a
wide variety of illnesses and age groups using an array of low and high technology
diagnostics and treatment, and a continually mounting base of evidence. Yet, there
is mounting evidence that points to serious problems in communication within
health care. Annually, 98,000 deaths are attributed to errors in health care (Kohn
et al. 2000), with an estimated 60 % attributed to avoidable communication failures
(Joint Commission on Accreditation of Healthcare Organizations 2005). Other
research using root cause analysis revealed that approximately 70 % of sentinel
events (serious negative consequences involving the unexpected occurrence or risk
of death or serious injury) are caused by poor communication (Cordero 2011) and
that poor information sharing and coordination is linked to patient mortality in
multiple settings (Kim et al. 2010; Knaus et al. 1986; Shortell et al. 1992; Williams
et al. 2007). These findings should not be surprising given the evidence that
miscommunication is an important contributor to errors in other complex and
high stakes domains such as aviation (Davison et al. 2003).

These failures are brought about by multiple challenges of communicating in the
high stakes health care domain. A key challenge is the high cognitive demands
associated with managing biological complexity in health care. This task requires

D.G. Morrow (✉)
Department of Educational Psychology, University of Illinois at Urbana-Champaign,
Education Building, 1310 S. 6th St., Champaign, IL, USA
e-mail: dgm@illinois.edu

K.D. Lopez
Department of Health Systems Science, College of Nursing, University of Illinois at Chicago,
845 S. Damen Ave., Chicago, IL, USA
e-mail: Kdunnl2@uic.edu

© Springer International Publishing Switzerland 2015   35
V.L. Patel et al. (eds.), *Cognitive Informatics for Biomedicine*, Health Informatics,
DOI 10.1007/978-3-319-17272-9_3

interpreting and sharing uncertain and dynamic patient information, including frequent unplanned and interruptive communication among clinicians from different disciplines who must collaborate despite discipline-specific terminologies and taxonomies. These challenges are exacerbated by rapid diffusion of health information and communication technologies that can increase communication complexity. In addition, the round-the-clock nature of health care requires frequent complete transfer of responsibility for patients within disciplines, or handoffs that increase the number of clinicians who take care of a single patient. Moreover, the high cost of health care leads to multiple federal regulations that directly impact how care is delivered. For all these reasons, communication challenges may be even greater in health care than in other complex domains that involve managing engineered systems. For example, in aviation, pilots' interaction with aircraft usually yield predictable consequences with swift feedback, while in health care the effects of clinicians' treatment of patients is much less predictable with more variable and sometimes delayed feedback about treatment success (Durso and Drews 2010).

Given the vast differences between patient-provider communication, communication about health in the media, communication within health care organizations between caregivers and non-caregivers, and communication between caregivers, we focus our discussion on the communication between clinicians who are involved in direct patient care. Despite the volume of research related to inter- and intra-disciplinary communication in patient care, this work is often not theoretically-based. For example, a recent systematic review of hand-off communication research found that only 34 % of studies were guided by theoretical frameworks (Abraham et al. 2014; also see Patterson and Wears 2010). Therefore, we will focus on existing theoretical foundations that can inform research to address these key challenges in health care that hold strong potential for improving the quality and safety of patient care. In the next section, we describe information processing and interactive theories of communication. We then summarize some important challenges related to communication in health care contexts and argue for the importance of communication theory for addressing these challenges.

3.2 Theories of Communication Relevant to Health Care

Several theoretical approaches help identify processes involved in health communication as well as factors that influence these processes and thus the success of communication. In this section, we review approaches that have influenced research about performance in complex domains such as aviation, and increasingly in health care.

3.2.1 *Information Processing*

A longstanding and fruitful approach assumes that communication can be explained in part in terms of mental processes involved in information exchange by producing and understanding messages. This approach has its origins in information theory, developed by Shannon and Weaver (1949). They distinguished technical communication (how accurately information is encoded, transmitted by sending them through a communication medium or channel, and decoded by interpreting the coded message), semantic communication (how well these codes convey meaning) and effectiveness (how well the message has the intended effect). Information theory most directly addressed the technical level. The approach has been successful in many ways, for example by guiding development of communication technology (e.g., speech synthesis and recognition systems) and explaining some aspects of communication success such as reducing the impact of channel capacity, noise, and related factors on speech comprehension (Wickens and Hollands 2000). Health care as well as other domains have greatly benefited from these improvements because of its reliance on many forms of voice communication (e.g., Interactive Voice Response systems, mobile phones, and dictation systems).

The information processing approach was elaborated during the cognitive revolution in which the mind was understood metaphorically in terms of the computer, and drawing upon linguistic theories of mental structures (Miller 2003). Communication was explained in terms of the cognitive processes required to produce and understand linguistic messages, as well as the cognitive abilities and resources that constrained these processes.

Speakers (or writers) generate ideas by activating concepts in long-term memory and assembling these concepts (and associated words) into ideas (represented as propositions) that are mapped onto syntactic structures to convey the ideas through speech (Levelt 1989). Word access and propositional encoding processes involved in speech planning are shaped by our cognitive architecture, such as the capacity of working memory, which constrains how much conceptual context can be active at one time, and thus the size of the planning unit, as revealed for example in patterns of pausing when talking (Levelt 1989). To understand these messages, listeners (readers) recognize spoken (printed) words, activate the corresponding lexical codes and concepts in long-term memory, and integrate these concepts into propositions or idea units. Understanding extended discourse involves identifying relationships among these ideas, often driven by identifying referents of co-referring expressions and drawing on knowledge to identify temporal, causal, and other relationships among the ideas (Kintsch 1998). Comprehension requires more than assembling concepts into propositions: the network of propositions (the textbase) must be interpreted in terms of what we know about the concepts in order to develop a situation model, or representation of the described events and scenes (Kintsch 1998; for application to issues of comprehension and knowledge representation in the medical domain, see Arocha and Patel 1994; Patel et al. 2002). Situation models may be concrete, reflecting our perceptual experience of the described situation (Zwaan and Taylor 2006), or more abstract, capturing the essential 'gist' of the message (Reyna 2008). Understanding as well as producing messages is constrained by limited cognitive resources. For example, readers tend to pause at the end of clauses and sentences, presumably to wrap up conceptual integration, so that the pattern of pausing when reading mirrors the pauses when producing the message (Stine-Morrow and Miller 2009).

Individual differences in cognitive resources such as working memory capacity help explain differences in successful communication. For example, age differences in comprehension of complex messages (e.g., conceptually dense text) often reflect age-related differences in cognitive resources (Stine-Morrow and Miller 2009). Knowledge, on the other hand, can facilitate comprehension, reducing need for effortful conceptual integration and inference processes (Kintsch 1998). Age differences in comprehension are often reduced for texts that are organized to match knowledge organization (Stine-Morrow and Miller 2009).

While the information processing approach has been successful both theoretically (supporting a large body of empirical research on language understanding and production processes and how they are shaped by cognitive resources) and practically (e.g., spurring development of communication technology), it is incomplete as an account of communication in complex domains. It is based on and guided by a conduit metaphor of communication, which assumes communication depends on how precisely linguistic codes match speaker ideas and how accurately listeners decode these ideas, or how well they 'take away' the message (Reddy 1979). Thus, the focus is more on participants' processes and resources than on communication medium, context, and purpose. Although this approach recognizes the importance of pragmatic as well as semantic views of language (e.g., explaining message effectiveness is an important goal of information theory), much of the work within this framework focused on how people represent message meaning, more than on the actions performed by speakers when using language; e.g., semantic rather than pragmatic effects of discourse (Austin 1960).

3.2.1.1 Persuasion/Risk Communication

Other theories within this tradition focus on affective as well as cognitive processes in communication, how these processes interact to influence addressees, and how speakers design messages to influence addressee beliefs and actions. For example, the elaboration-likelihood model argues that persuasive effects of messages depend on both a direct route (addressee's deliberative processing of message meaning) and on peripheral routes (addressee's responses to indirect, secondary aspects of the message context) (Petty and Cacioppo 1986). This research addressed social psychological problems related to attitude change, but the mechanisms presumed to underlie persuasive effects of messages were similar to information processing models of text processing. Similarly, cognitive models of risk communication focus both on how addressees represent message meaning and how these representations interact with beliefs and domain knowledge in order to influence behavior.

For example, mental model theory focuses on how to design messages to target addressees' conceptions of risk (Morgan et al. 2001). The fuzzy trace theory argues that addressees can understand risk at both verbatim and gist-based levels, which have different effects on decision making and action (Reyna 2008). A large body of research that builds on such theories investigates how to leverage technology to deliver health-related messages tailored to addressee characteristics (Kreuter and Wray 2003).

3.2.2 *Communication as Interaction*

Interactive theories analyze how meaning emerges from coordination of speaker and listener actions ("sense-making in the moment"), and how this activity is influenced by constraints imposed by communication media and context and by speakers' and addressees' cognitive resources. An important idea is that communicative success depends on the interaction of participants' cognitive resources, with joint attention as a key resource. Therefore, interactive theories can be interpreted within the framework of distributed cognition, which analyzes human performance, including communication, as emerging from cognitive resources distributed across social contexts such as conversational partners, and external contexts such as tools (Hutchins 1995; a detailed description can be found in Chap. 2 in this volume).

3.2.2.1 Common Ground

Conversational partners communicate by coordinating cognitive effort in order to construct meaning (Clark 1996). To do this, they 'ground' information, or agree that the information is mutually understood and acceptable (accurate and relevant to joint goals). Grounding rests on and contributes to shared situation models (Morrow and Fischer 2013). In this view, speakers not only ensure that they are understood, but collaborate with their addressees to create meaning. For example, speakers may implicitly invite their addressees to co-construct their message by presenting an intentionally 'underdeveloped' contribution, encouraging their addressees to help specify the content. For example, a resident might say "I checked that patient.", prompting a nurse to complete the contribution "The one with edema?" "Right. It's down". Speakers may also present a message they think is clear, but the addressee's request for clarification reveals that it is undeveloped (Clark 1996; Coiera 2000). Thus, ongoing feedback is essential to communication. For example, stories are more understandable when speakers receive immediate feedback from their addressees (Bavelas et al. 2000).

Communication depends on joint or collaborative effort, as well as the individual effort involved in producing and understanding messages (Clark 1996; Coiera 2000). Developing common ground itself requires effort. Pre-emptive grounding involves devoting effort ahead of time to develop shared knowledge about the message domain, communication strategies, and other aspects of communication (Coiera 2000). The upfront work involved in pre-emptive grounding facilitates communication as it occurs (e.g., little cost to grounding during communication). For example, aviation communication depends heavily on shared knowledge about aviation concepts, terminology, and communication procedures that is acquired by Air Traffic Controllers and pilots as part of their professional training. This shared knowledge enables rapid and efficient communication during flight operations (Morrow and Fischer 2013). Similarly, in health care, two providers may discuss patients before a formal hand-off in order to expedite the later conversation. Just-in-time grounding, on the other hand, involves devoting effort during, rather than before, communication. In this case, partners share less knowledge about the domain and/or the conventions of communication, and so must devote more effort 'on the fly' during communication (Coiera 2000). For example, communication between domain experts and novices or between experts from different subdomains (e.g., physicians and nurses) often requires partners to be more explicit, devoting more effort to ground contributions.

Common ground theory helps to refine the view of how cognitive resources constrain communication. Speakers *initiate* contributions by getting their addressee's attention using verbal or nonverbal (e.g., gestures) cues. They then *present* messages that are designed to be understood based on common ground (shared knowledge of the language, cultural context, as well as more specific concepts that are relevant based on the prior discourse and context of communication). Listeners not only understand the message (which involves activating and integrating concepts, as described above), but also signal to the speaker that they do or do not understand. In the latter case, they may implicitly (e.g., puzzled expression) or explicitly request clarification. The speaker and addressee *accept* the message as mutually understood, so that the contribution enters common ground. These phases typically overlap: speakers often initiate contributions by presenting messages, and listeners often signal acceptance by responding to the message with a relevant contribution (Clark 1996).

Interactive approaches emphasize that communication depends on partners' collaborative or joint effort. For example, Air Traffic Controllers communicate by radio with many aircraft in the same air space in order to manage the flow of traffic. They may try to reduce their own effort by presenting one long, rapidly delivered message to a pilot rather than breaking it into several shorter messages that require more radio time and complicates the task of talking to multiple pilots on a single radio line. However, this strategy may increase the addressed pilot's effort involved in understanding and accepting the long message (by 'reading back' or repeating key concepts from the message in order to demonstrate understanding and help establish common ground). It also increases the likelihood that the pilot misunderstands and requests clarification or that the pilot does not explicitly accept the message at all (responding with minimal or no acknowledgement). The controller in turn must spend more radio time in order to 'close the communication loop' by clarifying their message and seeking confirmation that the pilot understood. The upshot is increased collaborative effort (Morrow et al. 1994). In health care, outgoing ICU nurses who hand off patients to incoming nurses may overestimate common ground when the incoming nurses are already familiar with the patients, so that they present overly abbreviated reports. This strategy minimizes their own effort involved in hand-offs, but at the expense of the incoming nurse who is likely to misunderstand and to request clarification, resulting in increased collaborative effort (Carroll et al. 2012). In short, successful communication depends on partners' ability to coordinate contributions through shared attention and collaborative effort. Such communication problems in turn contribute to adverse events that reduce patient safety (The Joint Commission 2005).

3.2.2.2 Common Ground and HCI in Health Care

Common ground theory (and distributed cognition theories more generally) is important for identifying factors that influence communication in health care settings, which depends heavily on technology and is often distributed over space (synchronous remote) and time (asynchronous remote), as well as occurring face-to-face. Next, we consider how collaborative effort and communication success depend on resources related to communication media, participants (e.g., cognition), and health care tasks. We also consider the role of technology as an external resource that shapes communication.

Communication Media

Media differ in terms of the opportunities they afford for, and constraints they impose on, establishing common ground (Clark and Brennan 1991; Monk 2008). In face-to-face communication, partners are co-present and typically see and hear each other as well as the referent situation. They can use nonverbal (gesture and facial expression) as well as verbal resources in order to coordinate attention on linguistic information as well as the nonlinguistic context when presenting and accepting messages. Communication can be efficient, with less need for elaborate verbal description compared to other media (Convertino et al. 2008; Gergle et al. 2004). Turn-taking is rapid, with messages received almost as they are produced (contemporality), the possibility of signaling that a message is understood as it is presented (simultaneity), and the order of contributions easily determined (sequentiality) (Clark and Brennan 1991). Face-to-face communication is especially suited for coordinating to accomplish joint tasks such as performing surgery. Nonverbal cues are also critical for conveying emotion, which is important for provider-patient communication. For example, provider communication behaviors such as leaning toward the patient and using facial expressions that convey concern predict patient satisfaction (Ambady et al. 2002).

Face-to-face communication also has drawbacks. Communication at work is often complex, with partners having to keep track of interacting topics or conversational threads. This complexity requires partners to easily access concepts from prior discourse (reviewability) and revise contributions in light of the evolving discourse (revisability) (Clark and Brennan 1991). The transient nature of speech complicates comprehension of complex messages because of listeners' working memory limits. More generally, the time pressure of face-to-face communication may preclude the deliberation needed to craft complex messages, as well as to understand them.

Other media may impose more constraints on communication, providing fewer resources for grounding. Synchronous communication with partners at different locations (e.g., telephone), like face-to-face communication, allows rapid turn-taking, contemporality, and simultaneity that support grounding (e.g., immediately indicating and repairing comprehension problems), but eliminates visual cues (unless using videophone), which can increase collaborative effort involved in accepting contributions (Clark and Brennan 1991). Synchronous remote communication has become pervasive with mobile phone technology. When partners are not visually co-present, this medium may increase overall workload because speakers cannot modulate their communication as required by listener context. A good example comes from driver distraction research. Driver-passenger conversation is less likely to disrupt driving (e.g., lane control; likelihood of seeing highway exit) compared to cell phone conversation, in part because driver and passenger are co-present and the passenger can modulate their talk as required by the situation (Drews et al. 2008). Texting, like online chat, is similar to synchronous remote communication because proficient texters use compressed language that allows rapid turn-taking, although this medium does not allow contemporality. Texting also eliminates auditory (e.g., speech prosody) cues for grounding and affective messages, which may be remediated in part by innovative use of punctuation and other symbols that convey affect. Texting also provides a record of the message, which supports reviewability.

Grounding can be even more challenging for asynchronous remote communication such as email, which lacks contemporality, simultaneity, and sometimes sequentiality. More effort is needed to produce messages (typing vs speaking), which influences individual and collaborative effort involved in grounding. Asynchronous voice communication (such as exchanging pre-recorded messages) is often less effective than synchronous communication (telephone conversation). For example, introducing an EHR system in an Emergency Department may increase the use of EHR-based emails between nurses and physicians about patient treatment plans, which reduces face-to-face communication that helps to clarify and elaborate shared treatment plans. On the other hand, email supports message reviewability and revisability and affords time for deliberation, which may result in more comprehensive and understandable messages (Olson and Olson 2007).

Communication Media and Tasks

The effects of media-related constraints depend on the tasks that people communicate about (Zigurs and Buckland 1998). For example, remote communication may be more appropriate for tasks that hinge on message reviewability and revisability, such as integrating multiple sources of complex information in order to diagnose an illness or troubleshoot a problem. Face-to-face or synchronous remote media may be more effective for tasks requiring frequent interaction to accomplish goals or to resolve conflicting goals (negotiation, persuasion). For example, an unstable ICU patient receiving provisional treatment that requires close monitoring would be better served by a face-to-face nurse handoff rather than an asynchronous handoff based on a phone message from the outgoing nurse.

Participant Resources

While information processing theories focus on speaker and listener cognitive resources (e.g., attention, working memory) needed to produce and understand messages, interactive theories emphasize that resources are also essential for grounding contributions to build a shared situation model, so that communication success depends on collaborative effort. For example, speakers with fewer cognitive resources, either because of long-term effects such as aging or short-term effects such as fatigue or distraction, may take more short-cuts when producing messages (resulting in more elliptical or vague messages) potentially complicating message comprehension and grounding. Conversely, listeners with fewer resources are less likely to explicitly acknowledge contributions, providing less evidence for comprehension and undermining grounding. Older adults with fewer cognitive resources may be less adept at tailoring message presentation to listeners based on common ground (Horton and Spieler 2007). On the other hand, shared knowledge about language, the discourse topic, and other aspects of communication can reduce effort and support grounding. This knowledge arises from partner familiarity and membership in a variety of linguistic/cultural communities and includes social norms and conversational conventions (Clark 1996). Partners who share knowledge about the discourse topic more quickly establish co-reference (Isaacs and Clark 1987) and more effectively perform joint tasks by coordinating attention to key information (Richardson et al. 2007), suggesting knowledge reduces collaborative effort. Shared knowledge may also support retrieval of previously mentioned information (Ericsson and Kintsch 1995). These benefits may explain why experts benefit more than novices from collaboration (compared to working alone) when recalling and acting on domain-relevant information (Meade et al. 2009).

Technology and Communication

Technology shapes communication in many ways, especially by expanding the repertoire of media options that create new communication opportunities and constraints. In complex environments such as hospitals, where work is typically done by multiple distributed and interacting teams, technology provides many options for remote communication, both synchronous (chat, texting, videophone, electronic status boards) and asynchronous (voicemail, email, clinical messaging in EHRs).

Technology, broadly considered as "cognitive artifacts," includes paper-based tools such as notes or whiteboards (Hutchins 1995; Nemeth et al. 2004). Distributed cognition theories analyze how artifacts, a pervasive part of work environments, reduce the need for mental computation, memory search, and other effortful cognitive processes involved in producing and understanding messages. They can support grounding by providing easily shared external referents that reduce need for explicit description (Monk 2008). They also support reviewability in face-to-face communication (Gergle et al. 2004) and visibility in synchronous remote communication such as teleconferencing because speakers can gesture to guide attention to information on the tool (Monk 2008; Whittaker et al. 1993). They especially benefit older adults by reducing demands of speech production and comprehension on cognitive resources (Morrow et al. 2003).

However, it is important to note that the benefits of technology-based tools can be overestimated. For example, using video-conferencing or other technology to distribute information to remote team members does not in itself ensure that people work together to effectively ground and act on this information. More generally, such technology may tempt us to distribute large amounts of information to as many people as possible. This strategy may undermine communication and reduce safety if information distribution is not guided by strategies to manage joint attention to the information that is most relevant within an evolving mental model organized around shared goals.

There is much interest in designing health information technology that flexibly supports a range of communication and task goals in different workflow situations. An important challenge for communication theory and research is to understand and predict strengths and limitations of different communication media and tools in complex environments such as the ICU or primary care clinics. This requires integrating theories that identify how participant-related and media-related resources interact with tasks to influence work, with macro analysis of work processes in organizations. Macro-level theories focus on how system-level outcomes such as safety and efficiency emerge from the interaction of system levels, e.g., individuals interacting with devices in the context of teams, management, organizational policies and practices (Carayon et al. 2013; Kaufman et al. 2014). Such an approach would analyze communication in organizations, with technology-related factors at different system levels interacting to influence communication between dyads, teams, etc.

Another communication issue that becomes increasingly important as clinicians routinely collaborate with technology, rather than using technology to collaborate with each other, is how common ground is established between people and technology. People tend to take a 'social stance' toward technology and treat it as a communication partner (Reeves and Nass 1996). In addition, technology must be able to reciprocate by building up and acting on common ground with their human partners. This requires technology to update and reason from a model of the user's context during communication (Coiera 2000). A simple example comes from the literature on automated tutoring systems, which are most effective when providing prompts that scaffold student learning based on a model of the student's current state of knowledge about the target domain.

3.3 Key Challenges for Health Care Communication

3.3.1 The High Cognitive Demands Associated with Biological Complexity

Health care is an information intensive domain that includes knowledge of normal and abnormal physiology, pharmacology, multiple treatment options and health specialties, health system and organizational infrastructure, a high volume of new clinical evidence, and longitudinal information about patients, families and their communities. Delivering care to patients and communicating about care is therefore a highly complex endeavor characterized by both uncertain responses to treatment interventions and changing patient conditions (Glouberman and Mintzberg 2001). For acutely ill patients, each change in their condition requires the clinicians to reorganize and reinterpret multiple sources of data (e.g., lab values, physical exam, vital signs and patient's subjective responses) to inform their next decision (Coiera and Tombs 1998; Collins et al. 2007; Edwards et al. 2009; Grundgeiger and Sanderson 2009; Tucker and Spear 2006), which further increases cognitive demands. Thus the potential for information overload and its associated safety implications is very high (Beasley et al. 2011).

The cognitive complexity of health care both reflects, and in turn contributes to, the need to perform multiple, interleaved tasks that result in pervasive interruptions (Coiera and Tombs 1998; Collins et al. 2007). Interruptions increase clinicians' cognitive load because of the need to recall the interrupted tasks, introducing risk for confusion and error (Tucker and Spear 2006) and for forgetting critical tasks (Collins et al. 2007). Interruptions also increase the complexity of communication, making it more vulnerable to error during hand-offs (Behara et al. 2005), when caring for patients in ICUs (Grundgeiger and Sanderson 2009), and in many other clinical tasks. Cognitive load can be exacerbated by poorly designed information displays and electronic interfaces that fragment, rather than integrate, information needed to perform multiple tasks, which can increase the frequency and conse-quences of interruption. A multi-site study of EHRs found that health care workers waste much time sifting through multiple sources of the information to get a true picture of a patient's situation, which is needed for effective communication (Stead and Lin 2009). Similarly, a study of intensive care nurses found that information needed to perform many of the common nursing tasks were inaccessible, difficult to see, and/or located in multiple displays (Koch et al. 2012). In sum, problems associated with cognitive demands in health care have important implications for communication and lead to ineffective decision making, important tasks left undone and high potential for error. These implications are more easily seen when communication is analyzed as emerging from, as well as contributing to, clinical workflow (Kaufman et al. 2014).

Interactive theories of communication are essential for explaining how cognitive and communication complexity reduces work efficiency and safety, which in turn provides a foundation for improving communication. For example, the need to switch topics when discussing patient care, or to interleave communication with other clinical tasks, complicates processes involved in grounding information and developing a shared mental model of the task. In face-to-face communication, speakers may truncate contributions or listeners may fail to acknowledge these contributions in an attempt to manage their own workload, which ends up increasing the collaborative workload involved in effective communication, or increasing the chance of inaccurate or incomplete communication that undermines patient care. The impact of interruption on these grounding processes may be greater for remote (e.g., telephone) communication because speakers and listeners do not share a visual context, and therefore cannot modulate communication to accommodate each other's workload. Given the high cognitive demands in health care and its relationship to quality and safety in health care, the application of information processing and interactive theories can aid in the design of tools to help clinicians manage the demands of communication during complex work. For example, large electronic status boards in ICUs or other environments in which multiple clinicians must coordinate care can support the ability to jointly attend to critical information, a pre-requisite for grounding information to develop a shared mental model that supports team performance. Tools that allow communication partners to electronically share and update care plans can also support grounding during asynchronous remote communication. For example, electronic checklists that saliently indicate the currently performed subtask can remind clinicians where they left off in a task when they are interrupted.

3.3.2 The Pervasive Nature of Interdisciplinary Work

The promotion of health and treatment of illness often involves multiple members of a health care team. Ambulatory patient care is most often led by a "team" of clinicians from the medical or nursing discipline. Hospitalized patients also require the care of several health disciplines including medicine, nursing and pharmacy. In both ambulatory and hospitalized patients, the complexity and acuity of the patient's condition is often reflected by the number of disciplines involved in their care, which may also require one or more medical subspecialties (e.g., cardiology, endocrinology, hematology) as well as a combination of care from other disciplines such as physical, occupational and or respiratory therapy, dietary counseling, pharmacy and social service. This means that the most complex patients are more likely to have complex interdisciplinary teams that must communicate effectively in order to coordinate care by performing interdependent tasks.

Moreover, although members of the "team" have different roles, there is increasingly blurred boundaries between some disciplines that have overlapping expertise (Kilpatrick et al. 2012). Finally, because many patients have multiple chronic illnesses, this type of interdisciplinary work is pervasive in our health care system.

Unfortunately, the term "team" in health care often does not mean that the group involved in care effectively communicates, collaborates, and coordinates care together based on shared mental models and goals (Schoen et al. 2011). Despite calls for teamwork (Corrigan 2005; Kohn et al. 2000) and significant research to improve teamwork in healthcare (McCulloch et al. 2011), there are multiple barriers to effective teamwork (Rosen and Pronovost 2012). In practice, team members often partake in silo-ed work on the patient's behalf, sharing information passively through the health record or reactively interrupting a "team" member's work when there is an urgent need (Coiera and Tombs 1998; Stoller 2013). When "team" members have the opportunity to communicate, many clinicians favor face-to-face communication, perhaps because this medium affords rapid turn-taking and a wealth of nonverbal as well as verbal cues that support interpretation and grounding of information (Williams et al. 2007). However, this practice is challenged because the "team" members often work in geo-physically separate places (Dunn Lopez and Whelan 2009; Weller et al. 2014) and may work only temporarily together on a single patient during hospitalization or during the course of an illness. In addition, the composition of hospital teams are subject to frequent, sometimes daily, changes due to limitations in duty hours, changing schedules, and personnel rotations.

For ambulatory patients with chronic conditions, the "team" may be formed over longer periods of time, but may be assembled by the patient, such that the same team members, including different disciplines and subspecialists, may only have one patient in common. Another challenge of patient-assembled teams is that team members may work in different organizations with different medical record systems that do not readily share information across settings. Finally, ambulatory schedules are generally clinician-driven with little to no time for synchronous collaborative discussions.

Inadequate communication between health care team members can harm patients. For example, hospital resident physicians who experience communication problems with nurses report a greater number of serious medical errors and adverse patient outcomes than residents who did not report poor communication episodes with nurses (Baldwin and Daugherty 2008). Less frequent sharing of information in surgical patients has been shown to double the risk of post-operative complication rates (Mazzocco et al. 2009), perhaps because it is more difficult to develop shared accurate mental models of the task that enable cross-monitoring and other collaborative processes required for successful performance (Xiao et al. 2013).

Although more research on interdisciplinary teamwork is needed, there are some examples of positive outcomes related to teamwork training or interventions. Interventions to promote shared goals have been shown to reduce post-operative complication rates (Haynes et al. 2011). Improved delivery of care may reflect the use of tools (e.g., checklists) and explicit communication procedures that help team members from different disciplines coordinate their attention on critical information, reducing the collaborative effort required to update a shared mental model of the task at hand. However, effective use of checklists can sometimes itself require coordination that adds complexity to joint work (Drews 2013). Such tools are more effective when integrated with communication procedures (Gawande 2011). Specialized teams in hospitals with shared goals, training and tools, and that work together over time (e.g., rapid response teams) have been shown to improve some teamwork processes (Mackintosh et al. 2012).

3.3.3 Discipline-Specific Terminologies and Taxonomies

Given that interdisciplinary work is pervasive in health care, it is somewhat surprising that each discipline uses specific and different terminologies and taxonomies, which contributes to the challenge of effectively communicating and coordinating across disciplines. Some of these differences relate to discipline-specific knowledge, traditions, and education and training practices. Clinicians from different disciplines may interpret the same information differently or make different assumptions about which information is most relevant, reflecting these differences. For example, nurses and physicians (Johnson and Turley 2006) and even physicians from different subspecialties (Hashem et al. 2003) tend to interpret the same patient information differently. There is also a lack of history of interaction among team members that can create barriers to developing shared mental models because of limited shared experience related to communication conventions, and knowledge. In other words, there is less opportunity for pre-emptive grounding that would reduce effort during communication (Coiera 2000). Furthermore, each discipline focuses on interrelated but different information and aspects of patient care (DiEugenio et al. 2013). This has been demonstrated through natural language processing of nursing and physician discharge notes that revealed minimal overlap in terms mapped to similar or related concepts between nurses and physicians caring for the same patients (DiEugenio et al. 2013). Therefore, given that knowledge guides attention to and decisions about relevant information in complex situations, these knowledge and linguistic differences between disciplines can undermine grounding processes, making communication challenging unless it is very explicit, which may be too inefficient when health care work is demanding and urgent.

3.3.4 Rapid Diffusion of Health Information Technologies

Communication technologies are important for addressing some of these challenges, particularly the need for frequent interdisciplinary communication. These technologies allow rapid exchange of, and negotiation about, information among team members that address the challenges of both interdependence and uncertainty. While many clinicians favor face-to-face communication (Williams et al. 2007), this is often not possible in health care where individual work is highly mobile (Welton et al. 2006). Physicians in hospitals often divide their time among several units, resulting in limited direct contact with individual nurses throughout the day (Dunn Lopez 2008). In addition, to promote patient privacy, interaction with patients is most often in individual rooms such that clinician team members may be geo-physically close to each other, but unaware of their proximity, which would offer opportunity for care coordination discussions. As mentioned above, technologies such as EHR systems may reinforce discipline-based practices rather than bridge discipline-based differences in order to support coordinated care (Stoller 2013).

Recent research indicates that nurses and physicians use a variety of different types of communication technology in hospitals. Nurses and physicians reported believing that the exchange of patient information by email improves the speed and reliability of information exchange and results in faster and safer care (O'Connor et al. 2009). Nurses and physicians also agreed that text messaging, email, and electronic "tasking" (notification of tasks that need to be completed) help ensure that patient care tasks are not left undone and can improve efficiency (O'Malley et al. 2010). Both physician and nurse workflows were improved in an evaluation study of a web-based tool that triaged pages for physicians (Locke et al. 2009). In another study, wireless alerts to residents helped them prioritize their work and promote quicker response times (Reddy et al. 2005). A less commonly used hands-free wearable communication device was found to support efficient communication that improved overall workflow (Richardson and Ash 2010).

Although there is some evidence for benefits of communication technologies, there are also unintended consequences that promote errors and inefficiency (Ash et al. 2007, 2009; a detailed description regarding the role of unintended consequences in health care environments can be found in Chap. 11). Communication technologies have rapidly diffused into health care from other domains. There is a need for theoretically-based and empirically-derived guidelines to determine which technologies are most effective in differing clinical situations. Traditionally, clinicians have relied on synchronous communication modes such as face-to-face or telephone that occur in real-time (Coiera and Tombs 1998) and are perceived by many to offer more complete information transfer (Williams et al. 2007). While these modes offer many resources for grounding information in order to develop shared mental models that support collaboration (e.g., nonverbal as well as verbal cues, rapid turn-taking), synchronous communication in the fast-paced, multi-task health care domain can also be interruptive, inefficient, and distracting, which can increase cognitive workload, miscommunication, and risk for error (Coiera 2006; Coiera and Tombs 1998; Collins et al. 2007; Karsh et al. 2006; Tucker and Spear 2006). More recently, asynchronous modes (transmit messages to be received at a later time) are increasingly used. These include email and texting, and are less interruptive and more appropriate for non-urgent clinical matters (Coiera and Tombs 1998; also refer to Chaps. 10 and 13 in this volume). However, these asynchronous modes may also pose threats to patient safety, including uncertain delivery, texts sent to the wrong person (Wong et al. 2009), missed messages, and delays in transmission (O'Malley et al. 2010; Varpio et al. 2009). These media also narrow the range of information that can be easily communicated (e.g., affective as well as cognitive meaning). Tasks that require negotiation, such as consults to interpret complex and uncertain patient information in order to come to a diagnosis, may be especially vulnerable to such asynchronous communication. However, to the extent that technologies such as texting preserve aspects of face-to-face communication such as rapid turn-taking, they may combine flexibility of this communication while avoiding some drawbacks, such as limited message reviewability and revisability.

3.3.5 Frequent Complete Transfer of Responsibility Within Disciplines

The round-the-clock nature of health care makes it unsafe for individual clinicians to provide care every hour of every day. For this reason, patient care in acute settings is regularly and frequently (2–3 times per day for hospitalized patients) transferred between clinicians. This is commonly referred to as a "handoff", indicating that the responsibility and authority for care is transferred to another individual of the same discipline. These transitions are conducted between two people or in groups using a variety of communication media, including face-to-face, telephone, audio recording or electronic tools. They present a vulnerable time period for patient care (Arora et al. 2008) for a variety of reasons, including the fact that they often occur in noisy environments with frequent interruptions (Kitch et al. 2008). Communication problems during handoffs, including omission of key information, occur frequently and lead to redundant work, missed care, delays in diagnosis and treatment, and medical errors such as near misses and sentinel events (Horwitz et al. 2008).

Clinicians often prefer face-to-face handoffs, in part because of the rich nonverbal as well as verbal resources for grounding information. However, handoffs require communicating large amounts of patient information, which can hamper face-to-face communication because transient speech limits the ability to revise and review this complex information (Morrow and Fischer 2013). Multiple efforts to improve the quality of handoffs, in part by reducing demands on memory, include low tech memory aids such as mnemonics, checklists, or paper templates (Gogan et al. 2013). More recently, electronic handoff tools have emerged (Abraham et al. 2014; Anderson et al. 2010; Bernstein et al. 2010; Keenan et al. 2005; Van Eaton et al. 2004). These tools, when integrated into the electronic health record, may decrease clinical workload if information needed for handoff is incorporated in an automated manner into a handoff template.

Theories that articulate the impact of communication media and participant constraints guide analysis of how these support tools can improve or impair handoff communication. For example, electronic tools may impair communication accuracy and reduce the ability of incoming clinicians to assume responsibility for patient care to the extent they reduce the interactive synchronous communication needed to successfully ground information and negotiate shared goals. Moreover, some important functions of handoffs, such as discovering patient care errors when incoming clinicians review information, may be eliminated to the extent electronic tools reduce interaction during handoffs (Staggers and Blaz 2013).

3.4 Conclusion

Communication in the clinical environment has played a key role in health care for several decades. Over time, its importance has increased given the number of health care providers from many disciplines, specialties and sub-specialties working interdependently to provide discipline-specific care to patients. This importance is also reflected in the evidence that miscommunication often contributes to patient care errors and inefficiency. In response, there is increased attention on health care communication as a means to minimize inefficient and unsafe care related to poor communication processes. For example, it is hoped that the use of technology to increase the speed of information transfer and access to real time information among team members will reduce delays in care and shorten hospital stays, potentially saving substantial costs. However, because there are drawbacks as well as benefits to any technology, research is needed to evaluate the effects of clinical communication technologies.

With the crisis in health care costs in the United States, attention to the field of health care communication extends beyond academics to regulators. The Joint Commission has required implementation of a standardized handoff method since 2006, giving rise to the design and testing of tools for handoff communication (Agency for Healthcare Quality and Research 2012). To meet this requirement, many hospitals implemented measures that were not theoretically based. More recently, The Center for Medicare and Medicaid Services introduced significant financial incentives to implement electronic health records, with some of the emphasis on clinical communication and communication with patients (DesRoches et al. 2013). Again, the design, implementation, and evaluation of these tools are not often guided by communication theories.

In this chapter, we pointed out the need for, and value of, leveraging theories to guide research on communication in complex health care settings. These theories identify important characteristics of communication situations (e.g., media, participants, context) likely to impact the success of communication, as well as the processes underlying communication, which help explain why communication fails in particular situations. Such analyses in turn can guide development of design and training approaches to improve communication in clinical environments. These theories are especially important for explaining effects of technology on communication and delivery of patient care, and for anticipating potential effects of new technologies before they are implemented. Theories that have been most frequently applied to the health domain often derive from analysis of conversation (typically between two people; Clark 1996; see Monk 2008 for extensions to health care technology) and are used to analyze processes underlying exchange of information between patients and providers or between incoming and outgoing clinicians during handoffs (Abraham et al. 2013). An important challenge is to integrate such theories with more macro-level system theories in order to analyze processes and representations involved in communication among networks of people and technologies that coordinate to accomplish complex patient care tasks.

Discussion Questions
1. What are the key challenges to clinical communication?
2. What are the concepts and theories that can be applied to communication in healthcare?

Acknowledgements Preparation of this chapter was supported by the National Institute of Aging (Grant R01 AG31718) and the National Institute of Nursing Research (Grant R01 NR011300). Any opinions, findings, and conclusions or recommendations expressed in this publication are those of the authors and do not necessarily reflect the views of the NIH.

Additional Readings

Coiera, E. (2006). Communication systems in healthcare. *Clinical Biochemist Reviews, 27*(2), 89.
Collins, S. A., Bakken, S., Vawdrey, D. K., Coiera, E., & Currie, L. (2011). Clinician preferences for verbal communication compared to EHR documentation in the ICU. *Applied Clinical Informatics, 2*(2), 190.
O'Malley, A. S., Grossman, J. M., Cohen, G. R., Kemper, N. M., & Pham, H. H. (2010). Are electronic medical records helpful for care coordination? Experiences of physician practices. *Journal of General Internal Medicine, 25*(3), 177–185.

References

Abraham, J., Kannampallil, T., Almoosa, K. F., Patel, B., & Patel, V. L. (2013). Comparative evaluation of the content and structure of communication using two handoff tools: Implications for patient safety. *Journal of Critical Care, 29*(2), 311.e1–311.e7.
Abraham, J., Kannampallil, T., & Patel, V. L. (2014). A systematic review of the literature on the evaluation of handoff tools: Implications for research and practice. *Journal of the American Medical Informatics Association, 21*(1), 154–162.
Agency for Healthcare Quality and Research. (2012, October). Handoffs and signouts. *Patient Safety Primer.* Retrieved May 19, 2014, from http://psnet.ahrq.gov/primer.aspx?primerID=9
Ambady, N., Koo, J., Rosenthal, R., & Winograd, C. H. (2002). Physical therapists' nonverbal communication predicts geriatric patients' health outcomes. *Psychology and Aging, 17*(3), 443.

Anderson, J., Shroff, D., Curtis, A., Eldridge, N., Cannon, K., Karnani, R., . . . Kaboli, P. (2010). The veteran's affair shift change physician-to-physician hand off project. *The Joint Commission Journal on Quality and Patient Safety, 36*(2), 62–71.

Arocha, J. F., & Patel, V. L. (1994). Construction-integration theory and clinical reasoning. In C. A. Weaver III, S. Mannes, & C. R. Fletcher (Eds.), *Discourse comprehension: Essays in honor of Walter Kintsch* (pp. 359–381). Hillsdale: Lawrence Erlbaum Associates.

Arora, V., Johnson, J., Meltzer, D., & Humphrey, H. (2008). A theoretical framework and competency-based approach to improving handoffs. *Quality and Safety in Health Care, 17*(1), 11–14.

Ash, J., Sittig, D., Dyskstra, R., Guappone, K., Carpenter, J., & Seshadri, V. (2007). Categorizing the unintended sociotechnical consequences of computerized provider order entry. *International Journal of Medical Informatics, 76*(Suppl 1), S1–S27.

Ash, J., Sittig, D., Dyskstra, R., Campbell, E., & Guappone, K. (2009). The unintended consequences of computer provider order entry: Findings from a mixed methods exploration. *International Journal of Medical Informatics, 78*(Suppl 1), S69–S76.

Austin, J. (1960). *How to do things with words*. Oxford: Clarendon Press.

Baldwin, D., & Daugherty, S. (2008). Interprofessional conflict and medical errors: Results of a national multi-specialty survey of hospital residents in the US. *Journal of Interprofessional Care, 22*(6), 573–586.

Bavelas, J. B., Coates, L., & Johnson, T. (2000). Listeners as co-narrators. *Journal of Personality and Social Psychology, 79*(6), 941.

Beasley, J. W., Wetterneck, T. B., Temte, J., Lapin, J. A., Smith, P., Rivera-Rodriguez, A. J., & Karsh, B.-T. (2011). Information chaos in primary care: Implications for physician performance and patient safety. *The Journal of the American Board of Family Medicine, 24*(6), 745–751.

Behara, R., Wears, R. L., Perry, S. J., Eisenberg, E., Murphy, L., Vanderhoef, M. et al. (2005). *Advances in patient safety: From research to implementation* (2, AHRQ Publication Nos. 050021, pp. 1–4). Rockville: Agency for Healthcare Research and Quality. http://www.ahrq.gov/qual/advances/

Bernstein, J. A., Imler, D. L., Sharek, P., & Longhurst, C. A. (2010). Improved physician work flow after integrating sign-out notes into the electronic medical record. *Joint Commission Journal on Quality and Patient Safety, 36*(2), 72–78.

Carayon, P., Karsh, B.-T., Gurses, A., Holden, R., Hoonakker, P., Hundt, A., . . . Wetterneck, T. (2013). Macroergonomics in health care quality and patient safety. *Reviews of Human Factors and Ergonomics, 8*(1), 4–54.

Carroll, J. S., Williams, M., & Gallivan, T. M. (2012). The ins and outs of change of shift handoffs between nurses: A communication challenge. *BMJ Quality & Safety, 21*(7), 586–593.

Clark, H. (1996). *Using language*. Cambridge: Cambridge University Press.

Clark, H., & Brennan, S. (1991). Grounding in communication. *Perspectives on Socially Shared Cognition, 13*(1991), 127–149.

Coiera, E. (2000). When conversation is better than computation. *Journal of the American Medical Informatics Association, 7*(3), 277–286.

Coiera, E. (2006). Communication systems in healthcare. *Clinical Biochemistry Review, 27*, 89–98.

Coiera, E., & Tombs, V. (1998). Communication behaviors in a hospital setting: An observational study. *British Medical Journal, 316*, 673–677.

Collins, S., Currie, L., Patel, V., Bakken, S., & Cimino, J. (2007). Multitasking by clinicians in the context of CPOE and CIS use. *Studies of Health Technologies Information, 129*(part 2), 958–962.

Convertino, G., Mentis, H. M., Rosson, M. B., Carroll, J. M., Slavkovic, A., & Ganoe, C. H. (2008). *Articulating common ground in cooperative work: Content and process*. Paper presented at the proceedings of the SIGCHI conference on human factors in computing systems.

Cordero, C. (2011). *Advancing effective communication, cultural competence, and patient-and family-centered care: A roadmap for hospitals.* Oakbrook Terrace: The Joint Commission and National Association of Public Hospitals and Health Systems.

Corrigan, J. M. (2005). Crossing the quality chasm. In P. P. Reid, W. Dale Compton, J. H. Grossman, & G. Fanjiang (Eds.), *Building a better delivery system.* Washington, DC: National Academies Press.

Davison, J., Fischer, U., & Orasanu, J. (2003). *When language becomes a barrier instead of a bridge: Communication failures between pilots and air traffic controllers.* Paper presented at the proceedings of the 12th international symposium on aviation psychology, Columbus, OH.

DesRoches, C., Audet, A.-M., Painter, M., & Donelan, K. (2013). Meeting meaningful use criteria and managing patient populations: A national survey of practicing physicians. *Annals of Internal Medicine, 158*(11), 791–799.

DiEugenio, B., Lugaresi, C., Keenan, G., Lussier, Y., Li, J., Burton, M., … Boyd, A. (2013). *Integrating physician discharge notes with coded nursing care data to generate patient-centric summaries.* Paper presented at the American Medical Informatics Association, Washington, DC.

Drews, F. (2013). Human factors in critical care medical environments. *Reviews of Human Factors and Ergonomics, 8,* 103–148.

Drews, F. A., Pasupathi, M., & Strayer, D. L. (2008). Passenger and cell phone conversations in simulated driving. *Journal of Experimental Psychology: Applied, 14*(4), 392.

Dunn Lopez, K. (2008). *A mixed methods study of nurse-physician work relationships-oral presentation.* Paper presented at the Midwest Nursing Research Society annual meeting, Indianapolis, IN.

Dunn Lopez, K., & Whelan, C. (2009). A qualitative study of hospitalists and nonhospitalists work relationships with staff nurses. *Journal of Hospital Medicine, 4*(Supp 1), 39–40.

Durso, F. T., & Drews, F. A. (2010). Health care, aviation, and ecosystems a socio-natural systems perspective. *Current Directions in Psychological Science, 19*(2), 71–75.

Edwards, A., Fitzpatrick, L., Augustine, S., Trzebucki, A., Cheng, S., Presseau, C., … Kachnowski, S. (2009). Synchronous communication facilitates interruptive workflow for attending physicians and nurses in clinical settings. *International Journal of Medical Informatics, 78*(9), 629–637.

Ericsson, K. A., & Kintsch, W. (1995). Long-term working memory. *Psychological Review, 102* (2), 211.

Gawande, A. (2011). *The checklist manifesto: How to get things right.* New York: Holt & Co.

Gergle, D., Kraut, R. E., & Fussell, S. R. (2004). Language efficiency and visual technology minimizing collaborative effort with visual information. *Journal of Language and Social Psychology, 23*(4), 491–517.

Glouberman, S., & Mintzberg, H. (2001). Managing the care of health and the cure of disease: Part 1. *Health Care Management Review, 23*(1), 56–69.

Gogan, J. L., Baxter, R. J., Boss, S. R., & Chircu, A. M. (2013). Handoff processes, information quality and patient safety: A trans-disciplinary literature review. *Business Process Management Journal, 19*(1), 70–94.

Grundgeiger, T., & Sanderson, P. (2009). Interruptions in healthcare: Theoretical views. *International Journal of Medical Informatics, 78*(5), 293–307.

Hashem, A., Chi, M., & Friedman, C. (2003). Medical errors as a result of specialization. *Journal of Biomedical Informatics, 36*(1), 61–69.

Haynes, A. B., Weiser, T. G., Berry, W. R., Lipsitz, S. R., Breizat, A.-H. S., Dellinger, E. P., … Lapitan, M. C. M. (2011). Changes in safety attitude and relationship to decreased postoperative morbidity and mortality following implementation of a checklist-based surgical safety intervention. *BMJ Quality & Safety, 20*(1), 102–107.

Horton, W., & Spieler, D. (2007). Age-related differences in communication and audience design. *Psychology and Aging, 22*(2), 281.

Horwitz, L. I., Moin, T., Krumholz, H. M., Wang, L., & Bradley, E. H. (2008). Consequences of inadequate sign-out for patient care. *Archives of Internal Medicine, 168*(16), 1755–1760.

Hutchins, E. (1995). *Cognition in the wild* (Vol. 262082314). Cambridge, MA: MIT Press.

Isaacs, E. A., & Clark, H. H. (1987). References in conversation between experts and novices. *Journal of Experimental Psychology: General, 116*(1), 26.

Johnson, C., & Turley, J. (2006). The significance of cognitive modeling in building healthcare interfaces. *International Journal of Medical Informatics, 75*(2), 163–172.

Joint Commission on Accreditation of Healthcare Organizations. (2005). Root causes of medication errors (1995–2004). Retrieved November 2, 2005.

Karsh, B., Holden, R., Alper, S., & Or, C. (2006). A human factors engineering paradigm for patient safety: Designing to support the performance of the healthcare professional. *Quality and Safety in Health Care, 15*(Supp 1), i59–i65.

Kaufman, D. R., Mamykina, L., & Abraham, J. (2014). Communication and complexity: Negotiating transitions in critical care. In V. L. Patel, D. Kaufman, & T. Cohen (Eds.), *Cognitive informatics in health and biomedicine: Case studies on critical care, complexity and errors*. London: Springer.

Keenan, G., Yakel, E., & Marriott, D. (2005). HANDS: A revitalized technology supported care planning method to improve nursing handoffs. *Studies in Health Technology and Informatics, 122*, 580–584.

Kilpatrick, K., Lavoie-Tremblay, M., Ritchie, J. A., Lamothe, L., & Doran, D. (2012). Boundary work and the introduction of acute care nurse practitioners in healthcare teams. *Journal of Advanced Nursing, 68*(7), 1504–1515.

Kim, M., Barnato, A., Angus, D., Fleisher, L., & Kahn, J. (2010). The effect of multidisciplinary care teams on intensive care unit mortality. *Archives of Internal Medicine, 170*(4), 369–376.

Kintsch, W. (1998). *Comprehension: A paradigm for cognition*. Cambridge: Cambridge University Press.

Kitch, B. T., Cooper, J. B., Zapol, W. M., Marder, J. E., Karson, A., Hutter, M., & Campbell, E. G. (2008). Handoffs causing patient harm: A survey of medical and surgical house staff. *Joint Commission Journal on Quality and Patient Safety, 34*(10), 563–570.

Knaus, W. A., Draper, E. A., Wagner, D. P., & Zimmerman, J. E. (1986). An evaluation of outcome from intensive care in major medical centers. *Annals of Internal Medicine, 104*(3), 410–418.

Koch, S. H., Weir, C., Haar, M., Staggers, N., Agutter, J., Görges, M., & Westenskow, D. (2012). Intensive care unit nurses' information needs and recommendations for integrated displays to improve nurses' situation awareness. *Journal of the American Medical Informatics Association, 19*(4), 583–590.

Kohn, L. T., Corrigan, J. M., & Donaldson, M. S. (2000). *To err is human: Building a safer health system committee on quality of health care in America*. Washington, DC: Institute of Medicine.

Kreuter, M. W., & Wray, R. J. (2003). Tailored and targeted health communication: Strategies for enhancing information relevance. *American Journal of Health Behavior, 27*(Suppl 3), S227–S232.

Levelt, W. J. (1989). *Speaking: From intention to articulation* (ACL: MIT Press series in natural-language processing). Cambridge, MA: MIT Press.

Locke, K., Duffey-Rosenstein, B., De Lio, G., Morra, D., & Hariton, N. (2009). Beyond paging: Building a web-based communication tool for nurses and physicians. *Journal of General Internal Medicine, 24*(1), 105–110.

Mackintosh, N., Rainey, H., & Sandall, J. (2012). Understanding how rapid response systems may improve safety for the acutely ill patient: Learning from the frontline. *BMJ Quality & Safety, 21*(2), 135–144.

Mazzocco, K., Petitti, D. B., Fong, K. T., Bonacum, D., Brookey, J., Graham, S., . . . Thomas, E. J. (2009). Surgical team behaviors and patient outcomes. *The American Journal of Surgery, 197*(5), 678–685.

McCulloch, P., Rathbone, J., & Catchpole, K. (2011). Interventions to improve teamwork and communications among healthcare staff. *British Journal of Surgery, 98*(4), 469–479.

Meade, M., Nokes, T., & Morrow, D. G. (2009). Expertise promotes facilitation on a collaborative memory task. *Memory, 17*(1), 39–48.

Miller, G. A. (2003). The cognitive revolution: A historical perspective. *Trends in Cognitive Sciences, 7*(3), 141–144.

Monk, A. (2008). Common ground in electronically mediated conversation. *Synthesis Lectures on Human-Centered Informatics, 1*(1), 1–50.

Morgan, K. M., DeKay, M. L., Fischbeck, P. S., Morgan, M. G., Fischhoff, B., & Florig, H. K. (2001). A deliberative method for ranking risks (II): Evaluation of validity and agreement among risk managers. *Risk Analysis, 21*(5), 923.

Morrow, D. G., & Fischer, U. M. (2013). Communication in socio-technical systems. In J. D. Lee & A. Kirlik (Eds.), *The Oxford handbook of cognitive engineering* (pp. 178–199). Oxford: Oxford University Press.

Morrow, D., Rodvold, M., & Lee, A. (1994). Nonroutine transactions in controller-pilot communication. *Discourse Processes, 17*(2), 235–258.

Morrow, D., Ridolfo, H., Menard, W., Sanborn, A., Stine-Morrow, E., Magnor, C., . . . Bryant, D. (2003). Environmental support promotes expertise-based mitigation of age differences on pilot communication tasks. *Psychology and Aging, 18*(2), 268.

Nemeth, C. P., Cook, R. I., O'Connor, M., & Klock, P. A. (2004). Using cognitive artifacts to understand distributed cognition. *IEEE Transactions on Systems, Man and Cybernetics, Part A: Systems and Humans, 34*(6), 726–735.

O'Connor, C., Friedrich, J., Scales, D., & Adhikari, N. (2009). The use of wireless e-mail to improve healthcare communication. *Journal of the American Medical Informatics Association, 16*(5), 705–713.

O'Malley, A., Grossman, J., Cohen, G., Kemper, N., & Pham, H. (2010). Are electronic medical records helpful for care coordination? Experiences of physician practices. *Journal of General Internal Medicine, 25*(December, 3), 177–185.

Olson, G. M., & Olson, J. S. (2007). Computer-support cooperative work. In *Handbook of applied cognition* (pp. 497–526). Chichester: Wiley.

Patel, V. L., Arocha, J. F., & Kushniruk, A. W. (2002). Patients' and physicians' understanding of health and biomedical concepts: Relationship to the design of EMR systems. *Journal of Biomedical Informatics, 35*, 8–16.

Patterson, E. S., & Wears, R. L. (2010). Patient handoffs: Standardized and reliable measurement tools remain elusive. *Joint Commission Journal on Quality and Patient Safety, 36*(2), 52–61.

Petty, R. E., & Cacioppo, J. T. (1986). The elaboration likelihood model of persuasion. *Advances in Experimental Social Psychology, 19*, 123–205.

Reddy, M. (1979). The conduit metaphor: A case of frame conflict in our language about language. *Metaphor and Thought, 2*, 164–201.

Reddy, M., McDonald, D., Pratt, W., & Shabot, M. (2005). Technology, work, and information flows: Lessons from the implementation of a wireless alert pager system. *Journal of Biomedical Informatics, 38*, 229–238.

Reeves, B., & Nass, C. (1996). *How people treat computers, television, and new media like real people and places.* Stanford/New York: CSLI Publications/Cambridge University Press.

Reyna, V. F. (2008). A theory of medical decision making and health: Fuzzy trace theory. *Medical Decision Making, 28*(6), 850–865.

Richardson, J., & Ash, J. (2010). The effects of hands free communication devices on clinical communication: Balancing communication needs with clinical user control. *British Medical Journal, 17*(1), 91–98.

Richardson, D., Dale, R., & Kirkham, N. (2007). The art of conversation is coordination common ground and the coupling of eye movements during dialogue. *Psychological Science, 18*(5), 407–413.

Rosen, M. A., & Pronovost, P. J. (2012). Teamwork in healthcare: From training programs to integrated systems of development. In Eduardo Salas & Karen Frush (Eds.), *Improving patient safety through teamwork and team training* (p. 239). Oxford: Oxford University Press.

Schoen, C., Osborn, R., Squires, D., Doty, M., Pierson, R., & Applebaum, S. (2011). New 2011 survey of patients with complex care needs in eleven countries finds that care is often poorly coordinated. *Health Affairs, 30*(12), 2437–2448.

Shannon, C. E., & Weaver, N. (1949). *The mathematical theory of communication.* Urbana: University of Illinois Press.

Shortell, S. M., Zimmerman, J. E., Gillies, R. R., Duffy, J., Devers, K. J., Rousseau, D. M., & Knaus, W. A. (1992). Continuously improving patient care: Practical lessons and an assessment tool from the National ICU Study. *Quality Review Bulletin, 18*(5), 150–155.

Staggers, N., & Blaz, J. W. (2013). Research on nursing handoffs for medical and surgical settings: An integrative review. *Journal of Advanced Nursing, 69*(2), 247–262.

Stead, W., & Lin, H. (Eds.). (2009). *Computational technology for effective health care: Immediate steps and strategic directions.* Washington, DC: National Academies Press.

Stine-Morrow, E. A., & Miller, L. (2009). Aging, self-regulation, and learning from text. *Psychology of Learning and Motivation, 51,* 255–296.

Stoller, J. (2013). Electronic siloing: An unintended consequence of the electronic health record. *Cleveland Clinic Journal of Medicine, 80*(7), 406–409.

Tucker, A., & Spear, S. (2006). Operational failures and interruptions in hospital nursing. *Health Services Research, 41*(3), 643–662.

Van Eaton, E., Horvath, K., Lober, W., & Pellegrini, C. (2004). Organizing the transfer of patient information: The development of a computerized resident sign out system. *Surgery, 136,* 5–13.

Varpio, L., Schyer, C., & Lingard, L. (2009). Routine and adaptive expert strategies for resolving ICT mediated communication problems in the team setting. *Medical Education, 43,* 680–687.

Weller, J., Boyd, M., & Cumin, D. (2014). Teams, tribes and patient safety: Overcoming barriers to effective teamwork in healthcare. *Postgraduate Medical Journal, 90*(1061), 149–154. doi:10.1136/postgradmedj-2012-131168.

Welton, J., Decker, M., Adam, J., & Zone-Smith, L. (2006). How far do nurses walk? *Medsurg Nursing, 15*(4), 213–216.

Whittaker, S., Geelhoed, E., & Robinson, E. (1993). Shared workspaces: How do they work and when are they useful? *International Journal of Man-Machine Studies, 39*(5), 813–842.

Wickens, C., & Hollands, J. (2000). *Engineering psychology and human performance.* (3rd ed.). Upper Saddle River NJ: Prentice Hall. ISBN 0-321-04711-7.

Williams, R., Silverman, R., Schwind, C., Fortune, J., Sutyak, J., Horvath, K., … Dunnington, G. (2007). Surgeon information transfer and communication: Factors affecting quality and efficiency of inpatient care. *Annals of Surgery, 245*(2), 2007.

Wong, B., Quan, S., Cheung, C., Morra, D., Rossos, P., Sivjee, K., … Etchells, E. (2009). Frequency and clinical importance of pages sent to the wrong physician. *Archive of Internal Medicine, 169*(11), 1072–1073.

Xiao, Y., Parker, S. H., & Manser, T. (2013). Teamwork and collaboration. *Reviews of Human Factors and Ergonomics, 8*(1), 55–102.

Zigurs, I., & Buckland, B. (1998). A theory of task/technology fit and group support systems effectiveness. *MIS Quarterly, 22*(3), 313–334.

Zwaan, R. A., & Taylor, L. J. (2006). Seeing, acting, understanding: Motor resonance in language comprehension. *Journal of Experimental Psychology: General, 135*(1), 1.

Chapter 4
A New Socio-technical Model for Studying Health Information Technology in Complex Adaptive Healthcare Systems

Dean F. Sittig and Hardeep Singh

4.1 Introduction

The promise of health information technology (HIT) is safer, more efficient, and more effective healthcare systems. HIT (including electronic health records [EHRs]) has potential to improve care by reducing preventable errors, assisting healthcare providers with clinical decision-making, and enabling rapid communication among members of healthcare teams. In reality, implementation of HIT comes with innumerable challenges. Some of these challenges are foreseeable (e.g., maintaining safe and effective clinical operations during a transition between record systems). However, many others are unanticipated; examples include increased provider burden, inconsistent (or improper) user behavior, problems with interactions between systems, and errors in clinical content or function. Despite some successes, to date the realized benefits of HIT have fallen short of expectations. Hindsight suggests that many unintended consequences of HIT

Based on Sittig DF, Singh H. A New Socio-technical Model for Studying Health Information Technology in Complex Adaptive Healthcare Systems. Quality & Safety in Healthcare, 2010 Oct;19 Suppl 3:i68–74. doi:10.1136/qshc.2010.042085. PMID: 20959322

The views expressed in this article are those of the authors and do not necessarily represent the views of the Department of Veterans Affairs or the National Institutes of Health. No conflicts of interest

D.F. Sittig, Ph.D. (✉)
The UT-Memorial Hermann Center for Healthcare Quality & Safety, University of Texas School of Biomedical Informatics at Houston, 6410 Fannin St. UTPB 1100.43, Houston, TX 77030, USA
e-mail: Dean.F.Sittig@uth.tmc.edu

H. Singh, M.D., MPH
Houston VA HSR&D Center for Innovations in Quality, Effectiveness and Safety (IQuESt), The Michael E. Debakey Veterans Affairs Medical Center and the Section of Health Services Research, Department of Medicine, Baylor College of Medicine, Houston, TX, USA

© Springer International Publishing Switzerland 2015
V.L. Patel et al. (eds.), *Cognitive Informatics for Biomedicine*, Health Informatics, DOI 10.1007/978-3-319-17272-9_4

implementation are actually due to a lack of consideration of one or more facets of the systems into which HIT is introduced.

Implicit in some approaches to HIT implementation is the idea that new technologies are themselves the drivers of change and it is the responsibility of people and organizations to adapt to them. In contrast, socio-technical approaches posit that technologies operate within social and organizational contexts that are inseparable from the presence or influence of the technologies themselves. Such approaches have gained a foothold in research in the fields of organizational development and information systems, and have recently been applied specifically to the study of HIT.

An ongoing challenge to the design, development, implementation, and evaluation of HIT interventions is to operationalize their use within the complex adaptive healthcare system that consists of high-pressured, fast-paced, and distributed settings of care delivery. Given the dearth of models that are specifically designed to address safe and effective HIT development and use, we have developed a comprehensive, socio-technical model that provides a multidimensional framework within which any HIT innovation, intervention, application, or device implemented within a complex adaptive healthcare system can be studied. This model builds upon and bridges previous frameworks, and is further informed by our own work to study the safe and effective implementation and use of HIT interventions. In this chapter, we describe the conceptual foundations of our model and provide several examples of its utility for studying HIT interventions within real-world clinical contexts.

4.2 Background

Previous analyses of HIT interventions have been limited by a lack of conceptual models that have been specifically developed for this purpose. Examples of models previously applied by HIT investigators include:

- Rogers' diffusion of innovations theory (Rogers 2003), which has been used to help explain why some HIT innovations succeed while others fail (Ash 1997; Gosling et al. 2003). It outlines five characteristics that affect the likelihood that a particular innovation will be accepted: (1) relative advantage – how much "better" the new technology is compared to what it replaces; (2) compatibility – the extent to which the new technology is consistent with existing values, beliefs, previous experience, and current needs; (3) complexity – the level of difficulty involved in learning and using the new technology; (4) trialability – the feasibility of experimenting with the new technology; and (5) observability – the visibility of improvements resulting from the innovation. Unfortunately, none of these five characteristics address the design, development, or evaluation of HIT, nor the complexities involved in iteratively refining new technologies.

- Venkatesh's unified theory of acceptance and use of technology (UTAUT) (Venkatesh et al. 2003; Holden and Karsh 2010; Duyck et al. 2008; Kijsanayotin et al. 2009) synthesizes components of eight different models to describe determinants of users' acceptance of new technologies. The UTAUT model provides a powerful tool for HIT developers and implementers who face challenges in assessing whether a new technology intervention will succeed. It can also help them to understand what drives acceptance, and how to design and implement new interventions (e.g., novel training, marketing, or implementation methods) aimed at those who are less likely to use new systems successfully. However, this model fails to address any specific features or functions of HIT interventions; rather, it focuses solely on the users' reactions to these interventions.
- Hutchins' theory of distributed cognition (Hutchins 1996) identifies three key principles of cognitive processes, specifically that they are often distributed: (1) among members of a work team; (2) between internal human thought processes and items in the external physical world (e.g., on the computer screen or written notes); and (3) across time (i.e., later events are dependent on earlier events). Recently (Hazlehurst et al. 2003, 2007; Cohen et al. 2006; Patel et al. 2008), distributed cognition has been applied to study the design and utilization of HIT with a focus on how the combined human-HIT activity system can be improved. However, this theory does not explicitly include the specific technical details of the HIT system that we believe are critical to future success of HIT.
- Reason's Swiss Cheese Model (Reason 2000; van der Sijs et al. 2006; Lederman and Parkes 2005) describes a systematic approach to error reduction that relies on various defenses that improve the safety and effectiveness of the healthcare system. These defenses can be engineered into the HIT (examples include automated alerts, default values, or terminal placement). Errors may result from holes in these defenses due to active failures and/or latent conditions such as poorly trained individuals or inadequate policies and procedures. Although this model provides an excellent view of how errors might occur despite state-of-the-art HIT, it does not address specific aspects of the hardware, software, content or user interfaces of these systems.
- Norman's 7-step human-computer interaction model (Norman 1988; Malhotra et al. 2007; Sheehan et al. 2009) addresses one key element of any HIT system – the process by which a user interacts with a computer application. This model is very powerful for analyzing individuals as they interact with a computer. However, it does not explain the role of the hardware or software, or how the application fits into the user's larger workflow and organizational context.

Although all of these models account for one or more important facets of technology implementation, we believe that the scope of each model limits its utility to address the full range of factors that should be considered in the design, development, implementation, use, and evaluation of HIT interventions. For example, these models were not specifically designed to address the complex relationships between the HIT hardware, software, information content, and the human-computer interface. Furthermore, while most of these models provide general guidance to study the high-level aspects of HIT implementation within a given clinical environment, none of them include a measurement and monitoring infrastructure (e.g., methods to routinely collect data, create or review reports, or conduct surveillance of outcomes). Based on these limitations, our aim was to develop a more comprehensive model to integrate specific technological and measurement dimensions of HIT with other socio-technical dimensions (e.g., people, workflow, communication, organizational policies, external rules and regulations).

Four related socio-technical models have been particularly influential in providing the foundation of our proposed model. First, Henriksen's model focuses on the capabilities of the people involved in the complexity of the work, but does not delve into the technical characteristics of the hardware or software in use. Specifically, it addresses (1) individual provider characteristics; (2) the nature or complexity of the work or task performed; (3) the physical environment where care takes place; (4) the human-system interfaces involved; and (5) various characteristics of the organization (social, environment, and management) (Henriksen et al. 1993). Second, Vincent's 1998 framework for analyzing risk and safety proposes a hierarchy of patient, work, and environmental factors that can potentially influence clinical practice (Vincent et al. 1998), but fails to recognize the emerging role of computer-based systems that are now common in most healthcare settings. Third, Carayon's Systems Engineering Initiative for Patient Safety (SEIPS) model (Carayon et al. 2006) identifies three domains: (1) characteristics of providers, their tools and resources, and the physical/organizational setting; (2) interpersonal and technical aspects of healthcare activities; and (3) change in the patient's health status or behavior. Again, their model does an excellent job of characterizing the key actors and aspects of the healthcare work system, but falls short in its attention to the internal and external characteristics of the hardware and software that govern the human-computer interactions with the "technical" portion of their model. Finally, Harrison et al.'s Interactive Socio-technical Analysis (ISTA) framework provides an excellent broad overview of the complex, emergent interrelationships between HIT, clinicians, and workflows within any healthcare system (Harrison et al. 2007), but fails in its modelling of the specific aspects of the HIT (e.g., hardware configuration, clinical content available, aspects of the user interface, etc.) that play key roles in both the successes and failures within these complex interrelationships.

While these socio-technical models include a "technology" component, they fall short in their ability to break down the "technology" into its key components to enable researchers to dissect and better understand the causes, or at least the reasoning, that led to specific decisions related to particular HIT implementation or use problems, or to help identify specific technology-related solutions or areas for improvement. We have found that many HIT problems we are studying revolve around the interplay of hardware, software, content (e.g., clinical data and computer-generated decision support), and user interfaces. Failing to acknowledge these specific technology-specific elements or attempting to treat them separately can hinder overall understanding of HIT-related challenges. For example, the "content" dimension of our model accounts for much of what informaticians do, that is, studying the intricacies of controlled clinical vocabularies that provide the cognitive interface between the inexact, subjective, highly variable world of biomedicine and the highly structured, tightly controlled, digital world of computers (Rector 1999). A well-constructed, robust user interface vocabulary can make all the difference in the world to a busy clinician struggling to quickly and accurately enter a complex clinical order for a critically ill patient (Rosenbloom et al. 2006), and it is important to distinguish this aspect of technology from others that may contribute to additional challenges (e.g., a user interface that is difficult to navigate, an order entry application that is slow to respond, or computers that are only available at the main nursing station). Failure to do so, for example, leads to general statements such as "clinicians struggled with the new technology" or "it takes clinicians longer to complete their tasks using the new technology" without providing any insight into specific causes of the problems or their solutions. In this example, without a multidimensional understanding of the technological dimensions of the failed IT application, the researcher may incorrectly conclude that the hardware, application software, or user was responsible, when in fact a poorly designed or implemented clinical vocabulary might have been the root of the problem.

Finally, the preceding models do not account for the special monitoring processes and governance structures that must be put in place while designing and developing, implementing, or using HIT. For example, identifying who will make the decision on what, when, and how clinical decision support (CDS) interventions will be added (Wright et al. 2011); developing a process for monitoring the effect of new CDS on the systems' response time (Sittig et al. 2007); building tools to track the CDS that is in place (Sittig et al. 2010a); developing an approach for testing CDS; defining approaches for identifying rules that interact; developing robust processes for collecting feedback from users and communicating new system fixes, features, and functions; and building tools for monitoring the CDS system itself (Hripcsak 1993).

4.3 Moving Towards a New Socio-technical Model for HIT

To overcome the limitations of previous models, we propose a new socio-technical model to study the design, development, use, implementation, and evaluation of HIT (Fig. 4.1). Our comprehensive 8-dimensional model accounts for key factors that influence the success of HIT interventions. A major assumption of our model is that the 8 dimensions cannot be viewed as a series of independent, sequential steps. As with other components of complex adaptive systems, these 8 interacting dimensions must be studied in relationship to each other. Clearly, several of our model's components are more tightly coupled than others, for example, the hardware, software, content, and user interface are all completely dependent on one another.

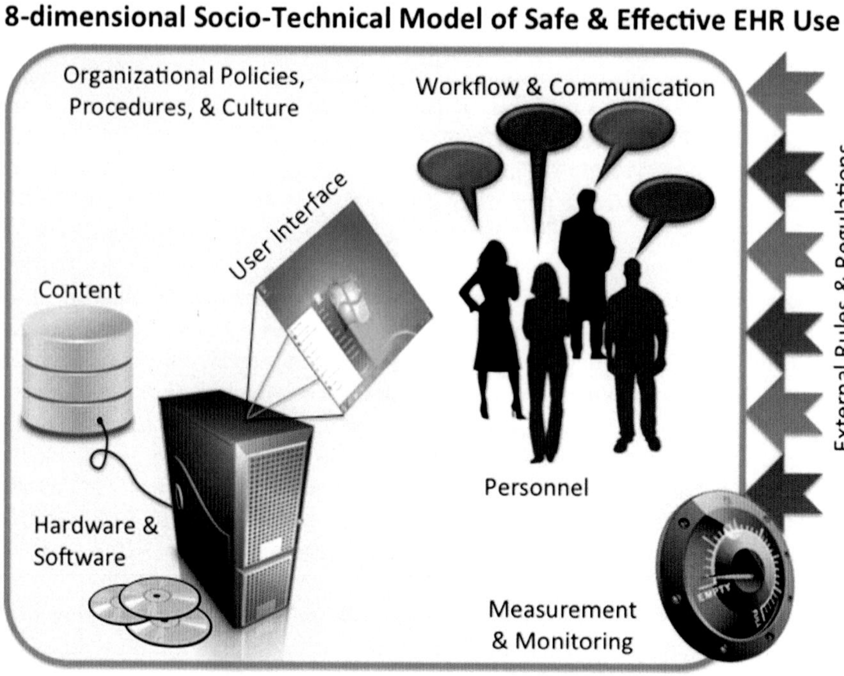

8-dimensional Socio-Technical Model of Safe & Effective EHR Use

Fig. 4.1 Illustration of the complex inter-relationships between the 8 dimensions of the new socio-technical model (Used with permission from: Menon et al. 2014)

However, all the other social components also exert strong influences on these technical components.

In our model, one cannot expect to gain an in-depth understanding of the intricacies of complex HIT interventions simply by integrating the results of studies performed within any single dimension of the model (Rasmussen 1997). Rather, HIT interventions must be understood in the context of their simultaneous effects across multiple dimensions of the model. For instance, a recent evaluation of a national program to develop and implement centrally stored electronic summaries of patients' medical records in the UK revealed their benefits to be lower than anticipated. The report cautioned that complex interdependencies between many socio-technical factors at the levels of the clinical encounter, organization, and the nation at large are to be expected in such evaluations (Greenhalgh et al. 2010). These study findings are illustrative of how and why our proposed model could be useful.

The 8 dimensions include:

1. **Hardware and Software Computing Infrastructure.** This dimension of the model focuses solely on the hardware and software required to run the applications. The most visible part of this dimension is the computer, including the monitor, printer, and other data display devices along with the keyboard, mouse,

and other data entry devices used to access clinical applications and medical or imaging devices. This dimension also includes the centralized (network-attached) data storage devices and all of the networking equipment required to allow applications or devices to retrieve and store patient data. Also included in this dimension is software at both the operating system and application levels. Finally, this dimension of the model subsumes all the machines, devices, and software required to keep the computing infrastructure functioning, such as the high-capacity air conditioning system, the batteries that form the uninterruptable power supply (UPS) that provides short-term electrical power in the event of an electrical failure, and the diesel-powered backup generators that supply power during longer outages.

   In short, this dimension is purely technical; it is only composed of the physical devices and the software required for keeping these devices running. One of the key aspects of this dimension is that, for the most part, the user is not aware that the majority of this infrastructure exists until it fails (Leveson and Turner 1993). For example, in 2002 the Beth Israel Deaconess Medical Center in Boston experienced a 4-day computer outage due to old, out-of-date computer equipment coupled with an outdated software program designed to direct traffic on a much less complex network. Furthermore, their network diagnostic tools were ineffective because they could only be used when the network was functioning (Kilbridge 2003).

2. **Clinical Content**. This dimension includes everything on the data-information-knowledge continuum that is stored in the system (i.e., structured and unstructured textual or numeric data and images that are either captured directly from imaging devices or scanned from paper-based sources) (Bernstam et al. 2010). Clinical content elements can be used to configure certain software requirements. Examples include controlled vocabulary items that are selected from a list while ordering a medication or a diagnostic test, and the logic required to generate an alert for certain types of medication interactions. These elements may also describe certain clinical aspects of the patients' condition (e.g., laboratory test results, discharge summaries, or radiographic images). Other clinical content, such as demographic data and patient location, can be used to manage administrative aspects of a patient's care. These data can be entered (or created), read, modified, or deleted by authorized users and stored either on the local computer or on a network. Certain elements of the clinical content, such as that which informs clinical decision support (CDS) interventions, must be managed on a regular basis (Sittig et al. 2010b).

3. **Human-Computer Interface**. An interface enables unrelated entities to interact with the system and includes aspects of the system that users can see, touch, or hear. The hardware and software "operationalize" the user interface; provided these are functioning as designed, any problems with using the system are likely due to human-computer interaction (HCI) issues. The HCI is guided by a user interaction model created by the software designer and developer (Shneiderman et al. 2009). During early pilot testing of the application in the target clinical environment, both the user's workflow and the interface are likely to need

revisions. This process of iterative refinement, wherein both the user and user interface may need to change, must culminate in an HCI model that matches the user's modified clinical workflow. For example, if a clinician wants to change the dose of a medication, the software requires the clinician to discontinue the old order and enter a new one, but the user interface should hide this complexity. This dimension also includes the ergonomic aspects of the interface (Svanæs et al. 2008). If users are forced to use a computer mouse while standing, they may have difficulty controlling the pointer on the screen because they are moving the mouse using the large muscles of their shoulder rather than the smaller muscles in the forearm. Finally, the lack of a feature or function within the interface represents a problem both with the interface and with the software or hardware that implements the interface.

4. **People**. This dimension represents the humans (e.g., software developers, system configuration and training personnel, clinicians, and patients) involved in all aspects of the design, development, implementation, and use of HIT. It also includes the ways that systems help users think and make them feel (Sittig et al. 2005a). Although user training is clearly an important component of the user portion of the model, it may not by itself overcome all user-related problems. Many "user" problems actually result from poor system design or errors in system development or configuration. In addition to the users of these systems, this dimension includes the people who design, develop, implement, and evaluate these systems. For instance, these people must have the proper knowledge, skills, and training required to develop applications that are safe, effective, and easy to use. This is the first aspect of the model that is purely on the social end of the socio-technical spectrum.

In most cases, users will be clinicians or employees of the health system. However, with recent advances in patient-centered care and development of personal health record systems and "home monitoring" devices, patients are increasingly becoming important users of HIT. Patients and/or their caregivers may not possess the knowledge or skills to manage new health information technologies, and this is of specific concern as more care shifts to the patient's home (Henriksen et al. 2009).

5. **Workflow and Communication.** This is the first portion of the model that acknowledges that people often need to work cohesively with others in the healthcare system to accomplish patient care. This collaboration requires significant two-way communication. The workflow dimension accounts for the steps needed to ensure that each patient receives the care they need at the time they need it. Often, the clinical information system does not initially match the actual "clinical" workflow. In this case, either the workflow must be modified to adapt to the HIT, or the HIT system must change to match the various workflows identified.

6. **Internal Organizational Policies, Procedures, Environment, and Culture.** The organization's internal structures, policies, environment, and procedures affect every other dimension in our model. For example, the organization's leadership allocates the capital budgets that enable the purchase of hardware and software, and internal policies influence whether and how offsite data

backups are accomplished. The organizational leaders and committees who write and implement IT policies and procedures are responsible for overseeing all aspects of HIT system procurement, implementation, use, monitoring, and evaluation. A key aspect of any HIT project is to ensure that the software accurately represents and enforces, if applicable, organizational policies and procedures. Likewise, it is also necessary to ensure that the actual clinical workflow involved with operating these systems is consistent with policies and procedures. Finally, internal rules and regulations are often created in response to the external rules and regulations that form the basis of the next dimension of the model.

7. **External Rules, Regulations, and Pressures.** This dimension accounts for the external forces that facilitate or place constraints on the design, development, implementation, use, and evaluation of HIT in the clinical setting. For example, the passage of the American Recovery and Reinvestment Act (ARRA) of 2009, which includes the Health Information Technology for Economic and Clinical Health (HITECH) Act, made available over 20 billion dollars for healthcare practitioners who become "meaningful users" of HIT. Thus, ARRA introduced the single largest financial incentive ever to facilitate electronic health record (EHR) implementation. Meanwhile, a host of federal, state, and local regulations govern the use of HIT. Examples include the 1996 Health Insurance Portability and Accountability Act (HIPAA), recent changes to the Stark Laws,[1] and restrictions on secondary use of clinical data. Finally, there are three recent national developments that have the potential to affect the entire healthcare delivery system in the context of HIT. These include: (1) the initiative to develop the data and information exchange capacity to create a national health information network (American Recovery and Reinvestment Act of 2009); (2) the initiative to enable patients to access copies of the clinical data via personal health records (Sittig 2002); and (3) clinical and IT workforce shortages (Detmer et al. 2010).

8. **System Measurement and Monitoring**. This dimension has largely been unaccounted for in previous models. We posit that the effects of HIT must be measured and monitored on a regular basis. An effective system measurement and monitoring program must address four key issues related to HIT features and functions (Leonard and Sittig 2007). First is the issue of availability – the extent to which features and functions are available and ready for use. Measures of system availability include response times and percent uptime of the system. A second measurement objective is to determine how clinicians are using the various features and functions. For instance, one such measure is the rate at which clinicians override CDS warnings and alerts. Third, the effectiveness of the system on healthcare delivery and patient health should be monitored to ensure that anticipated outcomes are achieved. For example, the mean HbA1c

---

[1] A federal law which prohibits a physician from referring a Medicare or Medicaid patient to an entity for specific health services if the physician (or an immediate family member) has a financial relationship with that entity.

value for all diabetic patients in a practice may be measured before and after implementation of a system with advanced CDS features. Finally, in addition to measuring the expected outcomes of HIT implementation, it is also vital to identify and document unintended consequences that manifest themselves following use of these systems (Ash et al. 2004). For instance, it may be worthwhile to track practitioner efficiency before and after implementation of a new clinical charting application (Bradshaw et al. 1989). In addition to measuring the use and effectiveness of HIT at the local level, we must develop the methods to measure and monitor these systems and assess the quality of care resulting from their use on a state, regional, or even national level (Sittig et al. 2005b; Sittig and Classen 2010).

4.4   Relationships and Interactions Among Components of the Socio-technical Model

Our research and experience has led us, and others, to conclude that HIT-enabled healthcare systems are best treated as complex adaptive systems (Begun et al. 2003). The most important result of this conclusion is that hierarchical decomposition (i.e., breaking a complex system, process, or device down into its components, studying them, and then integrating the results in an attempt to understand how the complete system functions) cannot be used to study HIT (Rouse 2008). As illustrated by the evaluation of centrally stored electronic summaries in the UK, complex interdependencies between various socio-technical dimensions are to be expected, and our HIT model (had it existed at the time) might have potentially predicted some of them and allowed them to be addressed prior to going-live rather than in the evaluation stages of the project. Therefore, one should not view or use our model as a set of independent components that can be studied in isolation and then synthesized to develop a realistic picture of how HIT is used within the complex adaptive healthcare system. Rather, the key to our model is how the 8 dimensions interact and depend on one another. They must be studied as multiple, interacting components with non-linear, emergent, dynamic behavior (i.e., small changes in one aspect of the system lead to small changes in other parts of the system under some conditions, but large changes at other times) that often appears random or chaotic. This is typical of complex adaptive systems, and our model reflects these interactions.

For example, a computer-based provider order entry (CPOE) system that works successfully in an adult surgical nursing unit within a hospital may not work at all in the nearby pediatric unit for any number of potential reasons, including: (1) hardware/software (e.g., fewer computers, older computers, poor wireless reception, poor placement); (2) content (e.g., no weight- or age-based dosing, no customized order sets or documentation templates); (3) user-interface (e.g., older workforce that has trouble seeing the small font on the screen); or (4) personnel (e.g., no clinical champion within the medical staff). However, each of these dimensions has a potential relationship with one or more of the other dimensions. For instance, computers may have been few or old because of some organizational limitations on financing, a constrained physical environment that results in limited space in the patient rooms or even the hallway for workstations, or a combination of these restrictions, there may be no customized order sets because clinician-users did not agree on how best to create them or on the medical evidence to support their decisions, and there was no clinical champion because the organization did not provide any financial incentive for the additional time this role would entail. Other reasons could include problems with the user interface and the communication and workflow related to how nurses process new medication orders using the EHR and record administration of medications using the new barcode medication administration system. These issues, in turn, may have been due to long-standing organizational policies and procedures that administrators were reluctant to reconsider. For example, the unit governance committee may have decided not to approve a request for mobile computers to help compensate for the lack of hardwired, stationary workstations in the patient rooms, with the result that nurses spent more time away from patients and therefore had a slower workflow related to processing new orders. The preceding example illustrates the interaction of six dimensions of our model: hardware/software, clinical content, user interface, people, workflow, and organizational policies. Additionally, some form of system measurement and monitoring could have detected these issues. In summary, our model provides HIT researchers with several new avenues of thinking about the interactions between key technology and social components of the HIT-enabled work system and how the interactions between the various socio-technical dimensions of our model must be considered in future research.

4.5   Applications of the Socio-technical Model in Real-World Settings

The following sections illustrate how we have used the socio-technical model of safe and effective HIT use within our research. In an attempt to describe how the model can be applied across the breadth of HIT research and development, and to provide examples of different systems and interventions that can be analyzed within this new paradigm, we highlight key elements of our model in the context of several recent projects.

4.5.1   HIT Design and Development

The design and development of CDS interventions within clinicians' workflow presents several challenges. We conducted several qualitative studies to gain insight into the 8 dimensions of our model during the development of a CDS tool within a CPOE application. This CDS intervention was designed to alert clinicians whenever they attempted to order a medication that was contraindicated in elderly patients or a medication that had known serious interactions with warfarin. For

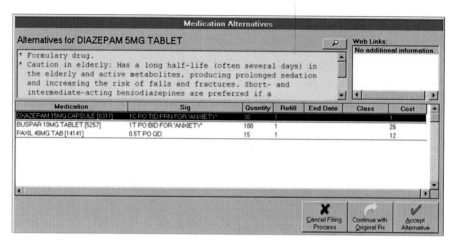

Fig. 4.2 An example pop-up alert warning a user that diazepam is not a preferred benzodiazepine for a patient 65 years or older (Used with permission from: Smith et al. 2006)

example, Fig. 4.2 shows a pop-up alert which appeared whenever a clinician attempted to order "diazepam" on a patient who was 65 years or older.

We used several methods, including focus groups, usability testing, and educational sessions with clinician users (Feldstein et al. 2004), to identify issues related to hardware/software, content, interface, people, measurement, workflow/communication, and internal policies and procedures. These efforts helped us, for example, to understand the need to meet with the organization's Pharmacy and Therapeutics committee (i.e., *internal policy*) to convince them to modify the medication formulary to include an alternative suggestion for specific medications contraindicated in the elderly. We also worked with the information technology professional (i.e., *people*) who was responsible for maintaining the textual appearance (i.e., font size – an element of the *user interface*) of the alerts as well as the *content* of the message, and the order of the messages. Fitting alert content within the constraints of the alert notification window (i.e., *user interface*) eliminated the need to train *clinicians* to use the horizontal scrolling capability. This is just one simple example of how use of the socio-technical model paid huge dividends during the development and implementation stages of this highly successful project (Feldstein et al. 2006; Smith et al. 2006).

4.5.2 HIT Implementation

In a separate study, we derived lessons that could be learned from CPOE implementation at another site (Sittig et al. 2006). One of the most important conclusions from this implementation was that problems could, and often do, occur in all 8 dimensions of the model. In addition, many of the problems resulted from interactions between two or more dimensions of the model (see Table 4.1) (Sittig and Ash 2010).

Table 4.1 Applications of the socio-technical model to analyze two HIT-related interventions

Socio-technical model dimension	Implementation of computer-based provider order entry	Follow-up of alerts related to abnormal diagnostic imaging results
Hardware and software	The majority of computer terminals were linked to the hospital computer system via wireless signal. Communication bandwidth was often exceeded during peak operational periods, which created additional delays between each click on the computer mouse	Alerts should be retracted when the patient dies or if the radiologist calls, or the patient is admitted before the alert is acknowledged. However, this can be done only through a centralized organizational policy
Clinical content	No ICU-specific order sets were available at the time of CPOE implementation. The hurried implementation timeline established by the leaders in the organization prohibited development of these order sets	Interventions to reduce alert overload and improve the signal to noise ratio should be explored. Unnecessary alerts should be minimized. However, people (physicians) may not agree which alerts are essential and which ones are not (van der Sijs et al. 2008)
Human computer interface	The process of entering orders often required an average of 10 clicks on the computer mouse per order, which translated to 1–2 min to enter a single order. Organizational leaders eventually hired additional clinicians to "work the CPOE system" while others cared for the patients	Unacknowledged alerts must stay active on the EHR screen for longer periods, perhaps even indefinitely, and should require the provider's signature and statement of action before they are allowed to drop off the screen. However, providers might not want to spend additional time stating their actions; who will make this decision?
People	Leaders at all levels of the institution made implementation decisions (re: hardware placement, software configuration, content development, user interface design, etc.) that placed patient care in jeopardy	Many clinicians did not know how to use many of the EHR's advanced features that greatly facilitated the processing of alerts, exposing a limitation in provider training. Adding to the problem, providers are only given 4 h of training time by the institution
Workflow and communication	Rapid implementation timeline did not allow time for clinicians to adapt to their new routines and responsibilities. In addition, poor hardware and software design and configuration decisions complicated the workflow issues	Communicating alerts to two recipients, which occurred when tests were ordered by a healthcare practitioner other than the patient's regular PCP, significantly increased the odds that the alert would not be read and would not receive timely follow-up action. No policy was available that states who is responsible for follow-up.

(continued)

Table 4.1 (continued)

Socio-technical model dimension	Implementation of computer-based provider order entry	Follow-up of alerts related to abnormal diagnostic imaging results
Organizational policies and procedures	Order entry was not allowed until after the patient had physically arrived at the hospital and been fully registered into the clinical information system	Every institution must develop and publicize a policy regarding who is responsible (PCP vs the ordering provider, who may be a consultant) for taking action on abnormal results. Such policies also help institutions meet external (i.e., Joint Commission) requirements
External rules, regulations, and pressures	Following the Institute of Medicine report *To Err is Human: Building a Safer Health System* and subsequent congressional hearings, the issue of patient safety has risen to a position of highest priority among health care organizations	Poor reimbursement and heavy workload of patients puts productivity pressure on providers. The nature of high-risk transitions between health care practitioners, settings, and systems of care makes timely and effective electronic communication particularly challenging
System measurement and monitoring	Monitoring identified a significant increase in patient mortality following CPOE implementation	An audit and performance feedback system should be established to give providers information on timely follow-up of patients' test results on a regular basis. However, providers may not want feedback or the institution does not have the persons required to do so

4.5.3   HIT Use

Safe and effective use of an EHR-based notification system involves many factors that are addressed by almost all dimensions of our model (Singh et al. 2009a, 2010a). For instance, many EHRs generate automated asynchronous "alerts" to notify clinicians of important clinical findings. We examined communication outcomes of over 2,500 such alerts that were specifically related to abnormal test results. We found that, despite assurance that abnormal test results were transmitted, 18.1 % of abnormal lab alerts and 10.2 % of abnormal imaging alerts were never acknowledged (i.e., were unread by the receiving provider). Additionally, 7–8 % of these alerts lacked timely follow-up, which was unrelated to acknowledgment of the alert. This study revealed complex interactions between users, the user interface, software, content, workflow/communication, and organizational policies related to who was responsible for abnormal test follow-up. Our findings thus highlighted the multiple dimensions, as well as the complex interactions between various dimensions, of our model that need to be addressed to improve the safety of EHR-based notification systems and perhaps other forms of CDS (see Table 4.1) (Hysong et al. 2009, 2010; Singh et al. 2010b; Singh and Vij 2010).

4.5.4 HIT Evaluation

Our model has provided guidance in evaluating HIT-related breakdowns in care, reminding us that however technologically savvy we make our patient care processes, we must also carefully monitor their impact, effectiveness, and unintended consequences. We recently evaluated why, despite implementation of an automated notification system to enhance communication of fecal occult blood test (FOBT) results, providers did not take follow-up actions in almost 40 % of cases (Singh et al. 2009b). Again, our findings highlighted multiple interacting dimensions within our socio-technical model. For instance, we found that clinician non-response to automated notifications was related to a software configuration error that prevented transmission of a subset of test results. However, we also found that if the institution was using certain types of workflows related to test performance, and if organizational procedures for computerized order entry of FOBTs were different, the problem may not have occurred. Thus, we found our multidimensional approach, which accounted for interactions, to be useful for comprehensive evaluation of HIT after implementation.

4.6 Model in Action: From Theory to Practice

Our preliminary studies of HIT safety and effectiveness have demonstrated the potential value of considering all 8 dimensions of our socio-technical model to anticipate, diagnose, and correct a variety of problems. Determining the broader impact and generalizability of this approach requires translating these concepts into more concrete and actionable guidance. To this end, our team recently developed a set of self-assessment tools for organizations and end-users who wish to evaluate the safety and effectiveness of HIT within their own settings (Sittig et al. 2014). Given the current emphasis on EHR implementation and upgrades in healthcare systems throughout the United States, we focused the content specifically on issues related to EHRs. The ultimate aim of these tools is to enhance system resilience, or the ability to continuously detect, correct, and prevent various risks related to EHRs.

Although EHR-related problems and risks are highly significant to organizations that are implementing new systems, vulnerabilities can persist or arise even within well-established systems. Thus, we developed our guides with the needs of users across the continuum of EHR implementation in mind. We coupled the socio-technical model with a three-phase model of safe EHR use that enumerates

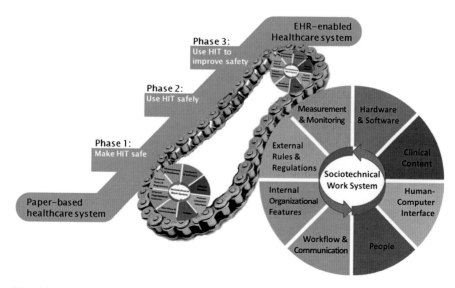

Fig. 4.3 Conceptual model for self-assessment of EHR safety and effectiveness (Used with permission from: Meeks et al. 2014)

specific risks across the "life cycle" of EHR implementation (Sittig and Singh 2012). According to the model, the first phase is concerned chiefly with addressing vulnerabilities that are unique and specific to EHRs and often emerge early in implementation (e.g., safety problems owing to unavailable or malfunctioning hardware or software). The second phase (using IT safely) addresses unsafe or inappropriate use of technology. The third phase (monitoring safety) addresses use of technology not only to deliver care, but also to monitor processes and outcomes and to identify potential safety hazards proactively. The socio-technical model and three-phase implementation model together formed the main conceptual basis for developing self-assessment tools (Fig. 4.3) (Meeks et al. 2014). The self-assessment tools were designed with the understanding that as EHR implementations mature, the demands and functions of the socio-technical system evolve as well.

The content of the self-assessment tools, known as the Safety Assurance Factors for EHR Resilience (SAFER) guides, was developed in multiple stages. From the outset, a multidisciplinary expert panel, with representation from the fields of informatics, patient safety, quality improvement, risk management, and human factors engineering, steered the initial generation of content. To maximize the utility and potential impact of the guides, the content was organized as a series of standalone guides that apply to nine high-risk areas:

- CPOE and e-prescribing
- Clinical decision support
- Test result reporting

- Communication between providers
- Patient identification
- EHR downtime events
- EHR customization and configuration
- System-system interface data transfer
- HIT safety-related human skills

For each topic, our team identified 10–25 recommended practices, which were chosen on the basis of our own research and that of others who study HIT safety and effectiveness. These practices were operationalized with concrete examples and written as checklist-type items so that the person(s) completing the checklist can indicate whether each practice is fully, partially, or not implemented in a given setting. During the validation process, our team visited several facilities and sought comments from a variety of potential users to ensure that items were consistently interpreted and meaningful across settings. Input from a variety of facility types, disciplines, and end-user roles is a strength of the SAFER guides. These guides are now available free of charge through the Office of the National Coordinator for HIT (www.healthit.gov/safer) in the hope they might help accelerate the discovery and development of best practices for training, patient care, policy, and use of EHRs for monitoring and patient safety.

4.7   Conclusions

This chapter has introduced a comprehensive paradigm for the study of HIT. We have successfully applied this model to study HIT interventions at different levels of design, development, implementation, use, and evaluation. In addition, we have applied the model to develop tools that organizations can use to self-assess the safety and effectiveness of HIT within their own settings. We anticipate that additional study of the 8 dimensions and their complex interactions will yield further refinements to this model and, ultimately, improvements in the quality and safety of HIT applications that translate to better health and welfare for our patients.

Discussion Questions
1. You have been asked to create a project plan for implementation of a new hand-held device that is designed to facilitate the process by which nurses record vital signs and clinical assessments of their patients. Describe 2–3 key considerations within each of the 8 dimensions of the socio-technical model that must be addressed to ensure success of the project.
2. What are some possible consequences of excluding frontline clinical personnel from decisions about HIT configurations and functions?

3. The leadership at a large healthcare facility have ordered a major update of the facility's EHR. Assuming a socio-technical approach to this project, what types of personnel might constitute an EHR implementation team?
4. You have been asked to evaluate the effectiveness of a recently implemented comparative effective research (CER) platform. List 2–3 measures that you could use within each of the 8 dimensions of the socio-technical model to assess the system's performance and utility.
5. Explain how an external rule or regulation (e.g., HIPAA, Meaningful Use requirements, or CMS conditions for participation) can affect the implementation and/or use of a new clinical computing device (e.g., voice-activated, handheld data review device) or application (e.g., an Internet-accessible, state-wide immunization registry).

Additional Readings

Meeks, D. W., Takian, A., Sittig, D. F., Singh, H., & Barber, N. (2014, February). Exploring the sociotechnical intersection of patient safety and electronic health record implementation. *Journal of the American Medical Informatics Association, 21*(e1), e28–e34. doi:10.1136/amiajnl-2013-001762. PMID: 24052536.

Sittig, D. F., & Singh, H. (2009, September 9). Eight rights of safe electronic health record use. *JAMA, 302*(10), 1111–1113. PMID: 19738098.

Sittig, D. F., & Singh, H. (2012a, September 18). Rights and responsibilities of users of electronic health records. *Canadian Medical Association Journal, 184*(13), 1479–1483. doi:10.1503/cmaj.111599. PMID: 22331971.

Sittig, D. F., & Singh, H. (2012b, November 8). Electronic health records and national patient-safety goals. *The New England Journal of Medicine, 367*(19), 1854–1860. doi:10.1056/NEJMsb1205420. PMID:23134389.

Sittig, D. F., Hazlehurst, B. L., Brown, J., Murphy, S., Rosenman, M., Tarczy-Hornoch, P., & Wilcox, A. B. (2012, July). A survey of informatics platforms that enable distributed comparative effectiveness research using multi-institutional heterogeneous clinical data. *Med Care, 50*(Suppl), S49–S59. PMID: 22692259.

Smith, M. W., Ash, J. S., Sittig, D. F., & Singh, H. (2014, September). Resilient practices in maintaining safety of health information technologies. *Journal of Cognitive Engineering and Decision Making, 8*(3), 265–282. doi:10.1177/1555343414534242.

References

American Recovery and Reinvestment Act. (2009). *State grants to promote health information technology planning and implementation projects.* Available at: https://www.grantsolutions.gov/gs/preaward/previewPublicAnnouncement.do?id=10534

Ash, J. (1997). Organizational factors that influence information technology diffusion in academic health sciences centers. *Journal of the American Medical Informatics Association, 4*(2, March–April), 102–111.

Ash, J. S., Berg, M., & Coiera, E. (2004). Some unintended consequences of information technology in health care: The nature of patient care information system-related errors. *Journal of the American Medical Informatics Association, 11*(2, March–April), 104–112.

Begun, J. W., Zimmerman, B., & Dooley, K. (2003). Health care organizations as complex adaptive systems. In S. M. Mick & M. Wyttenbach (Eds.), *Advances in health care organization theory* (pp. 253–288). San Francisco: Jossey-Bass.

Bernstam, E. V., Smith, J. W., & Johnson, T. R. (2010). What is biomedical informatics? *Journal of Biomedical Informatics, 43*(1, February), 104–110.

Bradshaw, K. E., Sittig, D. F., Gardner, R. M., Pryor, T. A., & Budd, M. (1989). Computer-based data entry for nurses in the ICU. *MD Computing, 6*(5, September–October), 274–280.

Carayon, P., Schoofs Hundt, A., Karsh, B. T., Gurses, A. P., Alvarado, C. J., Smith, M., & Flatley, B. P. (2006). Work system design for patient safety: The SEIPS model. *Quality & Safety in Health Care, 15*(Suppl 1, December), i50–i58.

Cohen, T., Blatter, B., Almeida, C., Shortliffe, E., & Patel, V. (2006). A cognitive blueprint of collaboration in context: Distributed cognition in the psychiatric emergency department. *Artificial Intelligence in Medicine, 37*(2, June), 73–83.

Detmer, D. E., Munger, B. S., & Lehmann, C. U. (2010). Medical informatics board certification: History, current status, and predicted impact on the medical informatics workforce. *Applied Clinical Informatics, 1*(1), 11–18. Available: http://www.schattauer.de/nc/en/magazine/sub ject-areas/journals-a-z/applied-clinical-informatics/issue/special/manuscript/12624/download. html

Duyck, P., Pynoo, B., Devolder, P., Voet, T., Adang, L., & Vercruysse, J. (2008). User acceptance of a picture archiving and communication system. Applying the unified theory of acceptance and use of technology in a radiological setting. *Methods of Information in Medicine, 47*(2), 149–156.

Feldstein, A., Simon, S. R., Schneider, J., Krall, M., Laferriere, D., Smith, D. H., Sittig, D. F., & Soumerai, S. B. (2004). How to design computerized alerts to safe prescribing practices. *Joint Commission Journal on Quality and Safety, 30*(11, November), 602–613.

Feldstein, A. C., Smith, D. H., Perrin, N., Yang, X., Simon, S. R., Krall, M., Sittig, D. F., Ditmer, D., Platt, R., & Soumerai, S. B. (2006). Reducing warfarin medication interactions: An interrupted time series evaluation. *Archives of Internal Medicine, 166*(9, May 8), 1009–1015.

Gosling, A. S., Westbrook, J. I., & Braithwaite, J. (2003). Clinical team functioning and IT innovation: A study of the diffusion of a point-of-care online evidence system. *Journal of the American Medical Informatics Association, 10*(3, May–June), 244–251.

Greenhalgh, T., Stramer, K., Bratan, T., Byrne, E., Russell, J., & Potts, H. W. (2010). Adoption and non-adoption of a shared electronic summary record in England: A mixed-method case study. *BMJ, 340*(June 16), c3111. doi:10.1136/bmj.c3111.

Harrison, M. I., Koppel, R., & Bar-Lev, S. (2007). Unintended consequences of information technologies in health care – An interactive sociotechnical analysis. *Journal of the American Medical Informatics Association, 14*(5, September–October), 542–549.

Hazlehurst, B., McMullen, C., Gorman, P., & Sittig, D. (2003). How the ICU follows orders: Care delivery as a complex activity system. In *AMIA annual symposium proceedings* (pp. 284–288).

Hazlehurst, B., McMullen, C. K., & Gorman, P. N. (2007). Distributed cognition in the heart room: How situation awareness arises from coordinated communications during cardiac surgery. *Journal of Biomedical Informatics, 40*(5, October), 539–551.

Henriksen, K., Kaye, R., & Morisseau, D. (1993). Industrial ergonomic factors in the radiation oncology therapy environment. In R. Nielsen & K. Jorgensen (Eds.), *Advances in industrial ergonomics and safety V* (pp. 325–335). Washington, DC: Taylor and Francis.

Henriksen, K., Joseph, A., & Zayas-Caban, T. (2009). The human factors of home health care: A conceptual model for examining safety and quality concerns. *Journal of Patient Safety, 5*(4, December), 229–236.

Holden, R. J., & Karsh, B. T. (2010). The technology acceptance model: Its past and its future in health care. *Journal of Biomedical Informatics, 43*(1, February), 159–172.

Hripcsak, G. (1993). Monitoring the monitor: Automated statistical tracking of a clinical event monitor. *Computers and Biomedical Research, 26*(5, October), 449–466.

Hutchins, E. (1996). *Cognition in the wild.* Cambridge, MA: MIT Press, 401 pp.

Hysong, S. J., Sawhney, M. K., Wilson, L., Sittig, D. F., Esquivel, A., Watford, M., Davis, T., Espadas, D., & Singh, H. (2009). Improving outpatient safety through effective electronic communication: A study protocol. *Implementation Science, 4*(1, September 25), 62. PMID: 19781075.

Hysong, S. J., Sawhney, M. K., Wilson, L., Sittig, D. F., Espadas, D., Davis, T. L., & Singh, H. (2010). Provider management strategies of abnormal test result alerts: A cognitive task analysis. *Journal of the American Medical Informatics Association, 17*, 71–77. PMID: 20064805.

Kijsanayotin, B., Pannarunothai, S., & Speedie, S. M. (2009). Factors influencing health information technology adoption in Thailand's community health centers: Applying the UTAUT model. *International Journal of Medical Informatics, 78*(6, June), 404–416.

Kilbridge, P. (2003). Computer crash–lessons from a system failure. *The New England Journal of Medicine, 348*(10, March 6), 881–882.

Lederman, R. M., & Parkes, C. (2005). Systems failure in hospitals–using reason's model to predict problems in a prescribing information system. *Journal of Medical Systems, 29* (1, February), 33–43.

Leonard, K. J., & Sittig, D. F. (2007). Improving information technology adoption and implementation through the identification of appropriate benefits: Creating IMPROVE-IT. *Journal of Medical Internet Research, 9*(2, May 4), e9.

Leveson, N. G., & Turner, C. S. (1993). An investigation of the Therac-25 accidents. *IEEE Computer, 26*(7), 18–41. Updated version available at: http://sunnyday.mit.edu/papers/therac.pdf

Malhotra, S., Jordan, D., Shortliffe, E., & Patel, V. L. (2007). Workflow modeling in critical care: Piecing together your own puzzle. *Journal of Biomedical Informatics, 40*(2, April), 81–92.

Meeks, D. W., Takian, A., Sittig, D. F., Singh, H., & Barber, N. (2014, February). Exploring the sociotechnical intersection of patient safety and electronic health record implementation. *Journal of the American Medical Informatics Association, 21*(e1), e28–e34. doi:10.1136/amiajnl-2013-001762. PMID: 24052536.

Menon, S., Smith, M. W., Sittig, D. F., Petersen, N. J., Hysong, S. J., Espadas, D., Modi, V., & Singh, H. (2014). How context affects electronic health record-based test result follow-up: A mixed-methods evaluation. *BMJ Open, 4*(11), e005985.

Norman, D. (1988). *The psychology of everyday things.* New York: Basic Books.

Patel, V. L., Zhang, J., Yoskowitz, N. A., Green, R., & Sayan, O. R. (2008). Translational cognition for decision support in critical care environments: A review. *Journal of Biomedical Informatics, 41*(3, June), 413–431.

Rasmussen, J. (1997). Risk management in a dynamic society: A modelling problem. *Safety Science, 27*(2), 183–213.

Reason, J. (2000). Human error: Models and management. *BMJ, 320*(7237, March 18), 768–770.

Rector, A. L. (1999). Clinical terminology: Why is it so hard? *Methods of Information in Medicine, 38*(4–5, December), 239–252.

Rogers, E. M. (2003). *Diffusion of innovations* (5th ed., p. 512). New York: Free Press.

Rosenbloom, S. T., Miller, R. A., Johnson, K. B., Elkin, P. L., & Brown, S. H. (2006). Interface terminologies: Facilitating direct entry of clinical data into electronic health record systems. *Journal of the American Medical Informatics Association, 13*(3, May–June), 277–288.

Rouse, W. B. (2008). Health care as a complex adaptive system: Implications for design and management. *The Bridge, 38*(1, Spring), 17–25.

Sheehan, B., Kaufman, D., Stetson, P., & Currie, L. M. (2009, November 14). *Cognitive analysis of decision support for antibiotic prescribing at the point of ordering in a neonatal intensive care unit.* In *AMIA annual symposium proceedings* (pp. 584–588).

Shneiderman, B., Plaisant, C., Cohen, M., & Jacobs, S. (2009). *Designing the user interface: Strategies for effective human-computer interaction* (5th ed., p. 672). Reading: Pearson Education.

Singh, H., & Vij, M. (2010). Eight recommendations for policies for communication of abnormal test results. *Joint Commission Journal on Quality and Patient Safety, 36*(5), 226–232.

Singh, H., Thomas, E. J., Mani, S., Sittig, D., Arora, H., Espadas, D., Khan, M. M., & Petersen, L. A. (2009a). Timely follow-up of abnormal diagnostic imaging test results in an outpatient setting: Are electronic medical records achieving their potential? *Archives of Internal Medicine, 169*(17, September 28), 1578–1586.

Singh, H., Wilson, L., Petersen, L. A., Sawhney, M. K., Reis, B., Espadas, D., & Sittig, D. F. (2009b). Improving follow-up of abnormal cancer screens using electronic health records: Trust but verify test result communication. *BMC Medical Informatics and Decision Making, 9* (December 9), 49.

Singh, H., Thomas, E. J., Sittig, D. F., Wilson, L., Espadas, D., Khan, M. M., & Petersen, L. A. (2010a). Notification of abnormal laboratory test results in an electronic medical record: Do any safety concerns remain? *The American Journal of Medicine, 123*(3, March), 238–244.

Singh, H., Wilson, L., Reis, B., Sawhney, M. K., Espadas, D., & Sittig, D. F. (2010b). Ten strategies to improve management of abnormal test result alerts in the electronic health record. *Journal of Patient Safety, 6*(2, June), 121–123.

Sittig, D. F. (2002). Personal health records on the internet: A snapshot of the pioneers at the end of the 20th century. *International Journal of Medical Informatics, 65*(1, April), 1–6.

Sittig, D. F., & Ash, J. S. (2010). *Clinical information systems: Overcoming adverse consequences.* Sudbury: Jones and Bartlett.

Sittig, D. F., & Classen, D. C. (2010). Safe electronic health record use requires a comprehensive monitoring and evaluation framework. *JAMA, 303*(5, February 3), 450–451.

Sittig, D. F., & Singh, H. (2012). Electronic health records and national patient-safety goals. *The New England Journal of Medicine, 367*(19, November 8), 1854–1860. doi:10.1056/NEJMsb1205420.

Sittig, D. F., Krall, M., Kaalaas-Sittig, J., & Ash, J. S. (2005a). Emotional aspects of computer-based provider order entry: A qualitative study. *Journal of the American Medical Informatics Association, 12*(5, September–October), 561–567.

Sittig, D. F., Shiffman, R. N., Leonard, K., Friedman, C., Rudolph, B., Hripcsak, G., Adams, L. L., Kleinman, L. C., & Kaushal, R. (2005b). A draft framework for measuring progress towards the development of a national health information infrastructure. *BMC Medical Informatics and Decision Making, 5*(Jun 13), 14.

Sittig, D. F., Ash, J. S., Zhang, J., Osheroff, J. A., & Shabot, M. M. (2006). Lessons from "Unexpected increased mortality after implementation of a commercially sold computerized physician order entry system". *Pediatrics, 118*(2, August), 797–801.

Sittig, D. F., Campbell, E. M., Guappone, K. P., Dykstra, R. H., & Ash, J. S. (2007). Recommendations for monitoring and evaluation of in-patient computer-based provider order entry systems: Results of a Delphi Survey. In *Proceedings of the American Medical Informatics Association Fall symposium* (pp. 671–675).

Sittig, D. F., Simonaitis, L., Carpenter, J. D., Allen, G. O., Doebbeling, B. N., Sirajuddin, A. M., Ash, S. J., & Middleton, B. (2010a). The state of the art in clinical knowledge management: An inventory of tools and techniques. *International Journal of Medical Informatics, 79*(1, January), 44–57.

Sittig, D. F., Wright, A., Simonaitis, L., Carpenter, J. D., Allen, G. O., Doebbeling, B. N., Sirajuddin, A. M., Ash, J. S., & Middleton, B. (2010b). The state of the art in clinical knowledge management: An inventory of tools and techniques. *International Journal of Medical Informatics, 79*(1, January), 44–57.

Sittig, D. F., Ash, J. S., & Singh, H. (2014). The SAFER guides: Empowering organizations to improve the safety and effectiveness of electronic health records. *The American Journal of Managed Care, 20*(5, May), 418–423. PMID: 25181570.

Smith, D. H., Perrin, N., Feldstein, A., Yang, X., Kuang, D., Simon, S. R., Sittig, D. F., Platt, R., & Soumerai, S. B. (2006). The impact of prescribing safety alerts for elderly persons in an electronic medical record: An interrupted time series evaluation. *Archives of Internal Medicine, 166*(10, May 22), 1098–1104.

Svanæs, D., Alsos, O. A., & Dahl, Y. (2008). Usability testing of mobile ICT for clinical settings: Methodological and practical challenges. *International Journal of Medical Informatics, 79* (4, September 10), e24–e34.

van der Sijs, H., Aarts, J., Vulto, A., & Berg, M. (2006). Overriding of drug safety alerts in computerized physician order entry. *Journal of the American Medical Informatics Association, 13*(2, March–April), 138–147.

van der Sijs, H., Aarts, J., van Gelder, T., Berg, M., & Vulto, A. (2008). Turning off frequently overridden drug alerts: Limited opportunities for doing it safely. *Journal of the American Medical Informatics Association, 15*(4, July–August), 439–448.

Venkatesh, V., Morris, M. G., Davis, F. D., & Davis, G. B. (2003). User acceptance of information technology: Toward a unified view. *MIS Quarterly, 27*, 425–478.

Vincent, C., Taylor-Adams, S., & Stanhope, N. (1998). Framework for analysing risk and safety in clinical medicine. *BMJ, 316*(7138, April 11), 1154–1157.

Wright, A., Sittig, D. F., Ash, J. S., Bates, D. W., Feblowitz, J., Fraser, G., Maviglia, S. M., McMullen, C., Nichol, W. P., Pang, J. E., Starmer, J., & Middleton, B. (2011). Governance for clinical decision support: Case studies and recommended practices from leading institutions. *Journal of the American Medical Informatics Association, 18*(2, March 1), 187–194. PMID: 21252052.

Chapter 5
Evaluation of Health Information Technology: Methods, Frameworks and Challenges

Thomas G. Kannampallil and Joanna Abraham

5.1 Introduction

The adoption and use of health information technology (HIT), especially Electronic Health Records (EHR), has increased over the last decade (Blumenthal 2009). This increase, at least in part, has been spurred by recent federal mandates as part of the American Reinvestment and Recovery Act (ARRA). These mandates have incentivized the use of HIT with the goal of improving the quality and safety of healthcare. Though there are several positive reports of significant benefits in cost savings, quality and safety, persuasive evidence of the substantial impact of HIT is currently lacking. Most often, HIT implementation is characterized by inconsistent and mixed results regarding their utility and value (Linder et al. 2007). A large body of research investigates the unintended and unanticipated consequences associated with the use of HIT that results in increased time spent on documentation, workarounds, communication failures, duplication and redundancy of information, and effort to maintain continuity of information and care (e.g., Ash et al. 2003; Koppel et al. 2005; McDonald et al. 2014; also see Chap. 11, on unanticipated consequences of HIT use). Furthermore, evaluation studies have also questioned the safety implications of EHR use (e.g., errors and adverse events) (Sittig and Classen 2010).

A recent Institute of Medicine (IOM) report (e.g., IOM 2011) has highlighted the lack of effective integration of appropriate evaluation methods during the design and development phases of HIT. The IOM committee has also called for a

T.G. Kannampallil (✉)
University of Illinois at Chicago, Chicago, IL, USA

The New York Academy of Medicine, New York, NY, USA
e-mail: tgk2@uic.edu

J. Abraham
Department of Biomedical and Health Information Sciences, College of Applied Health Sciences, University of Illinois at Chicago, Chicago, IL, USA
e-mail: abrahamj@uic.edu

© Springer International Publishing Switzerland 2015
V.L. Patel et al. (eds.), *Cognitive Informatics for Biomedicine*, Health Informatics,
DOI 10.1007/978-3-319-17272-9_5

systematic evaluation of not only the HIT systems, but also the context of clinical environments in which these systems would be used. Nevertheless, the challenge that is faced by developers and researchers alike is to *identify*, *select* and *use* appropriate methods of HIT evaluation. In this chapter, our aims are twofold: *first*, to provide an overview of the various methods that can be used for evaluating HIT systems. We have categorized evaluation methods under two general headings: (a) evaluation of systems, focusing on usability and other parameters related to human computer interaction (HCI) – these methods are analytic, and most often laboratory-based; (b) a more generic usability and situated testing of systems, focusing on a comprehensive perspective of the use of HIT systems within the context of clinical environments (e.g., the role of HIT on clinical workflow or its role in causing unintended consequences) – these methods are more open-ended, in-situ, and field-based. It is important to note that these categorizations are not mutually exclusive – evaluation of systems often involve the use of one or more methods from both categories. *Second*, we discuss the challenges of conducting comprehensive evaluation studies in the clinical environment, and approaches to potentially overcome these challenges. In addition, we provide examples of the use of the specific methods, and cross-references to other chapters in this volume that have utilized these methods in a clinical context.

5.2   Methods of Evaluation in Clinical Environments

A healthcare system is often considered a complex, socio-technical system consisting of many components – clinicians, patients, and HIT, to name a few (Kannampallil et al. 2011; Patel et al. 2014). Among these, HIT is a key component that is necessary to ensure the smooth and effective functioning of the modern healthcare system. HIT incorporation into a clinical environment often transforms the structure, processes or outcomes – hence appropriate evaluation is often necessary to determine its viability or effectiveness (Donabedian 1966). The pertinent question is *how do we study the effects of HIT on structure, processes or outcomes – both directly, and indirectly?* HIT evaluation is often built on components assessing the: (1) system functionality, (2) impact of the user interface on work activities, and (3) discovering specific interface and system issues that affect the contextual work activities of user (Kurosu 2014).

In general, an evaluation would involve questions of what, why, when and how: (a) *what* to evaluate (e.g., an interface); (b) *why* should it be evaluated – it should be noted that given the breadth of biomedical informatics research, the purpose of the evaluation can include the following: as a promotional activity (e.g., reassuring patients or clinicians that resources are safe), part of scholarly work (e.g., a research project), a pragmatic activity (e.g., to evaluate whether a device is cost effective to purchase), ethical activity (e.g., to evaluate whether a medical device is functional and can be used as an alternative to an existing device), or medico-legal (e.g., to reduce legal liability) (Friedman and Wyatt 2006); (c) *when* to evaluate (e.g., at what stage of the design or implementation process); and (d) *how* to evaluate (i.e., the methods and tools that should be used for evaluation).

In terms of "when to evaluate" a system, evaluation studies can be classified into two formative or summative. *Formative evaluation* is defined as "a rigorous assessment process designed to identify potential and actual influences on the progress and effectiveness of implementation efforts" (Stetler et al. 2006). These are performed during the early stages of system design, and continue throughout the system development lifecycle. These are conducted to receive early feedback from potential users, and are mostly conducted with prototypes (low-fidelity paper prototypes or hi-fidelity test interfaces). The purpose of these evaluations is to study the complexity of design and update the system before implementation through user feedback. In contrast, *summative evaluation* is performed at the completion of the design and development efforts. These are often considered comprehensive as it is expected to demonstrate the efficacy of a system in its environment of use.

In this chapter, we focus specifically on the "how to evaluate" aspect. We have classified evaluation methods into two categories: general analytic evaluation approaches and usability testing. This categorization was informally based on the type of participant in the evaluation. Analytic evaluation studies are, most often, using experts as participants – usability experts, domain experts, software designers – or in some cases, without participants. These techniques include task-analytic, inspection-based or model-based approaches and are most often conducted in laboratory-based (or controlled) settings.

In contrast, usability testing employs users and stakeholders in the evaluation process. Usability testing can be conducted in the field or in a controlled laboratory setting. For example, one can evaluate the use of a hand-held device in an Emergency Room (ER) using observational techniques. In contrast, EHR interfaces or other user interfaces can be tested in a laboratory environment where users are asked to complete specific simulated task scenarios. While certain methods of usability testing can be more effectively conducted in a laboratory setting, the settings are sometimes a matter of convenience (e.g., it is easier for a participant to complete a task with verbal think-aloud without interruptions in a laboratory setting than in a clinical setting). We have categorized usability testing into field-based studies (including general observational and other studies) that capture situated and contextual aspects of HIT use, and a general category of methods (e.g., interviews, focus groups, surveys) that solicit user opinions and can be administered in different modes (e.g., face-to-face or online). A brief categorization of the evaluation approaches can be found in Fig. 5.1. In the following sections, we provide a detailed description of each of the evaluation approaches along with research examples of its use.

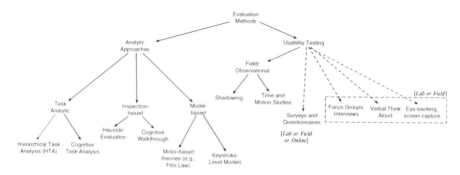

Fig. 5.1 Classification of evaluation methods

5.2.1 Analytical Approaches

Analytical approaches rely on analysts' judgments and analytic techniques to perform evaluations on user interfaces, and often do not directly involve the participation of end users. These approaches utilize experts – usability, human factors, or software – to conduct the evaluation studies. In general, analytical evaluation techniques involve *task-analytic* approaches (e.g., hierarchical and cognitive task analysis), *inspection-based* methods (e.g., heuristic evaluations and walkthroughs), and predictive *model-based* methods (e.g., keystroke models, Fitts Law). As will be described in the respective sections, the model-based techniques do not use any participants and relies on parameterized approaches for describing expert behavior. We describe each of these techniques, their applications, appropriate contexts of their use and examples from recent research literature.

5.2.1.1 Task Analysis[1]

Task analysis is one of most commonly used techniques to evaluate "existing practices" in order to understand the rationale behind people's goals of performing a task, the motivations behind their goals, and how they perform these tasks (Preece et al. 1994). As described by Vicente (1999), task analysis is an evaluation of the "trajectories of behavior." Hierarchical task analysis (HTA) and cognitive task analysis (CTA) are the most commonly used task-analytic methods in in biomedical informatics research.

---

[1] While GOMS (See Sect. 5.2.1.3) is considered a task-analytic approach, we have categorized it as a model-based approach for predictions of task completion times. It is based on a task analytic decomposition of tasks.

Hierarchical Task Analysis

HTA is the simplest task analytic approach and involves the breaking down of a task into sub-tasks and smaller constituted parts (e.g., sub-sub-tasks). The tasks are organized according to specific goals. This method, originally designed to identify specific training needs, has been used extensively in the design and evaluation of interactive interfaces (Annett and Duncan 1967). The application of HTA can be explained with an example: consider the goal of printing a Microsoft Word document that is on your desktop. The sub-tasks for this goal would involve finding (or identifying) the document on your desktop, and then printing it by selecting the appropriate printer. The HTA for this task can be organized as follows:

0. Print document on the desktop
1. Go to the desktop
2. Find the document

    2.1. Use "Search" function
    2.2. Enter the name of the document
    2.3. Identify the document

3. Open the document
4. Select the "File" menu and then "Print"

    4.1. Select relevant printer
    4.2. Click "Print" button

Plan 0: do 1–3–4; if file cannot be located by a visual search, do 2–3–4
Plan 2: do 2.1–2.2–2.3

In the above-mentioned task analysis, the task can be decomposed into the following: moving to your desktop, searching for the document (either visually or by using the search function and typing in the search criteria), selecting the document, opening and printing it using the appropriate printer. The order in which these tasks are performed may change based on certain situations. For example, if the document is not immediately visible on the desktop (or if the desktop has several documents making it impossible to identify the document visually), then a search function is necessary. Similarly, if there are multiple printer choices, then a relevant printer must be selected. The plans include a set of tasks that a user must undertake to achieve the goal (i.e., print the document). In this case, there are two plans: plan 0 and plan 2 (all plans are conditional on tasks having pertinent sub-tasks associated with it). For example, if the user cannot find a document on the desktop, plan 2 is instantiated, where a search function is used to identify the document (steps 2.1, 2.2 and 2.3). Figure 5.2 depicts the visual form of the HTA for this particular example.

HTA has been used significantly in evaluating interfaces and medical devices. For example, Chung et al. (2003) used HTA to compare the differences between 6 infusion pumps. Using HTA, they identified potential sources for the generation of human errors during various tasks. While exploratory, their use of HTA provided

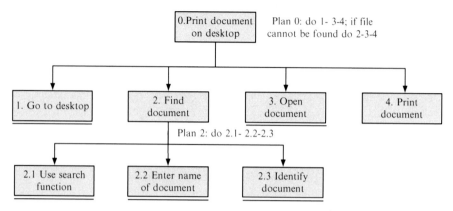

Fig. 5.2 Graphical representation of task analysis of printing a document: the tasks are represented in the *boxes*; the *line* underneath certain *boxes* represents the fact that there are no sub-tasks for these tasks

insights into how the HTA can be used for evaluating human performance and for predicting potential sources of errors. Alternatively, HTA has been used to model information and clinical workflow in ambulatory clinics (Unertl et al. 2009). Unertl et al. (2009) used direct observations and semi-structured interviews to create a HTA of the workflows. The HTA was then used to identify the gaps in existing HIT functionality for supporting clinical workflows, and the needs of chronic disease care providers.

Cognitive Task Analysis

CTA is an extension of the general task analysis technique to develop a more comprehensive understanding regarding the knowledge, cognitive/thought processes and goals that underlie observable task activities (Chipman et al. 2000). While the focus is on knowledge and cognitive components of the task activities and performance, CTA relies on observable human activities to draw insights on the knowledge based constraints and challenges that impair effective task performance.

CTA techniques are broadly classified into three groups based on how data is captured: (a) interviews and observations, (b) process tracing and (c) conceptual techniques (Cooke 1994). CTA supported by interviews and observations involve developing a comprehensive understanding of the tasks through discussions with, and task observations of experts. For example, a researcher observes an expert physician performing the task of medication order entry into a CPOE (Computerized Physician Order Entry) system and asks follow up questions regarding the specific aspects of the task. In a study on understanding providers' management of abnormal test results, Hysong et al. (2010) conducted interviews with 28 primary care physicians on how and when they manage alerts, and how they use the various features on the EHR system to filter and sort their alerts. The authors used the CTA approach supported by a combination of interviews and demonstrations. Participants were asked how they performed their alert management tasks and were asked to demonstrate these to the researcher. Based on the evaluation, they found that understanding of alert management differed (between 4 and 75 %) between providers and most did not use these features.

CTA supported by process-tracing approaches relies on capturing task activities through direct (e.g., verbal think aloud) or indirect (e.g., unobtrusive screen recording) data capture methods. Whereas the process-tracing approach is generally used to capture expert behaviors, it has also been used to evaluate general users. In a study on experts' information seeking behavior in critical care, Kannampallil et al. (2013) used the process-tracing approach to identify the nature of information-seeking activities including the information sources, cognitive strategies and shortcuts used by critical care physicians in decision making tasks. The CTA approach relied on the verbalizations of physicians, their access of various sources, and the time spent on accessing these sources to identify the strategies of information seeking. In a related study, the process-tracing approach was used to characterize the differences of information seeking practices of two groups of clinicians (Kannampallil et al. 2014).

Finally, CTA supported by conceptual techniques rely on the development of representations of a domain (and their related concepts) and the potential relationships between them. This approach is often used with experts and different methods are used for knowledge elicitation including concept elicitation, structured interviews, ranking approaches, card sorting, structural approaches such as multidimensional scaling, and graphical associations (Cooke 1994). While extensively used in general HCI studies, the use of conceptual techniques based CTA is much less prominent in biomedical informatics research literature. A detailed review of these approaches and their use can be found in Cooke (1994).

5.2.1.2 Inspection-Based Evaluation

Inspection methods involve one or more experts appraising a system, playing the role of a user in order to identify potential usability and interaction problems with a system (Nielsen 1994). Inspection methods are most often conducted on fully developed systems or interfaces, but may also be used on prototypes or beta versions. These techniques provide a cost-effective mechanism to identify the shortcomings of a system. Inspection methods rely on a usability expert, i.e., a person with significant training and experience in evaluating interfaces, to go through a system and identify whether the user interface elements conform to a pre-determined set of usability guidelines and design requirements (or principles). This method has been used as an alternative to recruiting potential users to test the usability of a system. The most commonly used inspection methods are heuristic evaluations (HE) and walkthroughs.

Heuristic Evaluation

HE techniques utilize a small set of experts to evaluate a user interface (or a set of interfaces in a system) based on their understanding of a set of heuristic principles regarding interface design (Johnson et al. 2005). This technique was developed by Jakob Nielsen and colleagues (Nielsen 1994; Nielsen and Molich 1990), and has been used extensively in the evaluation of user interfaces. The original set of heuristics was developed by Nielsen (1994) based on an abstraction of 249 usability problems. In general, the following ten heuristic principles (or a subset of these) are most often considered for HE studies: system status visibility; match between system and real world; user control and freedom; consistency and standards; error prevention; recognition rather than recall; flexibility and efficiency of use; aesthetic and minimalist design; help users recognize, diagnose and recover from errors; and help and documentation (retrieved from: http://www.nngroup.com/articles/ten-usability-heuristics/, on September 24, 2014; additional details can be found at this link). Conducting a HE involves a usability expert going through an interface to identify potential violations to a set of usability principles (referred to as the "heuristics"). These perceived violations could involve interface elements such as windows, menu items, links, navigation, and interaction.

Evaluators typically select a relevant subset of heuristics for evaluation (or add more based on the specific needs and context). The selection of heuristics is based on the type of system and interface being evaluated. For example, the relevant heuristics for evaluating an EHR interface would be different from that of a medical device. After selecting a set of applicable heuristics, one or more usability experts evaluate the user interface against the identified heuristics. After evaluating the heuristics, the potential violations are rated according to a severity score (1–5, where 1 indicates a cosmetic problem and 5 indicates a catastrophic problem). This process is iterative and continues till the expert feels that a majority (if not all) of the violations are identified. It is also generally recommended that a set of 4–5 usability experts are required to identify 95 % of the perceived violations or problems with a user interface. It should be acknowledged that HE approach may not lead to the identification of all problems and the identified problems may be localized (i.e., specific to a particular interface in a system). An example of an HE evaluation form is shown in Fig. 5.3.

In the healthcare domain, HE has been used in the evaluation of medical devices and HIT interfaces. For example, Zhang et al. (2003) used a modified set of 14 heuristics to compare the patient safety characteristics of two 1-channel volumetric infusion pumps. Four independent usability experts evaluated both infusion pumps using the list of heuristics and identified 89 usability problems categorized as 192 heuristic violations for pump 1, and 52 usability problems categorized as 121 heuristic violations for pump 2. The heuristic violations were also classified based on their severity. In another study, Allen et al. (2006) developed a simplified list of heuristics to evaluate web-based healthcare interfaces (printouts of each interface). Multiple usability experts assigned severity ratings for each of the identified violations and the severity ratings were used to re-design the interface.

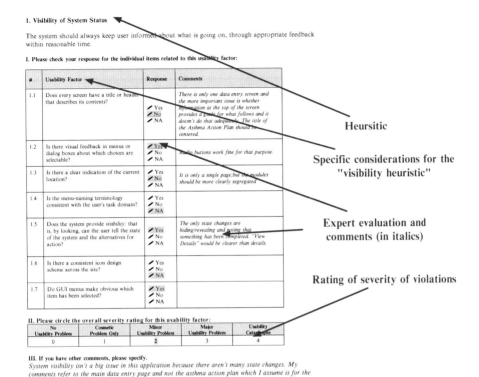

Fig. 5.3 Example of a HE form (for visibility) (Figure courtesy, David Kaufman, Personal communication)

HE has also been used for evaluating consumer-based pages (e.g., see the use of HE by Choi and Bakken (2010) on the evaluation of a web-based education portal for low-literate parents of infants). Variants of HE approaches have been widely used in the evaluation of HIT interfaces primarily because of its easy applicability. However, the ease of its application in a variety of usability evaluation scenarios often gives rise to inappropriate use. For example, there are several instances where only one or two usability experts (instead of the suggested 4–5 experts) are used for the HE. Other instances have used subject matter experts rather than usability experts for such evaluation studies.

Walkthroughs

Walkthroughs are another inspection-based approach that relies on experts to evaluate the cognitive processes of users performing a task. It involves employing a set of potential stakeholders (designers, usability experts) to characterize a sequence of actions and goals for completing a task. Most commonly used walkthrough, referred to as cognitive walkthrough (CW), involves observing, recording and analyzing the actions and behaviors of users as they complete a scenario of use. CW is focused on identifying the usability and comprehensibility of a system (Polson et al. 1992). The aim of CW is to investigate and determine whether the user's knowledge and skills and the interface cues are sufficient to produce an appropriate goal-action sequence that is required to perform a given task (Kaufman et al. 2003). CW is derived from the cognitive theory of how users work on computer-based tasks, using the exploratory learning approach, where system users continually appraise their goals and evaluate their progress against these goals (Kahn and Prail 1994).

While performing CW, the focus is on simulating the human-system interaction, and evaluating the fit between the system features and the user's goals. Conducting CW studies involves multiple steps. Potential participants (e.g., users, designers, usability experts) are provided a set of task sequences or scenarios for working with an interface or system. For example, for an interface for entering demographic and patient history details, participants (e.g., physicians) are asked to enter the age, gender, race and clinical history information. As the participants perform their assigned task, their task sequences, errors and other behavioral aspects are recorded. Often, follow up interviews or think aloud (described in a later section) are used to identify participants' interpretation of the tasks, how they make progress, and potential points of mismatches in the system. Detailed observations and recordings of these mismatches are documented for further analysis. While in most situations CWs are performed by individuals, sometimes groups of stakeholders perform the walkthrough together. For example, usability experts, designers and potential users could go through systems together to identify the potential issues and drawbacks. Such group walkthroughs are often referred to as pluralistic walkthroughs.

In biomedical informatics, it must be noted that CW has been used extensively in evaluating situations other than human computer interaction. For example, CW method (and its variants) has been used to evaluate diagnostic reasoning, decision-making processes and clinical activities. Kushniruk et al. (1996) used the CW method to perform an early evaluation on the mediating role of HIT in clinical practice. The CW was not only used to identify usability problems, but was instrumental in the development of a coding scheme for subsequent usability testing. Hewing et al. (2013) used CW to evaluate an expert ophthalmologist's reasoning regarding the plus disease (a condition of the eye) among infants. Using images, clinical experts were independently asked to rate the presence and severity of the plus condition and provide an explanation of how they arrived at their diagnostic decisions. Similar approaches were used by Kaufman et al. (2003) to evaluate the usability of a home-based, telehealth system.

While extremely useful in identifying the key usability issues, CW methods involve significant investments in cost and time for data capture and analysis.

5.2.1.3   Model-Based Evaluation

Model-based evaluation approaches use predictive modeling approaches to characterize the efficiency of user interfaces. Model-based approaches are often used for evaluating routine, expert task performance. For example, how can the keys of a medical device interface be optimally organized such that users can complete their tasks efficiently (and accurately)? Similarly, predictive modeling can be used to compare the data entry efficiency between interfaces with different layouts and organization. We describe two commonly used predictive modeling techniques in the evaluation of interfaces.

GOMS

Card et al. (1980, 1983) proposed the GOMS (Goals, Operators, Methods and Selection Rules) analytical framework for predicting human performance with interactive systems. Specifically, GOMS models predict the time taken to complete a task by a skilled/expert user based on "the composite of actions of retrieving plans from long-term memory, choosing among alternative available methods depending on features of the task at hand, keeping track of what has been done and what needs to be done, and executing the motor movements necessary for the keyboard and mouse" (Olson and Olson 2003). In other words, GOMS assumes that the execution of tasks can be represented as a serial sequence of cognitive operations and motor actions.

GOMS is used to describe an aggregate of the task and the user's knowledge regarding how to perform the task. This is expressed in terms of the *G*oals, *O*perators, *M*ethods and *S*election rules. *Goals* are the expected outcomes that a user wants to achieve. For example, a goal for a physician could be documenting the details of a patient interaction on an EHR interface. *Operators* are the specific actions that can be performed on the user interface. For example, clicking on a text box or selecting a patient from a list in a dropdown menu. *Methods* are sequential combinations of operators and sub-goals that need to be achieved. For example, in the case of selecting a patient from a dropdown list, the user has to move the mouse over to the dropdown menu, click on the arrow using the appropriate mouse key to retrieve the list of patients. Finally, *selection* rules are used to ascertain which methods to choose when several choices are available. For example, using the arrow keys on the keyboard to scroll down a list versus using the mouse to select.

One of the simplest and most commonly used GOMS approaches is the Keystroke-Level Model (KLM), which was first described in Card et al. (1983). As opposed to the general GOMS model, the KLM makes several assumptions regarding the task. In KLM, methods are limited to keystroke level operations and task duration is predicted based on these estimates. For the KLM, there are six types of operators: K for pressing a key; P for pointing the mouse to a target;

H for moving hands to the keyboard or pointing device; *D* for drawing a line segment; *M* for mental preparation for an action; and *R* for system response. Based on experimental data or other predictive models (e.g., Fitts Law), each of these operators is assigned a value or a parameterized estimate of execution time. We describe an example from Saitwal et al. (2010) on the use of the KLM approach.

In a study investigating the usability of EHR interfaces, Saitwal et al. (2010) used the KLM approach to evaluate the time taken, and the number of steps required to complete a set of 14 EHR-based tasks. The purpose of the study was to characterize the issues with the user interface and also to identify potential areas for improvement. The evaluation was performed on the AHLTA (Armed Forces Health Longitudinal Technology Application) user interface. A set of 14 prototypical tasks was first identified. Sample tasks included entering patient's current illness, history of present illness, social history and family history. KLM analysis was performed on each of the tasks: this involved breaking each of the tasks into its component goals, operators, methods and selection rules. The operators were also categorized as physical (e.g., move mouse to a button) or mental (e.g., locate an item from a dropdown menu). For example, the selection of a patient name involved 8 steps (*M* – mental operation; *P* – physical operation): (1) think of location on the menu [*M*, 1.2*s*], (2) move hand to the mouse [*P*, 0.4*s*], (3) move the mouse to "Go" in the menu [*P*, 0.4*s*], (4) extend the mouse to "Patient" [*P*, 0.4*s*], (5) retrieve the name of the patient [*M*, 1.2*s*], (6) locate patient name on the list [*M*, 1.2*s*], (7) move mouse to the identified patient [*P*, 0.4*s*] and (8) click on the identified patient [*P*, 0.4*s*]. In this case, there were a total of 8 steps that would take 5.2*s* to complete. In a similar manner, the number of steps and the time taken for each of the 14 considered AHLTA tasks were computed.

In addition, GOMS and its family of methods can be effectively used to make comparisons regarding the efficiency of performing tasks interfaces. However, such approaches are approximations and have several disadvantages. While GOMS provides a flexible and often reliable mechanism for predicting human performance in a variety of computer-based tasks, there are several potential limitations. A brief summary is provided here, and interested readers can find further details in Card et al. (1980). GOMS models can be applied only to the *error-free*, *routine* tasks of *skilled* users. Thus, it is not possible to make time predictions for non-skilled users, who are likely to take considerable time to learn to use a new system. For example, the use of the GOMS approach to predict the potential time spent by physicians in using a new EHR would be inaccurate – owing to relative lack of knowledge of the physicians regarding the use of the various interfaces, and the learning curve required to be up-to-speed with the new system. The complexity of clinical work processes and tasks, and the variability of the user population create significant challenges for the effective use of GOMS in measuring the effectiveness of clinical tasks.

Fitts Law

Fitts Law is used to predict human motor behavior; it is used to predict the time taken to acquire a target (Fitts 1954). On computer-based interfaces, it has been used to develop a predictive model of time it takes to acquire a target using a mouse (or another pointing device). The time taken to acquire a target depends on the distance between the pointer and target (referred to as amplitude, A) and the width of the target (W). The movement time (MT) is mathematically represented as follows:

$$MT = k.log_2\left(\frac{A}{W} + 1\right) where\ k\ is\ a\ constant, A - amplitude, W - width\ of\ the\ target$$

In summary, based on Fitts law, one can say that the larger objects are easier to acquire while smaller, closely aligned objects are much more difficult to acquire with a pointing device. While the direct application of Fitts law is not often found in the evaluation studies of HIT or health interfaces in general, it has a profound influence in the design of interfaces. For example, the placement of menu items and buttons, such that a user can easily click on them for selection, are based on Fitts law parameters. Similarly, in the design of number keypads for medical devices, the size of the buttons and their location can be effectively predicted by Fitts law parameters.

In addition to the above-mentioned predictive models, there are several other less common models. While a detailed description of each of them or their use is beyond the scope of this chapter, we provide a brief introduction to another predictive approach: Hick-Hyman choice reaction time (Hick 1951; Hyman 1953). Choice reaction time, RT, can be predicted based on the number of available stimuli (or choices), n:

$$RT = a + b.log_2(n); where\ a\ and\ b\ are\ constants$$

Hick-Hyman law is particularly useful in predicting text entry rates for different keyboards (MacKenzie et al. 1999), and time required to select from different menus (e.g., a linear vs. a hierarchical menu). In particular, the method is useful to make decisions regarding the design and evaluation of menus. For example, consider two menu design choices: 9 items deep/3 items wide and 3 items deep/9 items wide. The RT for each of these can be calculated as follows: $[3*(a + b.log_2(n)), <, 9, *(a + b.log_2(n))]$. This shows that the access to menus is more efficient when it is designed breadth-wise rather than depth-wise.

5.2.2 Usability Testing/User-Based Evaluation

In this section, we have grouped a range of approaches that are generally used for evaluating the usability of HIT systems. In general, we have classified them into field/observational studies, and general approaches for usability evaluation that can be utilized in both field and laboratory settings. While formal usability testing is often conducted in laboratory settings where user performance (and other selected variables) are evaluated based on pre-selected tasks, we have loosely classified the evaluation techniques that utilize users in the evaluation process into general approaches (those that can be used in both field and laboratory based studies) and field studies.

5.2.2.1 General Usability Testing Approaches

Interviews

Interviews are commonly used to elicit information about opinions and perspectives of participants and their work practices (Mason 2002). Within the context of HIT design and evaluation, interviews have been used to obtain clinicians' perspectives and their experiences within the context of the clinical workflow and its respective challenges and opportunities for design improvement. A study on physicians' use of EHR with particular emphasis on its barriers and solutions is a classic example of an interview study that investigates the impact of HIT on physician workflow. For example, Miller and Sim (2004) conducted over 90 interviews with physician champions and EHR managers. Through these interview sessions, they identified participant perceptions regarding barriers to EHR use including high initial set-up costs, slow and uncertain financial payoffs, high initial physician time costs related to challenges with the technology, attitudes and incentives to use the new system. Interview participants, when asked, suggested potential solutions such as performance incentives for achieving quality improvement, technical support for the system and incorporation of a community-wide data exchange.

Interviews are viewed as an approach to elicit additional information and are often used in concert with other field study methods (e.g., observation or shadowing). For example, Unertl et al. (2013) investigated the use of health information exchange (HIE) technology, and its impact on care delivery at an e-health organization. Multi-faceted data collection methods including observations, informal and formal interviews, were used to examine workflow and information flow among team members and patients. While the interview findings illustrated the benefits of HIE technologies for communication and care continuity, their adoption in practice was limited. The integrated analysis highlighted the importance of moving away from a data and information "ownership" model to a "continuity and context-aware" model for the design and implementation of HIE technology.

Often, the data obtained from interviews are used to analyze the contextual language and meaning as quoted by participants. For example, in a qualitative study on patient transfers, Abraham et al. (Abraham 2010; Abraham and Reddy 2008) observed breakdowns in information flow between clinical units, despite the effective use of a care coordination system. Using follow-up interviews, the authors captured participants' perspectives on the underlying cause for the information breakdowns. For example, in one of the interviews, an emergency department charge nurse was asked to describe the information sharing issues that affected the coordination of patient transfers from her unit. Her response was: "*A lot of times the attending residents don't know to put in medication or change orders, additional labs and if we are busy with other patients, we don't have time to go to the computer and even though these screens help, they still don't alleviate the problem.*" She further added that: "*I think basically they don't understand how the emergency department works, how difficult it is to hold patients, I don't think they understand the concept like I said we don't have the ancillary staff and so they have this expectation of what the patient is going to be like when they come up, you know they are disheveled or haven't had a bath or like you know they think that's horrible* (Abraham and Reddy 2008)."

Individual interviews can be classified into three major categories based on the format and level of standardization of the interview questions – structured, semi-structured and narrative (or unstructured). During *structured interviews*, all interviewees are asked the same questions in the same order. This allows for comparisons between responses across interviewees, which can be analyzed using qualitative and quantitative methods. *Semi-structured interviews*, unlike the structured interviews, are flexible and allow for probing of participants (i.e., with follow up questions) to discuss relevant issues.

In contrast to the structured methods of interviewing, narrative, open-ended, unstructured interviewing does not use any question-response structure. Instead, it adopts a storytelling and listening framework for obtaining participant perspectives. Narrative interviewing is typically comprised of four steps: (a) initiation (introduction of the topic for narration), (b) the main storytelling or narration, (c) questioning and clarification, and (d) concluding remarks (Farr 1982; Hermanns 1991). This particular type of interviewing allows participants to describe their story in their own spontaneous language. For instance, short HCI scenarios can be used to elicit participants' responses on how they react to a real-world situation. An example scenario can focus on the emergency medical service (EMS) personnel use of patient EHR to support handoff communication to an ER physician during a trauma patient drop-off. Some of the potential questions that follow the scenario could uncover the details of how the EMS and ED team respond to the trauma situation, and the EHR functions and features that can support such emergent communication during trauma resuscitation.

Most interviews are audio-recorded for a variety of reasons: (a) the data can be transcribed verbatim, with limited chances of missing key points made by participants, (b) provides the ability for the researcher to listen to the audio files and (c) features such as voice tone and frequency may be of interest for researchers. It is recommended that interviews be conducted at locations selected by the participants to ensure that they feel comfortable to freely talk, without being concerned about other colleagues overhearing their conversations.

Focus Groups

Focus group is a type of interactive interviewing method that involves an in-depth discussion of a particular topic of interest with a small group of participants. Focus group method has been described as "a carefully planned discussion designed to obtain perceptions on a defined area of interest in a permissive, non-threatening environment" (Krueger 2009). The central elements of focus groups as highlighted by Vaughn et al. (1996) include: (a) the group is an informal assembly of target participants to discuss a topic; (b) the group is small, between 6 and 12 members and is relatively homogeneous; (c) the group conversation is facilitated by a trained moderator with prepared questions and probes; and (d) given that the primary goal of a focus group is to elicit the perceptions, feelings, attitudes, and ideas of participants about a selected topic, it can be used to generate hypotheses for further research (Krueger 2009).

Unlike individual interviews, focus group discussions allow the researcher to probe responses to a particular research topic while capturing the underlying group dynamics of the participants. According to Kitzinger (1995), interaction is a crucial feature of focus groups as it captures their view of the world, the language they use about an issue and their values and beliefs about a situation (Gibbs 1997). For instance, a focus group involving usability experts, system designers and care providers can allow participants to share their varying perspectives on HIT system design based on their work role. This will enable them to voice the key issues on the fit or (lack thereof) between the functionalities of the system and the clinical workflow.

Many researchers have argued that focus group interviewing depends on the active discussion and engagement among participants, and therefore have strongly advocated for homogenous groups (similar participants) (e.g., Krueger 2009). Although the interaction between participants is considered a strength of the method, group participants and the setting can sometimes inhibit the group inter-action (Lewis 1992), especially during instances when sensitive personal issues are discussed. A decision regarding the composition should be based on the specific research (or design) question at hand. For example, a qualitative study supported by a series of seven focus group interviews with emergency medical services (EMS) and emergency room (ER) teams were conducted to investigate their coordination practices in a crisis response situation. The focus group participants were presented with a mass casualty incident situation, and were asked to respond to a series of events that unfolded. The questions were related to the decision making process during a large-scale emergency situation, with particular emphasis on (a) their information and communication needs, (b) their information and communication technology use, and (c) their roles and responsibilities during the crisis. During the focus group sessions, two researchers moderated the discussion, and took detailed notes. Barriers perceived to impact coordination activities between EMS and ED teams included ineffective information and communication technologies, lack of common ground, and breakdowns in information flow. Furthermore, the focus group interview participants also jointly identified several key socio-technical requirements for inter-team coordination systems such as situation awareness, context, and workflow (Paul et al. 2008; Reddy et al. 2009).

Another important factor that plays a vital role in focus group sessions is the presence of a skilled moderator (or facilitator) (Burrows and Kendall 1997) who manages the conversations and interactions between participants. Moreover, scheduling a convenient time and location for administering focus group interviews can be very difficult, given the number of participants that are involved.

Verbal Think Aloud

Verbal think aloud (or simply "think aloud") is often used to capture rich verbal data on the thought processes that underlie human actions. Analysis of these verbal reports can be used to characterize the underlying information and knowledge structures. Think aloud evaluations are generally characterized into two types: (1) concurrent and (2) retrospective (Ericsson and Simon 1980). A concurrent think aloud requires uninterrupted and direct verbalizations of participants as they perform a task, and is considered to be complete and consistent with their thought sequence. In contrast, a retrospective think aloud requires the researcher to ask and prompt subjects to recall their thought sequence while performing a task (or after completing a task). Ericsson and Simon (1984), the original proponents of the verbal think aloud method, suggested the value of think aloud data is based on the following assumptions: (1) the verbalizations capture only a subset of the cognitive processes underlying behavior; (2) human mind is an information processor; and (3) the verbalizations capture contents of working memory (i.e., information recently acquired is accessed).

Think aloud studies are typically conducted to identify and characterize cognitive processes such as reasoning, problem solving, and decision-making processes. For example, Patel and colleagues (Patel et al. 1994, 2001; Patel and Groen 1991a, b) have conducted several studies using verbal think aloud that investigated the nature of reasoning using electronic tools, its effects on expertise and decision-making. Most of these studies relied on verbalizations by a participant (e.g., a physician), and in-depth linguistic analysis of the verbalizations to identify inherent strategies in their reasoning and decision-making. Similarly, Fonteyn and Grobe (1994) utilized a think aloud study to understand the reasoning and decision-making behaviors of critical care nurses regarding unstable patients. Insights on the reasoning process of expert nurses informed the design of an expert system. Other examples of similar key studies can be found here (Fisher and Fonteyn 1995; Fowler 1997; Funkesson et al. 2007; Grobe et al. 1991; Simmons et al. 2003).

One of the concerns that have been raised in evaluation studies using verbal think aloud method is the issue of sample size. While many researchers have used a small sample size of five participants to focus on in-depth analysis of the cognitive processes, others have critiqued the sample size (e.g., Lewis 1994). Lundgrén-Laine and Salanterä (2010) have suggested that the characteristics of the study participants in terms of their verbalization skills and the appropriate application of the think aloud is more important than the sample size (Caulton 2001; Fonteyn et al. 1993; Hall et al. 2004). Measures of information and participant saturation are often used to determine study completion. A detailed description of the think aloud method and approaches for its analysis can be found here (Ericsson and Simon 1984).

5.2.2.2 Surveys and Questionnaires

Surveys and questionnaires are widely used in evaluation studies. Their widespread use is related to ease of administration (through multiple modes: online, face-to-face) and limited time required to complete (especially those that use Likert scale measures). In terms of usability evaluation, there are several surveys that are commonly used. A list of the commonly used usability surveys are provided below:

(a) *QUIS* (Questionnaire for User Interface Satisfaction: http://lap.umd.edu/quis/): measure user interface interaction and subjective satisfaction;
(b) *SUMI* (Software Usability Measurement Inventory: http://sumi.ucc.ie/): assess usability of software;
(c) *PSSUQ* (Post-Study System Usability Questionnaire), and *ASQ* (After Scenario Questionnaire: http://hcibib.org/perlman/question.cgi?form=ASQ) (Lewis 1991): address global usability of a system along with specific scenarios of use;
(d) *SUS* (System Usability Scale – http://www.usability.gov/how-to-and-tools/ methods/system-usability-scale.html) (Brooke 1996): a general survey of system usability;
(e) *Subjective workload assessment* (NASA-TLX Workload Instrument: http:// humansystems.arc.nasa.gov/groups/tlx/paperpencil.html) (Hart and Staveland 1988): a multi-item scale to determine the physical, temporal, mental, effort, frustration and performance while working with interfaces.

Although most of the above-mentioned surveys are validated for their reliability, researchers often use a variety of self-created surveys and questionnaires. Questionnaires, as opposed to the surveys that use a specific scale (e.g., a scale of 1–7), often use open-ended questions to elicit responses from participants regarding system use (e.g., "Describe some of the challenges that you faced while using the system?").

Surveys are often used along with other data collection methods and are considered a complementary data collection method in HIT evaluation. For example, Karahoca and colleagues (2010) used a generic survey along with system usage logs to characterize the usability of two mobile device prototypes. Similar open-ended questionnaires along with additional observational data was used by Holzinger and colleagues (2011) to characterize patient interactions with a mobile interface. Dalai and colleagues (in press) used the SUS scale and the NASA-TLX scales for comparing the effectiveness of two interfaces for comprehending psychiatric clinical narratives. These survey scales were used in concert with an analysis of verbal reports to evaluate the effectiveness of presented interfaces.

5.2.2.3 Field/Observational Approaches

In contrast to the analytic evaluation techniques that often yield objective data, there are several qualitative approaches that focus on the subjective and contextual assessments of system design and user interactions within the *context* of a real work environment (Kurosu 2014). These qualitative approaches are generally categorized as ethnographic-based methods and require an "immersion" in the field in order to understand the experiences and practices of the informants (Schatzberg 2008). Ethnography is a widely accepted method for data collection in the field of anthropology (Fetterman 1998). An ethnographer obtains a firsthand experience by immersing herself in the research setting for an extended period of time. This helps in gaining an understanding of the particular social and cultural practices of the setting. Ethnographic methods are used in a variety of domains to gain meaningful insights on the nuances and complexities of work practices (Forsythe 1999; Brixey et al. 2005).

Field studies using ethnographic methods allow for a situated, in-depth and in-situ evaluation of the clinical environments – providing insights on the use and interaction of care providers with the computer technologies and tools, situated within their organizational structures. Furthermore, field studies allow us to gain deeper insights on *not only* the interdependencies between the usability (ease of use, learnability and access) and the available functionality afforded by the technology, *but also*, the hidden tensions in the healthcare work practices arising from the contextual and environmental constraints that can potentially disrupt the user interaction with the technology. In other words, these methods provide an understanding of the effects of the user-system interaction on the end user *workflow* in actual practice. For instance, these methods can answer questions such as "how did the system change user behavior?"; "what are the reasons for poor task performance?"; "what are the unintended consequences or opportunities related to the system implementation in the work context?"; "what are the motivations behind the use of the system?" In contrast to the analytical approaches that are applicable only at an individual level, these empirical methods support the investigation of collaborative practices of work and the effect of technologies on coordination of work in these practices (e.g., Aarts et al. 2007; Horsky et al. 2006).

Field studies have been extensively used in studying the unique characteristics and nuances of clinical environments (e.g., Abraham and Reddy 2008; Malhotra et al. 2007), clinical and non-clinical activities and tasks surrounding clinical workflows such as information seeking practices of clinicians, coordination of patient transfer activities, decision making activities (e.g., Kannampallil et al. 2013, 2014; Patel and Kannampallil 2011; Patel et al. 2013), and HIT use in clinical environments (e.g., Abraham et al. 2009, 2012; Ash et al. 2004). Several of the chapters in this volume have used one or more of these methods. In the following sections, we describe two commonly used forms of structured field study approaches – shadowing, and time and motion studies.

Shadowing

Shadowing techniques involve a researcher closely following a participant over an extended period of time. In contrast to general observations of the entire unit and patient care team, shadowing techniques focus on collecting data about a single participant. The data obtained through shadowing are mainly related to the steps (e.g., process, activities or tasks) performed by the selected participant during the observational period. Specific to the use of HIT in clinical environments, shadowing can be used to gather data on the activities of different clinicians (attending physicians, residents, nurses) as they carry out their patient-care tasks, and their use of HIT. For example, in a study evaluating the use of EHR systems in an emergency care setting, Abraham et al. (2009; Abraham and Kannampallil 2014) shadowed attending physicians over multiple sessions. In addition to identifying the key activities around EHR use, they found that the use of the EHR led to additional "peripheral" activities that increased their work activities, consequently creating a fragmentation in the care process (e.g., the need to use multiple care artifacts, move across multiple locations and interact with several care providers). A similar shadowing study was conducted by Patterson et al. (2004) to investigate the barriers to effective use of clinical reminders supported by clinical decision support systems at multiple study sites. Using detailed shadowing notes and interview data, the authors identified six barriers: (a) workload during patient visits, (b) time to document when a clinical reminder was not clinically relevant, (c) inapplicability of the clinical reminder due to context-specific reasons, (d) limited training on how to use the clinical reminder software for rotating staff and permanent staff, (e) perceived reduction of quality of provider–patient interaction, and (f) the decision to use paper forms to enable review of resident physician orders prior to order entry.

Time and Motion Studies

Time and Motion study is a specific shadowing approach that helps in developing a deeper understanding of the impact of clinical work activities; for example, the changes on clinical efficiency, team coordination, rounds communication due to the implementation of a new health technology such as the computerized physician order entry system or an EHR system (Zheng et al. 2011). In routine time and motion studies, a researcher shadows the participant, capturing the sequence of a particular process/activity/task, in conjunction with the time spent by participant (on the process/activity/task). Time and motion studies help in examining the nature of emerging practices around care provider's adoption and use of the HIT system (e.g., Zheng et al. 2010). For instance, this method helps in understanding the role and the use of the EMR system for care activities such as developing an assessment and plan (in terms of distribution of time spent on clinical notes interface vs. patient labs interface). In addition to time, it is possible collect data on the locations traversed by the participant during the session. This provides an additional level of data on use and interaction of the HIT system within the context of its use, which can inform better design of HIT that are integrated within the clinical workflow. This method was used in a study that evaluated the impact of complexity on physician activities in an emergency care setting (Abraham and Kannampallil 2014). Based on the study, the authors characterized the nature of physician activities, the time allocated for these activities, how these activities were distributed across the unit and the susceptibility of these activities for interruptions, and found that approximately one-fourth (~25 %) of the physician activities (e.g., direct patient care) were localized at specific locations in the unit, while the rest of the activities (e.g., communication) were distributed across the unit and were less predictable. These non-localized activities also had a higher likelihood of interruptions. Based on the time and motion study, the authors highlight implications for mitigating the physician workload, and the design of technologies for monitoring such complex settings (Abraham and Kannampallil 2014).

Similar to shadowing, time and motion studies often require the use of a pre-defined taxonomy to record and document the observational data. The accuracy of the taxonomy, and its fit for the particular work environment is critical to the evaluation. Time and motion studies are very useful for assessing efficiency and effectiveness of HIT systems and also, human-centered characteristics of such technologies. An example of a validated taxonomy used by researchers in the medical informatics field was developed by Overhage et al. (2001), and later refined by Pizziferri et al. (2005). This taxonomy was recommended by the Agency for Healthcare Research and Quality (AHRQ) for collecting time-motion data in clinical workflow studies. This taxonomy has successfully been used to document the electronic documentation and note-writing practices of residents in a general medicine unit at a large teaching hospital (Mamykina et al. 2012). Using this taxonomy, they conducted a time and motion study on 11 resident physicians that provided insights on: (a) When and in what circumstances did residents use the EHR to write a note? (b) What were the general steps of EHR note composition? (c) Were there common patterns of transitions between these steps among residents? (d) How did the EHR documentation system facilitate or inhibit their clinical tasks such as developing a patient assessment and plan of care? The authors identified that seven of the 10 most common transitions between activities during note composition were between documenting, and gathering and reviewing patient data, and updating the plan of care. Through the fine-granular data collection on temporal properties of resident use of EHR system, the authors were able to find that clinical documentation on an EHR system was a *synthesis* activity, which was in contrast to the fundamental design of EHR systems that conceptualized clinical documentation as an uninterrupted composition. As highlighted in the above examples, time and motion studies solely depend on the observer to accurately document and record the participant time devoted to each task.

Shadowing and time and motion studies are labor-intensive and time-consuming, as they require continuous observation for extended periods of time by the researcher. Also, given that this method is a labor-intensive process, the sample size may be limited and may lead to questions regarding the generalizability of results. As with most observational studies, the presence of an observer can potentially impact the normal behavior of the participant due to awareness that he or she is being observed.

5.3   Considerations for Conducting HIT Evaluation Studies

In this chapter, we provided an overview of the range of methods that are available for conducting evaluation studies on HIT systems. The evaluation methods were classified into two general groups – analytical and user-based testing. While the methods are not truly mutually exclusive across these two groups, the classification provides a useful framework for selecting the appropriate method(s) for the evaluation of HIT systems. Additionally, given the complexities of the clinical environment, we have also adapted a more integrative perspective in terms of the applicable methods for HIT evaluation – acknowledging the importance of evaluation methods that capture the nuances of the work environment in which these systems are deployed. We highlight the role of field studies that capture the situated and contextual perspective of HIT including the effects of HIT implementations on clinical workflow, tasks and decision-making. Other chapters in this volume also provide extensions of these methods, both in terms of their use for evaluation and also for design. In Chap. 7, Kushniruk et al. introduces and explains user-centered design (UCD), a design approach that relies on some of the above-mentioned methods for the usability evaluation and design of HIT systems. Similarly, in Chap. 9, Kalenderian et al. describes the evaluation and re-design of a dental EHR interface.

In the rest of this section, we highlight some of the considerations for conducting HIT evaluation studies, directions of future evaluation studies and potential challenges for conducting these studies. One of the preliminary considerations for evaluations is to determine the environment in which the evaluation study will be conducted. As previously described, analytical evaluations are invariably conducted in a laboratory setting with experts. However, analytical evaluation studies would fail to capture the nuances and implications of the use of HIT within a clinical setting. For example, laboratory-based evaluations can identify most of the interface issues with a Computerized Physician Order Entry (CPOE) system, but long-term observational studies are possibly required for identifying the unintended effects of its use in clinical settings (as highlighted by Koppel et al. (2005) and Ash et al. (2004)). Similarly, remote usability evaluation studies are now routinely conducted using web-conference and screen sharing software (see for example, Kushniruk et al. 2008; also see Chap. 7, this volume, for low-cost simulation and tele-evaluation studies).

Another important consideration is the use of a framework to guide the evaluation process. These frameworks provide a theoretical and methodological scaffold for conducting an evaluation for improving the design of a system. While there are several such design and evaluation frameworks in general HCI (e.g., Scenario-based Design, Rosson and Carroll 2009), they are far less prominent in the healthcare research literature. One recent framework is TURF: Task, User, Representation, and Function (Zhang and Walji 2011). In addition to being a theoretical framework for describing and predicting usability differences between HIT systems, it also provides a framework for selecting appropriate evaluation methods, measuring the usability using these methods, and making design improvements based on the evaluation. Similar frameworks are likely to evolve with the widespread adoption of HIT and with the need for rapid evaluation protocols. Additionally, federally mandated programs such as the meaningful use (MU) of EHRs have furthered the adoption and use of HIT systems. However, with persistent concerns regarding EHRs (and HIT in general), further evaluation is very likely to continue. For example, EHR interfaces are still considered to have usability issues that require a redesign process. More research and development efforts, both from academia and healthcare industry partners, are likely to be forthcoming in this area.

Two other fast-growing fields within biomedical informatics are the use of mobile technology and consumer health informatics tools. The proliferation of mobile devices (phones, tablets) has provided a new approach for accessing and sharing health information between patients and their healthcare providers. Similarly, consumer health information tools have also been extensively used – for example, web-based social support tools, aggregated medical information tools and patient portals. These tools (both mobile and web-based) are still evolving and are likely an area of significant future design and evaluation (see Chaps. 12 and 13 in this volume for a detailed discussion of consumer informatics and mobile tools respectively).

Finally, it is also important to consider the challenges for conducting HIT evaluation studies. These require considerable investments in time, effort and planning, thoughtful considerations in selecting appropriate methods, and often require significant buy-ins from hospital administration and clinicians.

5.4   Conclusions

In this chapter, we described the traditional methods from usability engineering and HCI, and their applicability for HIT evaluation. The applicability of each of these methods for evaluation requires careful consideration. We have provided brief descriptions of these methods within the context of biomedical and healthcare applications. A detailed review is beyond the scope of this chapter (interested readers are encouraged to review the additional readings provided at the end of this chapter). Recently, more innovative techniques have been utilized for usability testing and evaluation. These have varied from general techniques such as eye-tracking, simulations and screen-capture tools to unobtrusive techniques that have used motion sensing (for a detailed review, see Chap. 6 in this volume by Zheng and colleagues). The scope of evaluation methods continues to expand in response to developing technologies, evolving health information tasks and changing circumstances (e.g., role of the health consumer).

Discussion Questions
1. Why is usability of systems a relevant topic for investigation? Why is evaluation of HIT a challenge to healthcare researchers?
2. When designing a new HIT system for a clinical vs. non-clinical setting, what are some of the considerations that must be made?
3. What are some of the considerations for evaluating a prototype vs. an actual, fully-developed system?
4. What methods will you use to evaluate a vendor-developed EHR?
5. How do usability issues manifest across professions? What can be done to mitigate them?

Additional Readings

Johnson, C. M., Johnston, D., & Crowle, P. K. (2011). *EHR usability toolkit: A background report on usability and electronic health records.* Rockville: Agency for Healthcare Research and Quality.

Kushniruk, A. W., & Patel, V. L. (2004). Cognitive and usability engineering methods for the evaluation of clinical information systems. *Journal of Biomedical Informatics, 37*(1), 56–76.

Preece, J., et al. (1994). *Human-computer interaction.* Addison-Wesley Longman Ltd.

Shortliffe, E. H., & Patel, V. L. (2011). Generation and formulation of knowledge: Human-intensive techniques. In R. A. Greenes (Ed.), *Clinical decision support: The road ahead.* Academic.

References

Aarts, J., Ash, J., & Berg, M. (2007). Extending the understanding of computerized physician order entry: Implications for professional collaboration, workflow and quality of care. *International Journal of Medical Informatics, 76*(Suppl 1), S4–S13.

Abraham, J. (2010). *Meta-coordination activities: Exploring articulation work in hospitals, in information sciences and technology (IST).* Doctoral dissertation, The Pennsylvania State University.

Abraham, J., & Kannampallil, T. G. (2014). Quantifying physician activities in emergency care: An exploratory study. In *Proceedings of the Human Factors and Ergonomics Society (HFES)*. Chicago: Sage.

Abraham, J., & Reddy, M. C. (2008). Moving patients around: A field study of coordination between clinical and non-clinical staff in hospitals. In *ACM conference on computer supported cooperative work (CSCW)*. ACM.

Abraham, J., Kannampallil, T. G., & Reddy, M. (2009). Peripheral activities during EMR use in emergency care: A case study. In *Proceedings of the American Medical Informatics Association (AMIA) annual symposium 2009*. San Francisco.

Abraham, J., Kannampallil, T., Patel, B., Almoosa, K., & Patel, V. L. (2012). Ensuring patient safety in care transitions: An empirical evaluation of a handoff intervention tool. In *Proceedings of the AMIA annual symposium*. Chicago.

Allen, M., Currie, L. M., Bakken, S., Patel, V. L., & Cimino, J. J. (2006). Heuristic evaluation of paper-based web pages: A simplified inspection usability methodology. *Journal of Biomedical Informatics, 39*(4), 412–423.

Annett, J., & Duncan, K. D. (1967). Task analysis and training design. *Occupational Psychology, 41*, 211–221.

Ash, J. S., Stavri, P. Z., & Kuperman, G. J. (2003). A consensus statement on considerations for a successful CPOE implementation. *Journal of the American Medical Informatics Association, 10*(3), 229–234.

Ash, J. S., Berg, M., & Coiera, E. (2004). Some unintended consequences of information technology in health care: The nature of patient care information system-related errors. *Journal of the American Medical Informatics Association, 11*(2), 104–112.

Blumenthal, D. (2009). Stimulating the adoption of health information technology. *New England Journal of Medicine, 360*(15), 1477–1479.

Brixey, J. J., Robinson, D. J., Tang, Z., Johnson, T. R., Zhang, J., & Turley, J. P. (2005). Interruptions in workflow for RNs in a level one trauma center. *AMIA Annual Symposium Proceedings, 2005*, 86.

Brooke, J. (1996). SUS: A 'quick and dirty' usabiliy scale. In P. W. Jordan, B. Thomas, & I. L. McClell (Eds.), *Usability evaluation in industry* (pp. 189–195). London: Taylor & Francis.

Burrows, D., & Kendall, S. (1997). Focus groups: What are they and how can they be used in nursing and health care research? *Social Sciences in Health, 3*, 244–253.

Card, S. K., Moran, T. P., & Newell, A. L. (1980). The keystroke-level model for user performance time with interactive systems. *Communications of ACM, 23*(7), 396–410.

Card, S. K., Newell, A., & Moran, T. P. (1983). *The psychology of human-computer interaction* (p. 469). Hillsdale: Lawrence Erlbaum Associates.

Caulton, D. A. (2001). Relaxing the homogeneity assumption in usability testing. *Behaviour & Information Technology, 20*, 1–7.

Chipman, S. F., Schraagen, J. M., & Shalin, V. L. (2000). Introduction to cognitive task analysis. In J. M. Schraagen, S. F. Chipman, & V. J. Shute (Eds.), *Cognitive task analysis* (pp. 3–23). Mahwah: Lawrence Erlbaum Associates.

Choi, J., & Bakken, S. (2010). Web-based education for low-literate parents in Neonatal Intensive Care Unit: Development of a website and heuristic evaluation and usability testing. *International Journal of Medical Informatics, 79*(8), 565–575.

Chung, P., Zhang, J., Johnson, T., et al. (2003). *An extended hierarchical task analysis for error prediction in medical devices*. In *Proceedings of the annual symposium of the American Medical Informatics Association 2003*.

Cooke, N. J. (1994). Varieties of knowledge elicitation techniques. *International Journal of Human-Computer Studies, 41*, 801–849.

Dalai, V. V., Khalid, S., Gottipati, D., Kannampallil, T. G., John, V., Blatter, B., Patel, V. L., & Cohen, T. I. P. (in press). Evaluating the effects of cognitive support on psychiatric clinical comprehension. *Aritificial Intelligence in Medicine, 62*(2), 91–104.

Donabedian, A. (1966). Evaluating the quality of medical care. *Milbank Memorial Fund Quarterly, 44*(2), 166–206.

Ericsson, K. A., & Simon, H. (1980). Verbal reports as data. *Psychological Review, 87*(3), 215–250.

Ericsson, K. A., & Simon, H. (1984). *Protocol analysis: Verbal reports as data.* Cambridge: MIT Press.

Farr, R. M. (1982). Interviewing: The social psychology of the inter-view. In F. Fransella (Ed.), *Psychology for occupational therapists* (pp. 151–170). London: Macmillan.

Fetterman, D. M. (1998). *Ethnography: Step by step* (2nd ed.). Thousand Oaks: Sage.

Fisher, A., & Fonteyn, M. E. (1995). An exploration of an innovative methodological approach for examining nurses' heuristic use in clinical practice. *Scholarly Inquiry for Nursing Practice, 9* (3), 263–276.

Fitts, P. M. (1954). The information capacity of the human motor system in controlling the amplitude of movement. *Journal of Experimental Psychology, 47*, 381–391.

Fonteyn, M. E., & Grobe, S. J. (1994). Expert system development in nursing: Implications for critical care nursing practice. *Heart & Lung: The Journal of Critical Care, 23*(1), 80–87.

Fonteyn, M., Kuipers, B., & Grobe, S. (1993). A description of think aloud method and protocol analysis. *Qualitative Health Research, 3*, 430–441.

Forsythe, D. E. (1999). "It's just a matter of common sense": Ethnography as invisible work. *Computer Supported Cooperative Work (CSCW), 8*(1–2), 127–145.

Fowler, L. P. (1997). Clinical reasoning strategies used during care planning. *Clinical Nursing Research, 6*(4), 349–361.

Friedman, C. P., & Wyatt, J. C. (2006). *Evaluation methods in biomedical informatics.* New York: Springer.

Funkesson, K. H., Anbäcken, E.-M., & Ek, A.-C. (2007). Nurses' reasoning process during care planning taking pressure ulcer prevention as an example. A think-aloud study. *International Journal of Nursing Studies, 44*, 1109–1119.

Gibbs, A. (1997). Focus groups. *Social Research Update, 19*, 1–7.

Grobe, S. J., Drew, J. A., & Fonteyn, M. E. (1991). A descriptive analysis of experienced nurses' clinical reasoning during a planning task. *Research in Nursing & Health, 14*(4), 305–314.

Hall, M., De Jong, M., & Steehouder, M. (2004). Cultural differences and usability evaluation: Individualistic and collectivistic participants compared. *Technical Communication, 51*(4), 489–503.

Hart, S., & Staveland, L. (1988). Development of NASA TLX (Task Load Index): Results of empirical and theoretical research. In P. Hancock & N. Meshkati (Eds.), *Human mental workload.* Amsterdam: North Holland Press.

Hermanns, H. (1991). Narratives interview. In U. Flick (Ed.), *Handbuch qualitative socialforschung* (pp. 182–185). Muenchen: Psychologie Verlags Union.

Hewing, N. J., Kaufman, D. R., Chan, R. P., & Chiang, M. F. (2013). Plus disease in retinopathy of prematurity: Qualitative analysis of diagnostic process by experts. *JAMA Ophthalmology, 131* (8), 1026–1032.

Hick, W. E. (1951). A simple stimulus generator. *Quarterly Journal of Experimental Psychology, 3*, 94–95.

Holzinger, A., Kosec, P., Schwantzer, G., Debevc, M., Hofmann-Wellenhof, R., & Frühauf, J. (2011). Design and development of a mobile computer application to reengineer workflows in the hospital and the methodology to evaluate its effectiveness. *Journal of Biomedical Informatics, 44*(6), 968–977.

Horsky, J., Gutnik, L., & Patel, V. L. (2006). Technology for emergency care: Cognitive and workflow considerations. In *American medical informatics association symposium proceedings.* Washington, DC.

Hyman, R. (1953). Stimulus information as a determinant of reaction time. *Journal of Experimental Psychology, 45*, 188–196.

Hysong, S. J., Sawhney, M. K., Wilson, L., Sittig, D. F., Espadas, D., Davis, T., & Singh, H. (2010). Provider management strategies of abnormal test result alerts: A cognitive task analysis. *Journal of the American Medical Informatics Association, 17*(1), 71–77.

IOM. (2011). *Health IT and patient safety: Building safer systems for better care.* Washington, DC: Institute of Medicine.

Johnson, C. M., Johnson, T. R., & Zhang, J. (2005). A user-centered framework for redesigning health care interfaces. *Journal of Biomedical Informatics, 38*, 75–87.

Kahn, M. J., & Prail, A. (1994). Formal usability inspections. In J. Nielson and R. L. Mack (Eds.) *Usability inspection methods* (pp. 141–171). New York: Wiley.

Kannampallil, T. G., Schauer, G. F., Cohen, T., & Patel, V. L. (2011). Considering complexity in healthcare systems. *Journal of Biomedical Informatics, 44*(6), 943–947.

Kannampallil, T. G., Franklin, A., Mishra, R., Cohen, T., Almoosa, K. F., & Patel, V. L. (2013). Understanding the nature of information seeking behavior in critical care: Implications for the design of health information technology. *Artificial Intelligence in Medicine, 57*(1), 21–29.

Kannampallil, T. G., Jones, L. K., Patel, V. L., Buchman, T. G., & Franklin, A. (2014). Comparing the information seeking strategies of residents, nurse practitioners, and physician assistants in critical care settings. *Journal of the American Medical Informatics Association, 21*, e249–e256.

Karahoca, A., Bayraktar, E., Tatoglu, E., & Karahoca, D. (2010). Information system design for a hospital emergency department: A usability analysis of software prototypes. *Journal of Biomedical Informatics, 43*(2), 224–232.

Kaufman, D. R., Patel, V. L., Hillman, C., Morin, P. C., Pevzner, J., Weinstock, R. S., Goland, R., Shea, S., & Starren, J. (2003). Usability in the real world: Assessing medical information technologies in patients' homes. *Journal of Biomedical Informatics, 36*(1), 45–60.

Kitzinger, J. (1995). Introducing focus groups. *British Medical Journal, 311*, 299–302.

Koppel, R., Metlay, J. P., Cohen, A., Abaluck, B., Localio, A. R., Kimmel, S. E., et al. (2005). Role of computerized physician order entry systems in facilitating medication errors. *JAMA, 293*(10), 1197–1203.

Krueger, R. A. (2009). *Focus groups: A practical guide for applied research.* Thousand Oaks: Sage.

Kurosu, M. (Ed.). (2014). *Human-computer interaction. Theories, methods, and tools* (pp. 469–480). Heidelberg: Springer.

Kushniruk, A. W., Kaufman, D. R., Patel, V. L., Levesque, Y., & Lottin, P. (1996). Assessment of a computerized patient record system: A cognitive approach to evaluating medical technology. *MD Computing, 13*, 406–415.

Kushniruk, A. W., Borycki, E. M., Kuwata, S., & Watanabe, H. (2008). Using a low-cost simulation for assessing the impact of a medication administration system on workflow. In *Studies in health technology and informatics* (pp. 567–572).

Lewis, J. R. (1991). Psychometric evaluation of an after-scenario questionnaire for computer usability studies: The ASQ. *ACM SIGCHI Bulletin, 23*(1), 78–81.

Lewis, A. (1992). Group child interviews as a research tool. *British Educational Research Journal, 18*, 413–421.

Lewis, J. R. (1994). Sample sizes for usability studies: Additional considerations. *Human Factors, 36*, 369–378.

Linder, J. A., Ma, J., Bates, D. W., Middleton, B., & Stafford, R. S. (2007). Electronic health record use and the quality of ambulatory care in the United States. *Archives of Internal Medicine, 167*(13), 1400–1405.

Lundgrén-Laine, H., & Salanterä, S. (2010). Think-aloud technique and protocol analysis in clinical decision-making research. *Qualitative Health Research, 20*(4), 565–575.

MacKenzie, I. S., Zhang, S. X., & Soukoreff, R. W. (1999). Text entry using soft keyboards. *Behaviour and Information Technology, 18*, 235–244.

Malhotra, S., Jordan, D., Shortliffe, E., & Patel, V. L. (2007). Workflow modeling in critical care: Piecing together your own puzzle. *Journal of Biomedical Informatics, 40*(2), 81–92.

Mamykina, L., Vawdrey, D., Stetson, P., Zheng, K., & Hripcsak, G. (2012). Clinical documenta-
   tion: Composition or synthesis? *Journal of the American Medical Informatics Association, 19*
   (6), 1025–1103.
Mason, J. (2002). *Qualitative researching*. London: Sage.
McDonald, C. J., Callaghan, F. M., Weissman, A., Goodwin, R. M., Mundkur, M., & Kuhn,
   T. (2014). Use of internist's free time by ambulatory care electronic medical record systems.
   JAMA Internal Medicine, 174(11), 1860–1863.
Miller, R. H., & Sim, I. (2004). Physicians' use of electronic medical records: Barriers and
   solutions. *Health Affairs (Millwood), 23*(2), 116–126.
Nielsen, J. (1994). Usability inspection methods. In *Conference companion on human factors in
   computing systems* (pp. 413–414). Boston: ACM.
Nielsen, J., & Molich, R. (1990). Heuristic evaluation of user interfaces. In *Proceedings of the
   SIGCHI conference on human factors in computing systems* (pp. 249–256). Seattle/Wa-
   shington, DC: ACM.
Olson, G. M., & Olson, J. S. (2003). Human-computer interaction: Psychological aspects of the
   human use of computing. *Annual Review of Psychology, 54*(1), 491–516.
Overhage, J., Perkins, S., Tierney, W., & McDonald, C. (2001). Controlled trial of direct physician
   order entry: Effects on physicians' time utilization in ambulatory primary care internal
   medicine practices. *Journal of the American Medical Informatics Association, 8*(4), 361–371.
Patel, V. L., & Groen, G. J. (1991a). The general and specific nature of medical expertise: A
   critical look. In K. A. E. J. Smith (Ed.), *Toward a general theory of expertise: Prospects and
   limits* (pp. 93–125). New York: Cambridge University Press.
Patel, V. L., & Groen, G. J. (1991b). Developmental accounts of the transition from medical
   student to doctor: Some problems and suggestions. *Medical Education, 25*(6), 527–535.
Patel, V. L., & Kannampallil, T. G. (2011). Cognitive approaches to clinical data management for
   decision support: Is it old wine in new bottle? In A. Holzinger & K.-M. Simonic (Eds.),
   Information quality in e-health (pp. 1–13). Berlin/Heidelberg: Springer.
Patel, V. L., Arocha, J. F., & Kaufman, D. R. (1994). Diagnostic reasoning and medical expertise.
   In L. M. Douglas (Ed.), *Psychology of learning and motivation* (pp. 187–252). San Diego:
   Academic.
Patel, V. L., Arocha, J. F., & Kaufman, D. R. (2001). A primer on aspects of cognition for medical
   informatics. *Journal of the American Medical Informatics Association, 8*(4), 324–343.
Patel, V. L., Kaufman, D. R., & Kannampallil, T. (2013). Diagnostic reasoning and decision
   making in the context of health information technology. *Reviews of Human Factors and
   Ergonomics, 8*, 149–190.
Patel, V. L., Kaufman, D. R., & Cohen, T. (2014). *Cognitive informatics in health and biomed-
   icine*. London: Springer.
Patterson, E. S., Nguyen, A. D., Halloran, J. P., & Asch, S. M. (2004). Human factors barriers to
   the effective use of ten HIV clinical reminders. *Journal of the American Medical Informatics
   Association, 11*(1), 50–59.
Paul, S. A., Reddy, M., Abraham, J., & DeFlitch, C. (2008). The usefulness of information and
   communication technologies in crisis response. In *AMIA annual symposium proceedings*.
   American Medical Informatics Association.
Pizziferri, L., Kittler, A., Volk, L., Honour, M., Gupta, S., & Wang, S. (2005). Primary care
   physician time utilization before and after implementation of an electronic health record: A
   time-motion study. *Journal of Biomedical Informatics, 38*(3), 176–188.
Polson, P. G., Lewis, C., Rieman, J., & Wharton, C. (1992). Cognitive walkthroughs: A method for
   theory-based evaluation of user interfaces. *International Journal of Man-Machine Studies, 36*
   (5), 741–773.
Preece, J., Rogers, Y., Sharp, H., Benyon, D., Holland, S., & Carey, T. (1994). *Human-computer
   interaction*. Essex: Addison-Wesley Longman Ltd.
Reddy, M. C., Paul, S. A., Abraham, J., McNeese, M., DeFlitch, C., & Yen, J. (2009). Challenges
   to effective crisis management: Using information and communication technologies to

coordinate emergency medical services and emergency department teams. *International Journal of Medical Informatics, 78*(4), 259–269.

Rosson, M. B., & Carroll, J. M. (2009). *Usability engineering: Scenario-based development of human-computer interaction.* Morgan Kaufman: Redwood City, CA.

Saitwal, H., Feng, X., Walji, M., et al. (2010). Assessing performance of an electronic health record (EHR) using cognitive task analysis. *International Journal of Medical Informatics, 79* (7), 501–506.

Schatzberg, M. (2008). Seeing the invisible, hearing silence, thinking the unthinkable: The advantages of ethnographic immersion. In *APSA 2008 annual meeting.* Boston: Hynes Convention Center.

Simmons, B., Lanuza, D., Fonteyn, M., Hicks, F., & Holm, K. (2003). Clinical reasoning in experienced nurses. *Western Journal of Nursing Research, 25*, 720–724.

Sittig, D. F., & Classen, D. C. (2010). Safe electronic health record use requires a comprehensive monitoring and evaluation framework. *JAMA, 303*(5), 450–451.

Stetler, C. B., Legro, M. W., Wallace, C. M., Bowman, C., Guihan, M., Hagedorn, H., . . ., Smith, J. L. (2006). The role of formative evaluation in implementation research and the QUERI experience. *Journal of General Internal Medicine, 21*(S2), S1–S8.

Unertl, K. M., Weinger, M. B., Johnson, K. B., & Lorenzi, N. (2009). Describing and modeling workflow and information flow in chronic disease care. *Journal of the American Medical Informatics Association, 16*(6), 826–836.

Unertl, K., Johnson, K., Gadd, C., & Lorenzi, N. (2013). Bridging organizational divides in health care: An ecological view of health information exchange. *JMIR Medical Informatics, 1*(2), e3.

Vaughn, S., Schumm, J. S., & Sinagub, J. (1996). *Focus group interviews in education and psychology.* Thousand Oaks: Sage.

Vicente, K. J. (1999). *Cognitive work analysis.* Mahwah: Lawrence Erlbaum Associates.

Zhang, J., & Walji, M. F. (2011). TURF: Toward a unified framework of EHR usability. *Journal of Biomedical Informatics, 44*(6), 1056–1067.

Zhang, J., Johnson, T. R., Patel, V. L., Paige, D. L., & Kubose, T. (2003). Using usability heuristics to evaluate patient safety of medical devices. *Journal of Biomedical Informatics, 36*(1), 23–30.

Zheng, K., Haftel, H. M., Hirschl, R. B., O'Reilly, M., & Hanauer, D. A. (2010). Quantifying the impact of health IT implementations on clinical workflow: A new methodological perspective. *Journal of the American Medical Informatics Association, 17*(4), 454–461.

Zheng, K., Guo, M. H., & Hanauer, D. A. (2011). Using the time and motion method to study clinical work processes and workflow: Methodological inconsistencies and a call for standardized research. *Journal of the American Medical Informatics Association, 18*(5), 704–710.

Chapter 6
Computational Ethnography: Automated and Unobtrusive Means for Collecting Data *In Situ* for Human–Computer Interaction Evaluation Studies

Kai Zheng, David A. Hanauer, Nadir Weibel, and Zia Agha

6.1 Introduction

Health information technology (HIT) holds great promise to cross the quality chasm of the US healthcare system and to bend the curve of ever-rising costs. However, many successfully deployed HIT systems have failed to generate anticipated benefits; (Bloomrosen et al. 2011) some are even associated with unintended adverse consequences (Kellermann and Jones 2013). It has been extensively documented that the lack of usability is one of the key factors accounting for the suboptimal outcomes of implementing the current generation of HIT systems (Bloomrosen et al. 2011). Human–computer interaction (HCI) evaluation studies, which help designers and researchers assess the effectiveness of competing designs

K. Zheng, Ph.D. (✉)
Department of Health Management and Policy, School of Public Health,
University of Michigan, Ann Arbor, MI, USA

School of Information, University of Michigan, Ann Arbor, MI, USA
e-mail: kzheng@umich.edu

D.A. Hanauer, M.D., M.S.
Department of Pediatrics, University of Michigan Medical School, Ann Arbor, MI, USA

School of Information, University of Michigan, Ann Arbor, MI, USA

N. Weibel, Ph.D.
Department of Computer Science and Engineering, Jacobs School of Engineering,
University of California, San Diego, La Jolla, CA, USA

Veteran Affairs Medical Research Foundation, HSRD VA San Diego Healthcare System,
San Diego, CA, USA

Z. Agha, M.D.
Department of Medicine, School of Medicine, University of California,
San Diego, La Jolla, CA, USA

West Health Institute, La Jolla, CA, USA

© Springer International Publishing Switzerland 2015
V.L. Patel et al. (eds.), *Cognitive Informatics for Biomedicine*, Health Informatics,
DOI 10.1007/978-3-319-17272-9_6

and identify potential usability pitfalls, are therefore of vital importance. HCI evaluation studies in healthcare have been traditionally conducted in the following four forms: (1) expert inspection (e.g., heuristic evaluation), (2) usability experiments carried out in laboratory settings, (3) field studies (e.g., ethnographical observation and contextual inquiries), and (4) perception solicitation through questionnaire surveys, interviews, or focus groups.

In *expert inspection*, evaluators—usually usability experts—execute scripted tasks through the target software system or device and determine its conformity to established principles of usability (the "heuristics"). This method is useful when widely recognized usability standards exist or when the goal of the evaluation is very specific, e.g., to improve the accessibility of the software or to eliminate potential patient safety hazards. *Usability experiments* are often used in formative evaluation to comparatively assess multiple design alternatives, or in summative evaluation to correct usability pitfalls before shipping the system/device to the hands of end users. Data collected through usability experiments can be both quantitative (e.g., time for task completion, number of keystrokes and mouse clicks required, and error rates) and qualitative (e.g., participant verbalization expressing their cognitive processes or commenting about the usability issues they encounter). Some usability experiments employ randomized controlled design to maximize the objectivity and generalizability of study results.

Both expert inspection and usability experiments are typically conducted in controlled environments wherein evaluators or test users perform predefined simulation tasks in a manipulated environment void of distractions. These tasks are carefully curated to best represent prospective end users' work, but they are by no means exhaustive. Further, simulation tasks often focus heavily on the user interface (UI) and are designed to assess an individual user working with a computer terminal in silos stripped of the context of a dynamic work setting involving multiple co-workers. As such, these approaches are widely criticized for their lack of consideration of complex task-dependencies in clinical work and the somewhat chaotic nature of clinical work environments ample of interruptions and communication failures.

Field studies conducted to collect *in situ* data describing how end users incorporate the system/device in their everyday job routines have thus become popular in recent years. These studies often involve shadowing clinicians in a medical facility to observe their individual work as well as their interactions with patients and other care providers. They draw upon principles from a variety of scientific fields such as computer-supported cooperative work (CSCW), distributed cognition, and social computing. For non-observable perceptional measures, such as satisfaction, stress, and perceived efficiency gains (and losses), questionnaire surveys and other direct *perception solicitation* methods are widely used (please refer to Chap. 5 in this volume for a detailed review).

While these traditional HCI approaches have great merit and are indispensable in studying and improving usability of software systems and medical devices in healthcare, they have several major limitations in common. First, recruiting research subjects or usability experts is an arduous task, as study participation requires significant time commitments. Second, the sample size of such studies (or size of the expert panel) is often small, constraining the generalization power of their research findings. Third, test users in a controlled environment, or subjects being shadowed by HCI researchers, may exhibit distinctive behaviors deviating from their normal work practice (i.e., the Hawthorne effect). Similarly, self-reported data collected via direct perception solicitation are susceptible to common cognitive biases and recall errors. For example, due to social desirability bias, informants may tend to answer questions in a manner that would be favorably received by others (e.g., to avoid being viewed as lacking competence in adapting to new technologies); or they may assess individual usability items based on their overall impression of the intervention, i.e., the Halo effect. Lastly, existing HCI methods usually produce discrete data representing only a very small fraction of user behaviors of interest, whereas computational ethnographical approaches are able to capture data continuously and at very low costs. For a review of common measurement issues associated with self-reported data, see Gonyea (2005).

In this chapter, we introduce *computational ethnography*, an emerging family of methods for conducting HCI studies in healthcare, which usually leverages automated and less obtrusive (or unobtrusive) means for collecting *in situ* data reflective of real end users' actual, unaltered behaviors using a software system or a device in real-world settings. These methods are based on the premise that user interactions with modern technologies always leave "digital traces" behind that can be utilized by HCI experts to fully or partially re-enact the activities. Typical examples of such digital traces include browsing history of webpages, keywords typed into a search engine, audit trails recording document access activities in electronic health records, and paging/phone logs stored in telecommunication systems.

In the next section, we will introduce the definition of computational ethnography, common types of digital trace data that are either being routinely collected in a healthcare environment or can be proactively collected by HCI experts, and commonly used analytical approaches for making sense of such data. We will conclude the chapter with two use cases illustrating how this new family of methods has been applied in healthcare to study end users' interactions with technological interventions in their everyday routines.

6.2 Computational Ethnography

6.2.1 Definition

The term *ethnography* originates from Greek ἔθνος ethnos ("folk, people, nation") and γράφω grapho ("I write"). It describes a method initially used by social science researchers, cultural anthropologists in particular, to closely examine the meaning in the lives of a cultural group. Researchers conducting ethnographical studies, or *ethnographers*, strive to develop 'thick' descriptions of everyday life and practice through a long-term engagement with the people they study and in the setting where their everyday lives take place. Participant observations and non-participant observations constitute the primary source of ethnographical data, which are often supplemented by other means of data collection such as artifact analysis and formal or informal interviews. Participant and non-participant observations differ on the degree to which researchers become active participants in the lives of the setting, or instead maintain a distance as 'detached' observers.

Ethnographical work by HCI researchers in healthcare produces vivid and nuanced accounts of how different players—clinicians, clerical staff, administrators, patients, and families—engage with technologies both during the early adoption and adaptation phases (the so called "burn-in period") as well as after the system or device has been used on a routine basis. Such work often pays extraordinary attention to the longitudinal and distributed nature of care processes and the complex interplay between people, technology, and the organization. Thus, ethnographical research accounts contain very subtle cultural and social contexts in a healthcare organization (or in a patient community) where technological systems are situated and what their designs ought to be rooted in. Many of the studies conducted in the field of CSCW are of this nature. For a review of these studies, see Fitzpatrick and Ellingsen (2013).

However, the limitations of ethnography are also widely acknowledged. Ethnographical fieldwork is extremely time consuming to conduct, sometimes taking many months, or even years, to complete. The lack of objectivity has always been and continues to be viewed as a threat to the legitimacy of ethnographical studies because generating an interpretive account of the lives of a study setting is inevitably influenced by ethnographers' own personal and professional experiences. This issue is particularly prominent in health sciences where controlled trials producing unambiguous and conclusive results are often deemed as the *de facto* standard of high-quality research. In addition, because of the complexity of medical work, it is often difficult for observers not trained in medicine, or in a particular medical specialty, to be able to understand what they are observing. Further, in modern healthcare organizations, a significant amount of work has become largely invisible or very difficult to observe by ethnographers. Interpersonal communications among healthcare workers for example are increasingly mediated by technologies (e.g., via pager messages or electronic notifications built into an order entry system), and a considerable proportion of clinical work (e.g., documentation) can be now done remotely or even after work.

Nonetheless, the widespread use of information systems and computer-mediated communication technologies in today's highly wired healthcare environments also creates an unprecedented opportunity for collecting ethnographical data through automated and electronic means. In fact, healthcare, perhaps more than any other industry, bears regulatory mandates (e.g., HIPAA[1] and Medicare Conditions of

[1] HIPAA, or the Health Insurance Portability and Accountability Act, defines policies, procedures, and guidelines for maintaining the privacy and security of protected health information as well as outlining offenses and sets civil and criminal penalties for violations.

Participation[2] in the US) that require them to truthfully record anything done to the patient, any communications surrounding the care for the patient, and any access to and modifications of the patient's medical records. Failing to do so is associated with significant financial and legal consequences. As a result, digital traces abound in healthcare organizations, providing an excellent source of data for ethnographers to retroactively reconstruct patient care activities at a fine level of granularity.

Combining the 'thickness' of ethnographical methods with the strength of automated computational approaches is thus a natural next step for HCI researchers. This new way of collecting behavioral and social data not only forms the basis of the computational ethnography methodology described this chapter, but also the emerging field of "computational social science" at large (Lazer et al. 2009; Giles 2012). In the context of this chapter, we define computational ethnography as "a family of computational methods that leverages computer or sensor-based technologies to unobtrusively or nearly unobtrusively record end users' routine, *in situ* activities in health or healthcare related domains for studies of interest to human–computer interaction." Because computational ethnography is based on data automatically captured through technological means, it by nature provides higher objectivity, less intrusion, more inclusiveness (i.e., into spaces and time where/when direct observation by human observers is not possible), and better scalability for data collection, aggregation, and analysis. Note that while recording user interactions with a computer system such as keystrokes (Card et al. 1980) and analyzing the behavioral data thus obtained (Ritter and Larkin 1994) have been a widely used study approach in HCI, unless their data are collected in users' everyday settings via unobtrusive or nearly unobtrusively means (i.e., as opposite to a controlled laboratory environment), such studies do not meet the definition of computational ethnography. Similarly, quantitative observational studies involving independent human observers (e.g., in a time and motion observation) to collect interaction or behavioral data also do not meet the definition of computational ethnography.

6.2.2 Common Sources of Computational Ethnographical Data

As mentioned earlier, in a modern healthcare organization, clinician, staff, and patient activities always leave behind abundant digital traces that can be leveraged to study interesting HCI problems. Such data are already being routinely collected or can be proactively collected by deploying specific tracking devices. In this section, we introduce five sources of computational ethnographical data that have been commonly used in HCI evaluation studies in healthcare.

---

[2] § 482.24 Condition of Participation: Medical Record Services. http://www.gpo.gov/fdsys/granule/CFR-2011-title42-vol5/CFR-2011-title42-vol5-sec482-24/content-detail.html

6.2.2.1 Computer Logs

Most modern computer systems are capable of generating log files for purposes such as helping engineers monitor a system's performance or helping administrators gauge the usage of newly deployed software. In the US, there is a federal mandate by both HIPAA and the HITECH Act[3] demanding all HIT systems have the security auditing capability. For example, the HIT Certification Program overseen by the Office of the National Coordinator for Health Information Technology (ONC)[4] requires that all electronic health records (EHR) systems certified through the program to implement security audit logs (commonly referred to as audit trails). The certification criteria contain detailed specifications on (*1*) what constitutes auditable events (e.g., creation, modification, deletion, or printing of electronic health information); (*2*) metadata that must be recorded for each auditable event (e.g., date, time, patient identification, and user identification); and (*3*) tamper-resistance measures in place to ensure the auditing function is enabled by default and audit trails are immutable. Having an EHR system equipped with these security-auditing features is a prerequisite to meeting the meaningful use criterion in order to "protect electronic health information created or maintained by the certified EHR technology through the implementation of appropriate technical capabilities" (Eligible professional meaningful use core measures). The certification criteria further recommend all EHR systems adopt an American Society for Testing and Materials (ASTM) International standard, ASTM E2147-01,[5] as the format to record and store audit trail data. This means that in the not too distant future audit trial logs generated by different HIT vendor systems at different institutions could be easily merged and jointly analyzed.

Table 6.1 exhibits a sample security audit log. As illustrated in the sample, security log entries contain rich information describing medical work. These log entries not only reveal the occurrence of a clinical event (when, by whom, related to which patient), but also what the event was about (e.g., chart access vs. placing orders) as well as the identifier of the medical record describing the event allowing for further drill-down analyses. In addition, audit trails contain the IP address of the device from which the data access/writing request originated and potentially also

---

[3] The Health Information Technology for Economic and Clinical Health Act, or the HITECH Act, sets meaningful use of EHRs as a critical national goal and allocates incentive funds to accelerate their adoption. The HITECH Act contains specific privacy and security requirements, mainly through software certification, to ensure adequate protection of protected health information stored in EHRs.

[4] The Office of the National Coordinator for Health Information Technology (ONC) is the principal federal entity responsible for coordinating nationwide efforts to support the adoption of HIT and the promotion of nationwide health information exchange. It was created in 2004 and is organizationally located within the Office of the Secretary for the U.S. Department of Health and Human Services. http://www.healthit.gov

[5] ASTM E2147-01: Standard Specification for Audit and Disclosure Logs for Use in Health Information Systems. http://www.astm.org/Standards/E2147.htm

Table 6.1 A sample security audit log

TIMESTAMP	EVENT_NAME	EVENT_TYPE	TASK	PARTICIPANT_ID
09/01/2013 07:21:21 UTC	Logon Attempt	Security		0
09/01/2013 07:21:22 UTC	Inbox	View List		0
09/01/2013 07:21:45 UTC	Query List	Patient	QUERY Read Patient List	0
09/01/2013 07:21:48 UTC	Maintain Reference Data	Organization Groups	Tasks that contain only requests that read or query	0
09/01/2013 07:21:48 UTC	View Encounter	Open Chart	patient context	4070370
09/01/2013 07:21:50 UTC	Problems	Read	OUTPUT Prompt Programs	4070370
09/01/2013 07:21:51 UTC	Query Clinical Events	Results		4070370
09/01/2013 07:21:51 UTC	Clinical Diagnoses	Read	OUTPUT Prompt Programs	4070370
09/01/2013 07:22:36 UTC	Maintain Person	Chart Access Log	RUN Preferences	4070370
09/01/2013 07:22:36 UTC	Flowsheet	View		4070370
09/01/2013 07:22:36 UTC	Maintain Person	Chart Access Log	RUN Preferences	4070370
09/01/2013 07:22:36 UTC	Query Clinical Events	Results	QUERY - Clinical Event Query	4070370
09/01/2013 07:23:02 UTC	Maintain Person	Chart Access Log	RUN Preferences	4070370
09/01/2013 07:23:02 UTC	Flowsheet	View		4070370
09/01/2013 07:23:19 UTC	Maintain Person	Chart Access Log	RUN Preferences	4070370
09/01/2013 07:23:29 UTC	Maintain Clinical Document	Attempt to View Document		4070370
09/01/2013 07:23:47 UTC	Maintain Clinical Document	Attempt to View Document		7485199
09/01/2013 07:24:53 UTC	Maintain Person	Chart Access Log	RUN Preferences	4070370
09/01/2013 07:24:54 UTC	UPDATE Orders	Order	10 mg = 1 tab(s), PO, qDay, # 30 tab(s), Refill(s) 0	4070370
09/01/2013 09:00:58 UTC		Order	5 mg = 1 tab(s), PO, qDay, # 30 tab(s), Refill(s) 11	4070370
09/01/2013 09:00:59 UTC	Genview	View	IRUN Patient List Management	4070370
09/01/2013 09:37:40 UTC	Logout Attempt	Security		0

geocoding data supplied by mobile devices. Such information can be combined with timestamps to reconstruct the spatiotemporal distribution of clinical work in a medical facility. Audit trail logs thus provide rich sources of data for HCI experts to conduct workflow and temporal rhythm studies, studies on distributed cognition and social information processing, and studies on information and patient handoffs. For example, Hripcsak et al. (2011) used audit logs captured in an EHR system to characterize the amount of time clinicians spent authoring clinical notes and the proportion of such notes that was viewed by others (Hripcsak et al. 2011). For a review of HCI studies conducted in both healthcare and non-healthcare contexts using computer log data, see Hilbert and Redmiles (2000) and Dumais et al. (2014).

A significant limitation of using security audit logs in HCI research is that some transitory screen activities (e.g. user moving a window around to reduce the amount of visual clutter on the screen) are not logged which nevertheless could be of considerable interest to HCI experts. Further, timestamps recorded in a security audit log file only indicate when a clinical action occurred. This information is not adequate to answer important usability questions such as how long it took the user to perform the action (e.g., to fill out a medication ordering form), or if the user chose the optimal options when using the system (since the original clinical context may also be unknown). Additional tools are therefore needed for HCI experts to acquire supplemental data on screen activities, described in the next section.

6.2.2.2 Screen Activities

Screen activities, such as mouse cursor trails, mouse clicks/drags, keystrokes, and window activation and window movements, have been popularly used in HCI research to study user interactions with a software system to detect potential usability pitfalls. Screen activities reveal rich details of user behaviors that may not be otherwise available, e.g., user clicking a "+" sign to expand a tree view to see a full list of medications, or clicking the "Close" button to skip a popup window presenting a computer-generated clinical decision-support reminder. This additional level of detail is very important for HCI research in healthcare because many commercial HIT systems may not log user actions that do not involve direct accesses of or modifications to patient charts.

Screen activities may be recorded as a sequence of screen snapshots or as a video stream. Figure 6.1 illustrates a sample frame from a video clip capturing a user session took place in an outpatient exam room. When a front-mounted camera is available, additional contextual video/audio data (shown in the bottom right window) may also be recorded along with screen activities providing an opportunity for HCI experts to study the clinician's (as well as the patient's) facial expressions, body gestures, and conversations between the clinician and the patient.

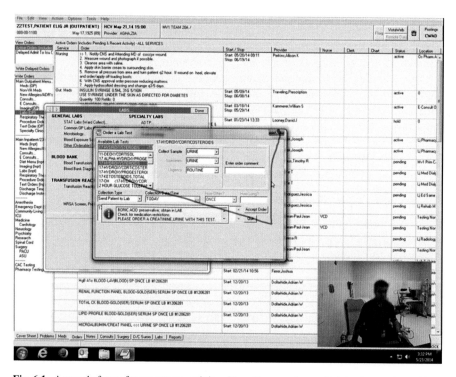

Fig. 6.1 A sample frame from a screen activity video clip recording a clinician interacting with an EHR system. The superimposed *dark grey* path shows the trail of the mouse cursor over the 1 s prior to the capture of this frame

Table 6.2 A sample screen activity log

ELAPSED_TIME	EVENT	DETAIL	APPLICATION_OWNER	WINDOW_TITLE	EXTRA
00:13.3	Keystrokes	D (Shift)			
00:13.5	Keystrokes	y			
00:13.6	Keystrokes	Backspace			
00:20.4	Mouse Clicks	L Button Down			
00:20.5	Mouse Clicks	R Button Down			
00:20.8	Window/Dialog Events	Focus	Context	Cut	Ctrl+X
00:21.9	Mouse Clicks	L Button Down		Reminders	
00:34.8	Window/Dialog Events	Focus		HTN Lifestyle Education	
00:35.5	Window/Dialog Events	Move	Reminder Resolution: HTN Lifestyle Education	Reminder Resolution: HTN Lifestyle Education	
00:36.4	Mouse Clicks	L Button Down	Reminder Resolution: HTN Lifestyle Education	Finish	
00:36.6	Window/Dialog Events	Focus	Sign Note		
00:36.6	Mouse Clicks	L Button Down	Sign Note	OK	
00:36.7	Window/Dialog Events	Focus	Order Menu		
00:36.9	Mouse Clicks	Wheel (-)			

Screen activities may also be recorded as log data containing a chronological list of user interaction events that can be computationally analyzed. Screen footage and contextual videos, on the other hand, are much harder to analyze which often requires prolonged and laborious manual coding processes. As illustrated in a sample screen activity log shown in Table 6.2, a variety of usability metrics can be readily derived from the structured log data including time efficiency (how much time it takes to complete a given task), operation efficiency (how many mouse clicks or keystrokes it requires to complete a given task), and error rates (e.g., frequency of user clicking a wrong button or the ratio of unnecessary mouse/keyboard activities that did not contribute to the accomplishment of a given task). For example, Magrabi et al. (2010) used screen activities to examine how task complexity and interruption affect clinician performance in terms of error rates, resumption lag, and task completion time in creating and updating electronic medication charts (Magrabi et al. 2010). Screen activity logs, especially when combined with other sources of data (e.g., security auditing logs), can also reveal other interaction behaviors of high interest to HCI researchers such as how clinicians copy/paste text from various sources in a an EHR system to construct a narrative note.

Many software tools are available for capturing and analyzing computer screen activities. Morae (TechSmith Corporation, Okemos, MI), for example, is a commercial product widely used in usability studies and market research that allows for observing, recording, and analyzing user interactions with software systems such as websites.[6] Both the video footage shown in Fig. 6.1 and the screen activity log shown in Table 6.2 were generated using Morae. In healthcare, screen activity capturing tools have been developed specifically to work with HIT systems such as

---

[6] http://www.techsmith.com/morae.html

EHRs. Turf (an acronym for "Task, User, Representation, Function"), for example, is an EHR usability assessment tool developed at the National Center for Cognitive Informatics and Decision Making funded by the ONC's Strategic HIT Advanced Research initiative.[7] Turf is an integrated toolkit that allows for screen capturing, UI markups, and heuristic evaluation (e.g., experts can use the system to indicate potential usability issues on a screen and label them as minor, moderate, major or catastrophic). The evaluation criteria incorporated in Turf are based on the National Institute of Standards and Technology's (NIST) EHR usability evaluation protocol, NISTIR 7804.[8]

6.2.2.3 Eye Tracking

Screen activity data capture how users interact with a software system using mouse and keyboard. However, user activities that do not trigger a traceable screen event are not captured. These activities may include, for example, a clinician reading from an EHR system to digest a patient's earlier discharge summary before meeting the patient in an exam room, or examining the content of a computer-generated drug safety alert before acting upon it. Head and eye movements captured through eye-tracking devices can thus become an important source of data enabling HCI experts to study interesting topics such as how clinicians seek information and make sense of a patient case out of a large volume of patient records and whether there is a tendency among clinicians to skip computer-generated advisories without carefully reading them.

An eye-tracking device measures a person's head position (gaze) and eye movements relative to the head that reveal the person's visual and overt attention processes. Modern eye-tracking technologies are often based on optical sensors that capture the vector between the pupil center and the corneal reflections created by casting a beam of infrared or near-infrared non-collimated light on the eye. In HCI, the eye-tracking technique has been commonly used in assessing the usability of websites e.g. to study which portion(s) of the screen that web surfers' attention tends to focus on more often so as to optimize the placement of online advertisements (Poole and Ball 2005). It has also been used in healthcare particularly in the areas of autism research (Falck-Ytter et al. 2013), anxiety and depression (Armstrong and Olatunji 2012), and training and assessing the skills of surgeons (Tien et al. 2014).

Figure 6.2 shows an eye-tracking device mounted below a computer monitor in an outpatient exam room. This configuration is not intrusive and can detect both head and eye movements, and is thus more practical to use in everyday healthcare settings. Eye-tracking data obtained through the device can be synchronized with

---

[7] https://turf.shis.uth.tmc.edu/turfweb/

[8] NISTIR 7804: Technical Evaluation, Testing and Validation of the Usability of Electronic Health Records. http://www.nist.gov/manuscript-publication-search.cfm?pub_id=909701

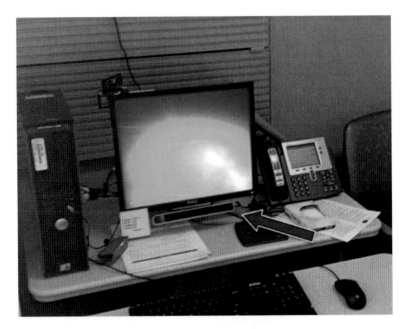

Fig. 6.2 A table-mounted eye tracker in an outpatient exam room

screen activity recordings to reveal which part of the computer screen the user was looking at moment-by-moment during a use session. The end result can be plotted as heat-maps showing hotspots on an application's UI or eye trails traversing different parts of the screen, as illustrated in Fig. 6.3a, b, respectively. In addition, the eye-tracking data provide hints as to when the user gazes away from the computer to attend to other stimuli in the room, e.g., the patient. This allows HCI experts to study how the presence of computers in an exam room might interfere with patient–provider communications. Many manufactures produce eye-tracking devices and analytical software are produced. Leading vendors include Tobii Technology[9] and SensoMotoric Instruments (SMI).[10]

6.2.2.4 Motion Capture

A considerable body of the HCI literature in healthcare concerns how introduction of computerized systems changes the dynamics of patient–clinician interactions in an exam room. It has been extensively documented that computer use during clinical consultations could be associated with adverse impact such as diminished quality of patient–clinician communications and elevated levels of patient disengagement and dissatisfaction. Some frequently reported reasons include loss of eye

---

[9] http://www.tobii.com/

[10] http://www.smivision.com/

a

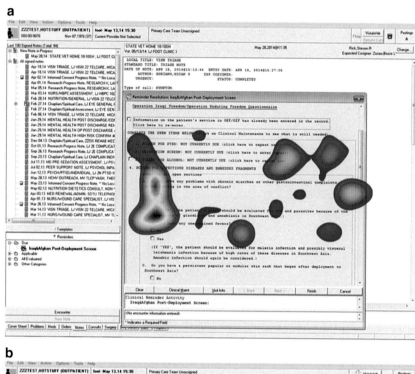

b

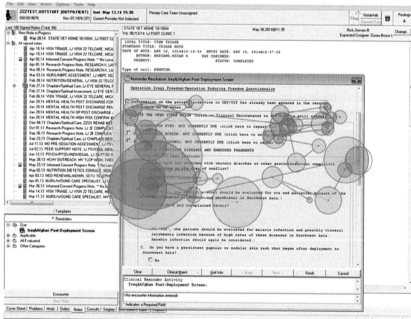

Fig. 6.3 Heat-map and eye trails produced by eye-tracking data

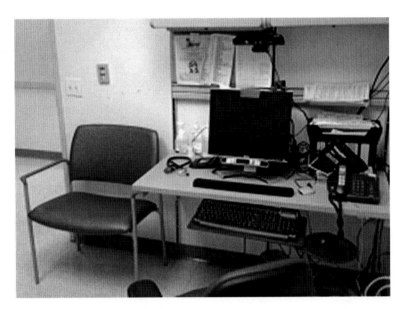

Fig. 6.4 Microsoft Kinect™ installed in an outpatient exam room and monitoring a physician's movements

contact, rapport, and provision of emotional support; interference with conversations due to the clinician gazing back-and-forth at the computer screen; reduced emphasis on psychosocial questioning and relationship maintenance; and irrelevant computer-prompted inquiries diluting the focus on the patient's current issues. For a review of these potential issues, see Kazmi (2013).

Besides the methods for capturing computer activities and eye movements, HCI experts in healthcare are also experimenting with novel sensor-based technologies that allow for automated collection and analysis of additional dimensions of patient–clinician interaction data such as vocalization, body orientation, and body gestures. Microsoft Kinect™,[11] for example, is an affordable yet effective solution that includes an infrared depth sensor for tracking depth data (i.e., participants' distance and angle relative to the position of the camera), body movements (kinetics through motion of body joints e.g. head, should center, shoulder left/right, elbow left/right, wrist left/right, hand left/right, etc.), and head orientation (e.g., pitch, roll, yaw). It also has a built-in microphone array that detects the angle of multiple audio sources which makes it possible to perform automated segmentation of voice data to identify vocalization sequences, clinician's visual attention (EHR vs. patient), as well as characterize turn-talking behaviors in terms of whether the clinician or the patient was talking. Such data can thus enable HCI experts to answer daunting questions e.g. the body language that clinicians use when interacting with patients while simultaneously using computerized systems such as EHRs. Figure 6.4 shows a Kinect mounted above and behind a computer monitor in an outpatient exam

---

[11] http://kinectforwindows.org

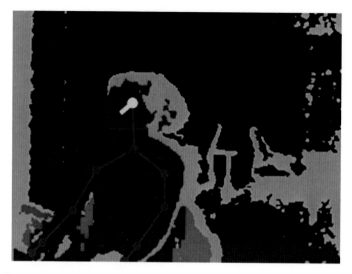

Fig. 6.5 Skeletal and depth data recorded by Kinect. The *red* overlay indicates that a body has been recognized; the *purple dots* indicate body joints connected through *purple lines*; the *yellow line* indicates the gaze vector as inferred from pitch yaw and roll

room. Figure 6.5 illustrates a sample frame from a depth and skeleton image sequence recorded by Kinect's depth camera.

A distinctive advantage of using sensor-based technologies such as Kinect is that the data collected can be programmatically analyzed eliminating the need to have human coders to manually review hours of video/audio data. Microsoft provides a non-commercial Kinect Software Development Kit (SDK) freely available to HCI experts to develop customized analytical programs to perform post-processing tasks such as background removal, gesture recognition, facial recognition, and voice recognition.[12]

For example, the depth, skeletal, and voice direction data are all recorded as digitized coordinates which can be easily computed to determine the relative positions of the participants in the room (typically a clinician and a patient if it is an outpatient primary care exam room) at each given time during a clinical encounter. This allows HCI experts to automatically segment the progression of a clinical consultation into distinct stages e.g. greetings, physical exam, conversing in seated positions, and patient and/or clinician leaving the room. Nonverbal communications such as head orientation and body gestures can also be automatically recognized and studied, and can be further synchronized with eye-tracking data to precisely profile the clinician's gazing behavior when using the EHR to enter or retrieve information while talking to the patient. Large-scale deep analyses of patient–clinician interactions are thus possible at reasonably costs without involving laborious manual coding processes. For a more in-depth discussion on how to

---

[12] http://www.microsoft.com/en-us/kinectforwindowsdev/

use sensor-based technologies to study the dynamics of patient–clinician interactions in exam rooms and potential practical obstacles, see Weibel et al. (2015).

6.2.2.5 Real-Time Locating Systems (RTLS)

Clinicians as well as patients move around constantly in a medical facility to provide/receive care and to interact with other stakeholders (e.g., families, specialists, pharmacists). While the other computational ethnographical methods described in this section help HCI experts examine the interactions between clinicians, patients, and computerized systems, they do not allow for comprehensive collection of motion-location data that may lead into novel insights. For example, with motion-location data, HCI researchers are in a better position to answer questions such as whether the physical layout of an outpatient clinic or an inpatient ward is optimally designed to facilitate patient care delivery, and whether the introduction of HIT systems might result in a reduction of face time among healthcare coworkers. Sensor-based RTLS systems, most commonly based on the radio-frequency identification (RFID) technology,[13] provide a solution to capturing such motion-location data. RFID has a long history of being used in healthcare for supply chain management purposes (e.g., asset tracking of medical devices) and patient safety purposes (e.g., patient identification), and has been increasingly used in HCI studies to determine the whereabouts of clinicians or patients. For a review of applications of RFID in healthcare, see Wamba et al. (2013) and Rosen et al. (2014).

An RFID tag or badge contains an electronic transponder that emits or responds to electromagnetic signals to both identify itself and triangulate its position relative to base stations installed in the environment. The locating precision depends on vendor and configuration, but is generally adequate for studying problems concerned in HCI such as whether two or a group of healthcare providers are in close spatial proximity (e.g., the same room), which provides an opportunity for them to engage in interpersonal communications. Joined with timestamps, the spatiotemporal data collected via an RTLS system allow HCI experts to explore a variety of interesting topics, for example, clinicians' movement patterns, the dynamics of team aggregation and dispersion, and potential workflow deficiencies.

6.2.2.6 Other Types of Computational Ethnographical Data

Besides the five major types of computational ethnographical data discussed in this section, there are also other sources of digital traces that HCI experts may potentially tap into, such as paging/phone logs tracked by telecommunication systems,

---

[13] Wifi, cellular, and ZigBee triangulation technologies have also been developed and used for RTLS.

email messages delivered or received by email servers, internet traffic monitored by proxy servers and firewall systems, and data and metadata collected by barcode scanners and by medical devices e.g. intelligent infusion pumps. Combining these data sources together allows HCI experts to study everyday activities taking place in a healthcare environment at an unprecedented level of comprehensiveness, depth, and accuracy.

6.2.3 Analyzing Computational Ethnographical Data

6.2.3.1 Coding Computational Ethnographical Data

To analyze computational ethnographical data, a coding schema must be first identified or developed for properly labeling and categorizing the events recorded. For example, to make sense of security audit logs, researchers need to first determine the taxonomies used for "event name" and "event type" (see Table 6.1), which can often be found in software documentation or obtained directly from the vendor. Over the years, the HCI and the health informatics research communities have created many task taxonomies to characterize clinicians' work in different care areas or different medical specialties. For example, Tierney et al. (1993) developed a clinical task taxonomy comprised of tasks commonly performed by inpatient internists (Tierney et al. 1993) and subsequently adapted it to use in ambulatory primary care settings (Overhage et al. 2001). Wetterneck et al. (2012) developed a comprehensive primary care task list for evaluating clinic visit workflow which incorporates more granular task and task category definitions such as looking up the referral doctor from an EHR system or from a paper chart (Wetterneck et al. 2012). Similar taxonomies have been established to characterize the work by anesthesiologists (Hauschild et al. 2011), ICU nurses (Douglas et al. 2013), clinicians working on general medicine floors (Westbrook and Ampt 2009), as well as clinical activities specifically related to medication ordering and management (Westbrook et al. 2013).

If an HCI study mainly concerns clinicians' documentation behavior, it is advised that the researchers base their analysis on a formal classification of EHR functions and record structures, such as ASTM International's "Standard Practice for Content and Structure of the Electronic Health Record (EHR), ASTM E1384-07,"[14] "Standard Specification for Healthcare Document Formats, E2184-02",[15] or "Data Elements for EHR Documentation" curated by the American Health Information Management Association (Kallem et al. 2007). These standards define basic functions of EHR systems, common types of clinical documents, and the structure of each document type (e.g., sections and data elements that should be contained in

---

[14] http://www.astm.org/Standards/E1384.htm

[15] http://www.astm.org/Standards/E2184.htm

a discharge summary). Using these standards properly can help standardize the conduct and results reporting of documentation behavior research.

6.2.3.2   Analyzing Computational Ethnographical Data

Data collected using computational ethnographical methods can be analyzed in many ways depending on the objective and the context of an HCI study. For example, researchers interested in patient throughput may perform time series analyses to determine the intensity of clinical activities in different units in a hospital during different hours of the day and different days of the year; researchers interested in time efficiency may compute descriptive statistics to determine average turnaround between a medication order is placed and the medication is fulfilled/administered using a new computerized order entry system; and researchers interested in optimizing a UI design may use the amount of eyeball and mouse movements as a surrogate measure of the effectiveness of the organization of information and UI elements on the screen. Error rates, documentation patterns, and formation and dismissal of care teams are also frequently studied research topics (Magrabi et al. 2010; Bohnsack et al. 2009; Vawdrey et al. 2011). In this section, we describe a few unique analytical approaches that are particularly useful in analyzing computational ethnographical data.

First, *temporal data mining* is commonly used in computational ethnography. This is because computational ethnographical data are always recorded in the form of, or can be easily transposed into, *time-stamped event sequences* exhibiting the temporal (and potentially spatial) distribution of occurrences of a series of events. Because temporal data mining identifies temporal interdependencies between events, this family of methods is ideal for discovering hidden regularities from computational ethnographical data that may have significant clinical or behavioral implications. For example, HCI researchers studying the impact of HIT on clinical workflow may be interested in identifying clinical activities that are usually carried out in a given sequential order to examine whether the design of a HIT system may facilitate or hinder the ordered execution of a series of clinical tasks.

Sequential pattern analysis is one such temporal data mining method for characterizing how interrelated events are chronologically arranged. Sequential pattern analysis was initially developed by Agrawal and Srikant (1995) to study customers' shopping behavior, e.g., predicting a customer's future merchandise purchases based on the person's past shopping record. Consider the following three event sequences wherein each symbol representing a clinical activity: $\underline{ab}e\underline{gcd}hf$, $e\underline{abhcd}$, $\underline{abhcdfg}$. It can be easily observed that $ab...cd$ is a frequently occurring pattern supported by all three sequences. If the implementation of a new HIT system requires cd to be performed prior to ab, or another task to be performed between a and b or between c and d, it is possible that the new system may introduce considerable disruptions to the established workflow as well as clinicians' cognitive processes. For a review of sequential data analysis and temporal mining, see Sanderson and Fisher (1994) and Laxman and Sastry (2006).

Second, time-stamped events sequences derived from computational ethno-graphical data can be used for *transition analyses*. For example, from the three sample event sequences above, it can be easily calculated that the probability of observing event *b* following event *a* is 1, and the probabilities of observing *e* and *h* following *b* are 0.25 and 0.5, respectively. This information enables HCI researchers to characterize the nature of task transitions in clinical care. It may also allow HCI researchers to associate 'cost' with each task transition and assess whether the introduction of a new software system might increase or decrease such cost. Here, 'cost' may consist of cognitive load of switching between tasks as well as the physical effort that the task switching may incur. Studying the cost associated with task transitions is important because it has been shown in the cognition literature that frequent task switching is often associated with increased mental burden on the performer (e.g., task prioritizing and task activation). Additionally, switching between tasks that are of distinct natures could result in a higher likelihood of cognitive slips and mistakes; for example, the loss-of-activation error manifesting as forgetting what the preceding task was about in a task execution sequence.

Lastly, transition probabilities hereby obtained allow HCI researchers to conduct Markov chain analysis (Grinstead and Snell 1997) to determine that in a series of events which event might most likely appear in which step. These Markov chains, based on empirical contexts, may represent activities that a primary care physician performs during an outpatient patient visit or care procedures that a patient must go through before a surgical operation. Such information helps HCI researchers quantify the nature of established workflow in a healthcare environment and design software systems accordingly that best align with such workflow.

6.2.4 Limitation of Computational Ethnography

Comparing to traditional approaches for conducting HCI fieldwork, computational ethnographical methods provide an automated and less intrusive means for HCI researchers to study software systems or medical devices deployed in the field and used in naturalistic settings. However, computational ethnography also has notable shortcomings. A critical limitation of computational ethnographical methods is that while automatically captured digital trace data help HCI researchers tell what happened in the field, they are often inadequate to shed light on why clinicians demonstrated the observed behaviors. Mixed methods, which combine the merits of computational ethnography with qualitative research designs such as interviews, context inquiry and ethnographically based observations, are therefore highly encouraged. Further, computational ethnographical data are not necessarily com-plete for characterizing clinicians' certain behaviors. For example communication analyses solely based on computer logs (paging/phone, email, messaging, etc.) may fail to consider other important channels of communication among clinicians such as hallway or bedside conversations. Thus, when conducting computational ethnographical investigations, researchers shall be always mindful whether such data are a truly comprehensive reflection of clinicians' work of interest. Lastly, computational ethnographical data may originate from multiple sources posing great challenges to synchronization and integrative analysis. In addition, computational ethnographical data may be originally collected to support operational purposes (e.g., security auditing), rather than research. Preparing such data for research reuse could therefore be resource consuming and may require sophisticated analytical skills.

6.3 Case Studies

6.3.1 Understanding Clinicians' Navigation Behavior in EHRs

In their paper "*An Interface-Driven Analysis of User Interactions with an Electronic Health Records System*," Zheng et al. (2009) applied the computational ethnographical approach to study primary care physicians' usage behavior of an ambulatory care EHR system (Zheng et al. 2009). In the study, a homegrown EHR system was reengineered to allow real-time capture of comprehensive UI interaction events such as mouse clicks and keystrokes. These UI interaction events, along with audit trails recording EHR document retrieval, creation, and modification events, provided data for computational ethnographical analyses.

Figure 6.6 illustrates the UI of the EHR system studied. Listed in Table 6.3 are 17 major EHR features provided in the system to allow clinicians to perform various documentation or chart viewing tasks. Based on the digital trace data and timestamps, event sequences were constructed representing how these 17 EHR features were sequentially accessed, which might represent how the corresponding clinical tasks were sequentially carried out. *HMXAD*, for example, represents a task sequence of "History of Present Illness" (H) → "Medication" (M) → "Physical Examination" (X) → "Assessment & Plan" (A) → "Diagnosis" (D). The empirical study was conducted in an ambulatory primary care clinic and lasted 10 months. Data were recorded in a total of 973 distinct patient encounters seen by 30 resident physicians.

The computational ethnographical data recorded in the empirical study were analyzed using a sequential pattern analysis, which uncovers hidden navigational patterns in the resident physicians' use of the EHR system; and a Markov chain model, which characterizes the sequential dependencies among the 17 EHR features based on transition probabilities. The sequential patterns identified in the study are shown in Table 6.4. These patterns satisfied a minimum support threshold of 15 %, i.e., each appeared in at least 15 % of the patient encounters studied.

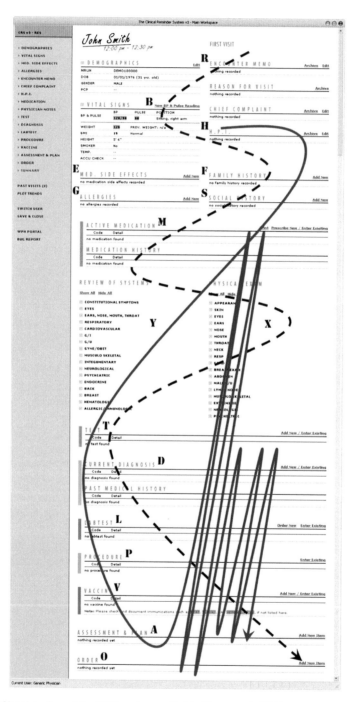

Fig. 6.6 User interface of the EHR system studied in Zheng et al. (2009)

Table 6.3 Major EHR features studied

Label	Feature	Label	Feature
A	Assessment & Plan	O	Order
B	Retaking BP	P	Procedure
D	Diagnosis (problem list)	R	EncounteR Memo
E	Medication Side Effects	S	Social History
F	Family History	T	Office Test
G	AllerGies	V	Vaccination
H	History of Present Illness (HPI)	X	Physical EXamination
L	Laboratory Test	Y	Review of SYstems
M	Medication		

Table 6.4 Sequential patterns identified

Pattern	Level of support (%)
ADAD	51.16
DADA	43.97
XADA	40.17
OMOM	32.77
MOMO	29.39
YXAD	21.78
HS	19.03
OL	18.6
OMY	16.7
LO	15.64
HO	15.01

As shown in Table 6.4, *ADAD* and *DADA* were the most common recurring feature combinations sequentially carried out, which suggests that when the resident physicians used the EHR system to document or view patient data, they often accessed the "Assessment & Plan" and "Diagnosis" sections of the EHR consecutively, and frequently switched between these two features back and forth. "Medication" and "Order" are another pair of EHR features that appeared to be often used together.

Figure 6.7 illustrates the results obtained from the Markov chain analysis where feature transitions with a probability above 0.5 are highlighted using bold arcs. Prominent transitions can be easily observed from the figure; for example, after a resident physician completed "Physical Examination", the chance that she or he would immediately move on to document "Assessment & Plan" (0.687) is higher than the probabilities of using all other EHR features combined. Similarly, "Assessment & Plan" → "Diagnosis" (0.764) is a frequent task transition, suggesting that immediately after documenting in the "Assessment & Plan" section in the EHR system, a resident physician would most likely begin working on "Diagnosis." Likewise, "Order" has a high probability of transitioning to "Medication" (0.57), as does "Family History" → "Social History" (0.538).

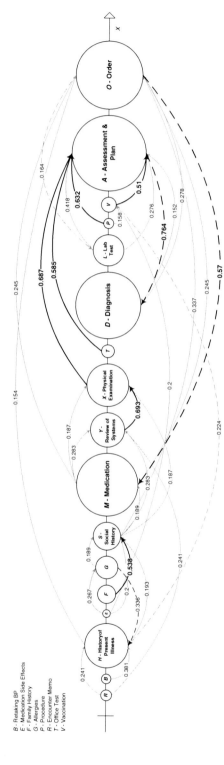

Fig. 6.7 Tasks and task transition probabilities during an outpatient primary care visit (Reproduced from Zheng et al. 2009). Size of a node is proportional to the activity's frequency of occurrence as empirically observed. *Bold edges*: transitions with a probability over 0.5; *Dashed edges*: task transitions running counter to the anticipated workflow. Transitions with a probability lower than 0.15 are not shown

Figure 6.7 illustrates the Markov chain constructed based on the feature transition probabilities. This information reveals that after a user logged into the EHR system, in which step a particular EHR feature would most likely be accessed. As exhibited in the figure, "History of Present Illness" was usually the first stop after a user started to use the system. Then, the most likely accessed next EHR feature was "Social History," followed by "Assessment & Plan." From Fig. 6.7, it becomes clear how resident physicians in the study practice tended to organize their clinical work chronologically during a typical outpatient primary care encounter.

The results of this computational ethnographical study led to the discovery of the resident physicians' navigational patterns in using the ambulatory care EHR system in the study clinic. This discovery may in turn lead to a better understanding of their cognitive processes when providing patient care. For HCI researchers, this learning may directly inform improvement opportunities to ameliorate the usability of the EHR system, e.g., usability deficiencies may surface if certain UI design of the system might require an excessive number of mouse clicks in order to accomplish frequent task transitions.

For example, the empirical data recorded in this study show that "History of Present Illness" was one of the most frequently used features and was usually accessed immediately after a user logged into the system. This feature should therefore be placed in a distinctive, salient onscreen position in the UI. Further, the study identified several pairs of features (e.g., "Assessment & Plan" $\leftrightarrows$ "Diagnosis" and "Order" $\leftrightarrows$ "Medication") that were often accessed together. This prompts EHR designers to place these features in adjacent locations on the screen, or provide certain navigational aids (e.g. hyperlink shortcuts), to facilitate these frequent feature switches. The result would be a more optimized designs better aligned with clinicians' workflow as well as their mental model of accessing/documenting information and providing patient care.

6.3.2 Analyzing the Dynamics of Provider–Patient Interactions

The second case study, "Interpreter-mediated physician–patient communication: opportunities for multimodal healthcare interfaces," was conducted by Weibel et al. (2013). This study examined physician–patient communications mediated by medical interpreters with patients who have low English proficiency. The fieldwork was conducted at a community health center that provides comprehensive care for low income and multiethnic patient populations. A majority of these patients show limited English proficiency (LEP); most of them require the assistance of an interpreter during physician–patient consultations.

In the study, the researchers analyzed multiparty and multimodal interactions in the exam room from a distributed cognition perspective. The study employed a novel computational ethnographical approach to simultaneously capture multiple data streams to examine physician, patient, and interpreter interactions. This allowed the researchers to investigate beyond speech—what has been traditionally considered the primary modality for communication—to include other types of nonverbal exchanges such as eye contact, gestures, and body orientation.

To capture multiparty multimodal interactions, the study deployed an experimental recording system using two Microsoft Kinects that allowed the capture of body positioning, directional audio, video footage, and depth-imaging of the scene. The analysis leveraged a suite of analysis techniques that the researchers previously developed called ChronoViz (shown in Fig. 6.8),[16] a tool that aids visualization and analysis of multimodal sets of time-coded information with a focus on the analysis of video in combination with other data sources. In this study, ChronoViz was used to facilitate the analysis of simultaneous bodily action, voice, and gaze (head position) of multiple participants (Fouse et al. 2011).

Figure 6.9 also shows the position of patient, doctor, and interpreter in the exam room. The physician and the patient usually sit side-by side. The physician sits in a rolling desk chair, with the EHR directly in front of her on a rolling, height-adjustable platform. The patient sits next to the physician on the front edge of a traditional exam table. The interpreter typically sits in a simple chair backed against the exam room wall, next to the door, approximately six feet directly in front of the patient. The empirical study recorded 12 outpatient encounter sessions (half requiring the service of an interpreter). Each generated two video streams, two directional audio streams, two depth data streams, and derived body joint positions (calculated by the Kinect algorithms).

A group of five researchers analyzed the data with the assistance of ChronoViz. Given the richness and complexity of interaction between individuals and with the EHR, as well as the distinct physician–patient interactions while an interpreter was present in the room, two encounters were selected for an in-depth drilldown analysis. One session involved an English-fluent patient; the other involved an LEP patient who required an interpreter. Body position, head position, right and left hand position, and speech instances (not transcriptions of them) of both patient and physician across the entire sessions were coded. Speech, body position, and head position were also annotated for the interpreter in the second session.

The drilldown analysis revealed differing multiparty communication patterns. Not surprisingly, the interpreter functioned as a middleman who spoke directly after both the patient and the physician (Fig. 6.10). This pattern was only interrupted when the interpreter was not able to directly translate the physician or the patient's speech due to usage of other artifacts (e.g., paper, the EHR system). Further, gesture communication patterns differed between the interpreter and non-interpreter sessions. In both sessions, a variety of gesture types were observed, including deictic (e.g. pointing at EHR or paper), iconic (e.g. hand in shape of cyst), and beat gestures (e.g. hand palm up). When the interpreter was not present, the physician's gestures were distributed fairly evenly across the three gesture types; and the patient

---

[16] http://chronoviz.com/

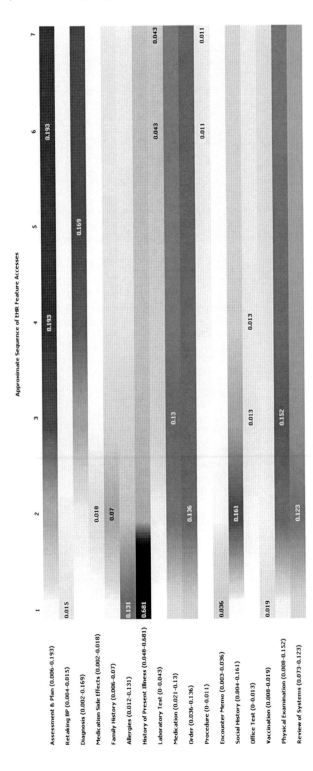

Fig. 6.8 A diagram that visualizes the Markov chain constructed based on transition probabilities (Reproduced from Zheng et al. 2009). Gray-scale gradient is proportional to the probabilities of observing a row activity in each of the Markov chain steps. Darker areas indicate higher probabilities. Numbers in parentheses: the range of probabilities of observing an activity in these Markov chain steps; Numeric labels on gray-scale stripes: the maximum probability of observing a row activity

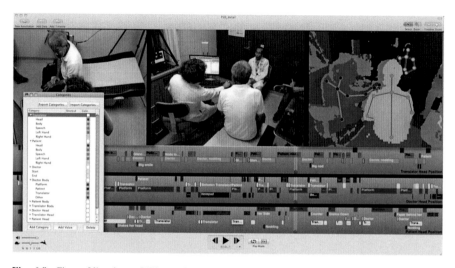

Fig. 6.9 ChronoViz view of Kinect data (Reproduced from Weibel et al. 2013). The *top half* shows video feeds (two video and one depth-image) from two Kinects. The *center* video and *right* depth-image show the interpreter facing the physician (*left*) and the patient (*right*). The *bottom half* shows three timelines with annotations of a 5-min medical session indicating information such as who is talking (patient, interpreter, doctor), their body positions, and what they are interacting with

Fig. 6.10 Speech analysis of an interpreter-mediated communication session (Reproduced from Weibel et al. 2013). The timeline displays three levels, each representing the speech of one member of the team: the *top line* is the patient's speech (*green*), the *middle line* is the interpreter's speech (*blue*), and the *lowest line* displays the physician's speech (*red*). A *line* is superimposed to connect utterances of the three individuals. *Yellow lines* represent common physician–interpreter–patient interaction patterns; *purple lines* identify the rare physician–patient interaction patterns

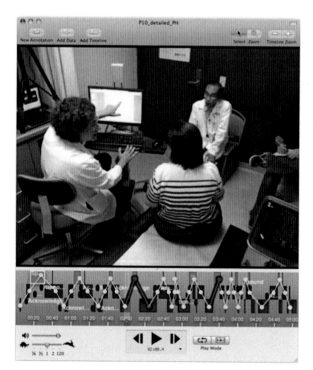

communicated with more beat gestures (approximately 36 % deictic, 10 % iconic, 55 % beat). The presence of the interpreter radically changed the gesture pattern: the physician used iconic gestures much more often (approximately 31 % deictic, 44 % iconic, 25 % beat), while all of the interpreter's and patient's gestures were iconic (gesture were used exclusively to communicate the shape, size, and location of an injury).

Another key observation from the study is that often one of the parties involved was "left in the dark." The patient often did not understand what the physician was saying and must await the interpreter's translation, and the physician could not understand what the interpreter was saying to the patient nor be sure of translation accuracy. In addition, there were challenges of where to direct attention when various parties were talking. While facial expressions and gesture play a significant in facilitating communication, the patient might be looking at the interpreter when the physician was talking, or the physician at the interpreter when the patient was talking and as a result missed important cues. The communication process was further challenged when the interpreter was left out of the loop because of inability to attend to the EHR display or some other artifact, such as paper. In the study, the physician commonly pointed to the information displayed on the EHR and patients, according to their gestures and body position, suggested that they were also interested in looking at the data. A key problem, however, was that neither the patient nor the interpreter could effectively see the display. This is evident as when the interpreter was present in the room, no pointing gestures to the EHR by the patient or the interpreter were identified from the empirical data. This suggests that the value of using the EHR as a shared communication tool could diminish significantly with LEP patients.

6.4 Conclusions

In summary, comparing to traditional HCI approaches, computational ethnographical methods provide an automated and less obtrusive means for measuring and analyzing the multimodal nature of patient–clinician–computer interactions. Computational ethnography can thus be conducted at an unprecedented level of scale to uncover end users' true, unaltered behaviors interacting with technological systems in healthcare. However, while computational ethnographical data abound in modern healthcare organizations (e.g., routinely tracked audit trails and communication logs), their power for enabling HCI evaluation studies is yet to be fully unleashed. We therefore encourage students, HCI researchers, and healthcare administrators, to carefully consider using computational ethnographical data captured in everyday healthcare settings to generate new knowledge that could inform strategies for improving the usability of technological systems, and ultimately operation efficiency, quality of care, and patient safety.

Discussion Questions

1. The sample audit trail log shown in Table 6.1 exhibits a clinician's use session with an EHR system. In the "PATIENT_ID" column, it can be observed that the clinician worked primarily on patient "4070370" throughout the session but she or he, rather abruptly, viewed a document belonging to patient "7485199" at 07:23:19 UTC.

   (a) What might be the possible explanation(s) of this EHR use behavior? Provide one scenario of "inappropriate" use and one scenario of "beneficial" use.
   (b) How might the EHR system be redesigned to prevent "inappropriate" use, or to facilitate "beneficial" use?
   (c) If the audit trail log were not available, propose an alternative method of recording data that can capture this behavior.

2. Provide an example wherein your everyday activities leave behind some "digital traces" that can be analyzed using computational ethnographical methods.

   (a) Identify the data type that best characterizes these digital traces;
   (b) Propose an analytical method discussed in this chapter to analyze the data;
   (c) Also discuss what potential insights may be drawn from the analysis. These could be insights for better understanding the user behavior or for informing better design of certain technological systems.

Acknowledgement We are grateful to Steven Rick who contributed the photos used in this chapter to illustrate computational ethnographical data recording devices deployed in exam rooms.

Additional Readings

Dumais, S., Jeffries, R., Russell, D. M., Tang, D., & Teevan, J. (2014). Understanding user behavior through log data and analysis. In J. S. Olson & W. Kellogg (Eds.), *Ways of knowing in HCI* (pp. 349–372). New York: Springer.

Laxman, S., & Sastry, P. S. (2006). A survey of temporal data mining. *Sadhana-Academy Proceedings in Engineering Sciences, 31*(2), 173–198.

Weibel, N., Emmenegger, C., Lyons, J., Dixit, R., Hill, L. L., & Hollan, J. D. (2013). Interpreter-mediated physician-patient communication: Opportunities for multimodal healthcare interfaces. In *Proceedings of the 7th international conference on Pervasive Computing Technologies for Healthcare (PervasiveHealth'13)* (pp. 113–120).

Weibel, N., Rick, S., Emmenegger, C., Ashfaq, S., Calvitti, A., & Agha, Z. (2015). LAB-IN-A-BOX: Semi-automatic tracking of activity in the medical office. *Personal and Ubiquitous Computing, 19*(2), 317–334.

Zheng, K., Padman, R., Johnson, M. P., & Diamond, H. S. (2009). An interface-driven analysis of user interactions with an electronic health records system. *Journal of the American Medical Informatics Association, 16*(2), 228–237.

Zheng, K., Haftel, H. M., Hirschl, R. B., O'Reilly, M., & Hanauer, D. A. (2010). Quantifying the impact of health IT implementations on clinical workflow: A new methodological perspective. *Journal of the American Medical Informatics Association, 17*(4), 454–461.

References

Agrawal, R., & Srikant, R. (1995). Mining sequential patterns. In *Proceedings of the 11th international conference on data engineering* (pp. 3–14).

Armstrong, T., & Olatunji, B. O. (2012). Eye tracking of attention in the affective disorders: A meta-analytic review and synthesis. *Clinical Psychology Review, 32*(8), 704–723.

Bloomrosen, M., Starren, J., Lorenzi, N. M., Ash, J. S., Patel, V. L., & Shortliffe, E. H. (2011). Anticipating and addressing the unintended consequences of health IT and policy: A report from the AMIA 2009 Health Policy Meeting. *Journal of the American Medical Informatics Association, 18*(1), 82–90.

Bohnsack, K. J., Parker, D. P., & Zheng, K. (2009). Quantifying temporal documentation patterns in clinician use of AHLTA—The DoD's ambulatory electronic health record. In *AMIA Annual Symposium Proceeding* (pp. 50–54).

Card, S. K., Moran, T. P., & Newell, A. (1980). The keystroke-level model for user performance time with interactive systems. *Communications of the ACM, 23*(7), 396–410.

Douglas, S., Cartmill, R., Brown, R., Hoonakker, P., Slagle, J., Schultz Van Roy, K., Walker, J. M., Weinger, M., Wetterneck, T., & Carayon, P. (2013). The work of adult and pediatric intensive care unit nurses. *Nursing Research, 62*(1), 50–58.

Dumais, S., Jeffries, R., Russell, D. M., Tang, D., & Teevan, J. (2014). Understanding user behavior through log data and analysis. In J. S. Olson & W. Kellogg (Eds.), *Ways of knowing in HCI* (pp. 349–372). New York: Springer.

Eligible professional meaningful use core measures. Measure 14 of 14, Stage 1. http://www.cms.gov/Regulations-and-Guidance/Legislation/EHRIncentivePrograms/downloads/15_Core_ProtectElectronicHealthInformation.pdf. Accessed 20 May 2014.

Falck-Ytter, T., Bölte, S., & Gredebäck, G. (2013). Eye tracking in early autism research. *Journal of Neurodevelopmental Disorders, 5*(1), 28.

Fitzpatrick, G., & Ellingsen, G. (2013). A review of 25 years of CSCW research in healthcare: Contributions, challenges and future agendas. *Computer Supported Cooperative Work, 22* (4–6), 609–665.

Fouse, A., Weibel, N., Hutchins, E., & Hollan, J. D. (2011). ChronoViz: A system for supporting navigation of time-coded data. In *Proceedings of the 2011 ACM conference on Human Factors in Computing Systems, Extended Abstracts (CHI EA '11)* (pp. 299–304).

Giles, J. (2012). Computational social science: Making the links. *Nature, 488*(7412), 448–450.

Gonyea, R. M. (2005). Self-reported data in institutional research: Review and recommendations. *New Directions for Institutional Research, 127*, 73–89.

Grinstead, C. M., & Snell, J. L. (1997). Markov chains. In *Introduction to probability* (pp. 405–470). Providence: American Mathematical Society.

Hauschild, I., Vitzthum, K., Klapp, B. F., Groneberg, D. A., & Mache, S. (2011). Time and motion study of anesthesiologists' workflow in German hospitals. *Wiener Medizinische Wochenschrift, 161*(17–18), 433–440.

Hilbert, D. M., & Redmiles, D. F. (2000). Extracting usability information from user interface events. *ACM Computing Surveys, 32*(4), 384–421.

Hripcsak, G., Vawdrey, D. K., Fred, M. R., & Bostwick, S. B. (2011). Use of electronic clinical documentation: Time spent and team interactions. *Journal of the American Medical Informatics Association, 18*(2), 112–117.

Kallem, C., Burrington-Brown, J., & Dinh, A. K. (2007). Data elements for EHR documentation. *Journal of AHIMA, 78*(7):web extra.

Kazmi, Z. (2013). Effects of exam room EHR use on doctor-patient communication: A systematic literature review. *Informatics in Primary Care, 21*(1), 30–39.

Kellermann, A. L., & Jones, S. S. (2013). What it will take to achieve the as-yet-unfulfilled promises of health information technology. *Health Affairs (Millwood), 32*(1), 63–68.

Laxman, S., & Sastry, P. S. (2006). A survey of temporal data mining. *Sadhana-Academy Proceedings in Engineering Sciences, 31*(2), 173–198.

Lazer, D., Pentland, A., Adamic, L., Aral, S., et al. (2009). Social science. Computational social science. *Science, 323*(5915), 721–723.

Magrabi, F., Li, S. Y., Day, R. O., & Coiera, E. (2010). Errors and electronic prescribing: A controlled laboratory study to examine task complexity and interruption effects. *Journal of the American Medical Informatics Association, 17*(5), 575–583.

Overhage, J. M., Perkins, S., Tierney, W. M., & McDonald, C. J. (2001). Controlled trial of direct physician order entry: Effects on physicians' time utilization in ambulatory primary care internal medicine practices. *Journal of the American Medical Informatics Association, 8*(4), 361–371.

Poole, A., & Ball, L. J. (2005). Eye tracking in human-computer interaction and usability research: Current status and future. In C. Ghaoui (Ed.), *Encyclopedia of human-computer interaction.* Hershey: Idea Group, Inc.

Ritter, F. E., & Larkin, J. H. (1994). Developing process models as summaries of HCI action sequences. *Human Computer Interaction, 9*(4), 345–383.

Rosen, M. A., Dietz, A. S., Yang, T., Priebe, C. E., & Pronovost, P. J. (2014, July 22). An integrative framework for sensor-based measurement of teamwork in healthcare. *Journal of the American Medical Informatics Association.* pii: amiajnl-2013-002606. doi:10.1136/amiajnl-2013-002606. [Epub ahead of print].

Sanderson, P. M., & Fisher, C. (1994). Exploratory sequential data analysis: Foundations. *Human-Computer Interaction, 9*(4), 251–317.

Tien, T., Pucher, P. H., Sodergren, M. H., Sriskandarajah, K., Yang, G. Z., & Darzi, A. (2014). Eye tracking for skills assessment and training: A systematic review. *Journal of Surgical Research, 191*(1), 169–178.

Tierney, W. M., Miller, M. E., Overhage, J. M., & McDonald, C. J. (1993). Physician inpatient order writing on microcomputer workstations effects on resource utilization. *JAMA, 269,* 379–383.

Vawdrey, D. K., Wilcox, L. G., Collins, S., Feiner, S., Mamykina, O., Stein, D. M., Bakken, S., Fred, M. R., & Stetson, P. D. (2011). Awareness of the care team in electronic health records. *Applied Clinical Informatics, 2*(4), 395–405.

Wamba, S. F., Anand, A., & Carter, L. (2013). A literature review of RFID-enabled healthcare applications and issues. *International Journal of Information Management, 33*(5), 875–891.

Weibel, N., Emmenegger, C., Lyons, J., Dixit, R., Hill, L. L., & Hollan, J. D. (2013). Interpreter-mediated physician-patient communication: Opportunities for multimodal healthcare interfaces. In *Proceedings of the 7th international conference on Pervasive Computing Technologies for Healthcare (PervasiveHealth'13)* (pp. 113–120).

Weibel, N., Rick, S., Emmenegger, C., Ashfaq, S., Calvitti, A., & Agha, Z. (2015). LAB-IN-A-BOX: Semi-automatic tracking of activity in the medical office. *Personal and Ubiquitous Computing, 19*(2), 317–334.

Westbrook, J. I., & Ampt, A. (2009). Design, application and testing of the Work Observation Method by Activity Timing (WOMBAT) to measure clinicians' patterns of work and communication. *International Journal of Medical Informatics, 78*(Suppl 1), S25–S33.

Westbrook, J. I., Li, L., Georgiou, A., Paoloni, R., & Cullen, J. (2013). Impact of an electronic medication management system on hospital doctors' and nurses' work: A controlled pre-post, time and motion study. *Journal of the American Medical Informatics Association, 20*(6), 1150–1158.

Wetterneck, T. B., Lapin, J. A., Krueger, D. J., Holman, G. T., Beasley, J. W., & Karsh, B. T. (2012). Development of a primary care physician task list to evaluate clinic visit workflow. *BMJ Quality Safety, 21*(1), 47–53.

Zheng, K., Padman, R., Johnson, M. P., & Diamond, H. S. (2009). An interface-driven analysis of user interactions with an electronic health records system. *Journal of the American Medical Informatics Association, 16*(2), 228–237.

Chapter 7
User-Centered Design and Evaluation of Clinical Information Systems: A Usability Engineering Perspective

Andre Kushniruk, Helen Monkman, Elizabeth Borycki, and Joseph Kannry

7.1 Introduction

Designing useful and usable clinical information systems continues to be a major healthcare challenge. There are numerous reports of clinical information systems that have failed to be fully used by clinicians, deemed to be unusable by end users or do not fit the workflow of the clinical settings where they are deployed. In addition to this, it has been recognized that poorly designed clinical information systems and their user interfaces can pose significant hazards to patient safety, in some cases, leading to medical errors (Beuscart-Zéphir et al. 2005; Borycki and Kushniuk 2008; Koppel et al. 2005; Kushniruk et al. 2005). In this chapter, we describe approaches for the design and evaluation of user interfaces for clinical information systems based on methods from the usability engineering literature that have been adapted for the design and evaluation of clinical information systems. Several examples involving the application of user centered design (UCD) approaches will be described, including the application of rapid low-cost usability engineering methods and the use of clinical simulations. Challenges in designing and deploying usable interfaces for clinical information systems will be considered. The content of this chapter should be of interest to a wide audience, ranging from those who design and evaluate health information systems, to end users of such systems (i.e., doctors, nurses and patients) who would like an appreciation of how system usability can be assessed and improved in their organizations.

Usability can be defined as a measure of use and ease of system use in terms of the following dimensions: (1) effectiveness, (2) efficiency, (3) learnability,

A. Kushniruk (✉) • H. Monkman • E. Borycki
School of Health Information Science, University of Victoria, Victoria, BC, Canada
e-mail: andrek@uvic.ca

J. Kannry
Icahn School of Medicine at Mount Sinai, New York, NY, USA

© Springer International Publishing Switzerland 2015

V.L. Patel et al. (eds.), *Cognitive Informatics for Biomedicine*, Health Informatics,
DOI 10.1007/978-3-319-17272-9_7

(4) safety, and (5) enjoyability (Preece et al. 2011). Usability engineering involves the application of scientific methods for the evaluation of usability of information systems. Usability engineering methods can be applied throughout system development process, from early system prototyping to system deployment and post-implementation (Kushniruk et al. 1996; Kushniruk and Patel 2004; Nielsen 1993; Patel and Kushniruk 1998; Patel and Kaufman 2006; Kaufman et al. 2003). Usability engineering emerged as a field of study in the 1980s and aims to improve the usability of existing or proposed user interfaces, feeding recommendations back to designers. Initially, the field emerged from the disciplines of Computer Science and Psychology, but has now led to the development and training of professional practitioners who work in the area of usability engineering and applies methods such as usability testing and inspection. As will be described, usability engineering methods involve two main approaches: (1) usability testing, where users of systems or user interfaces are observed (and typically recorded) as they interact with the system under study to carry out tasks, and (2) usability inspection methods, which involve trained usability analysts systematically "stepping through" a user interface or system, comparing it against a set of usability principles and noting usability problems (Nielsen 1993). We argue that UCD in conjunction with rapid usability evaluation is more likely to lead to systems that are both useful and usable (Borycki et al. 2013).

We begin with a discussion of a topic central to effective design and evaluation of health information systems, namely the incorporation of user input into the design and refinement of clinical information systems through UCD. Closely related to this is a discussion of the application of methods that have emerged from the field of usability engineering that can be employed in conjunction with UCD in order to develop and test systems. As will be described, such approaches can be applied at a low cost in settings ranging from fixed usability laboratories to real-world settings and contexts. Extension of the approaches involving the use of clinical simulations will be described along with the importance of applying usability engineering methods to ensure system safety.

7.2   Assessing User Needs

UCD has been defined as "a multi-disciplinary design approach based on active involvement of users for a clear understanding of the user and task requirements, and the iteration of design and evaluation" (Mao et al. 2005, p. 51). UCD aims to develop systems that are useful and usable (Karat 1997) by applying tenets of human factors (i.e., to enhance human capabilities and overcome human limitations) to the design of products and systems to promote user acceptance and adoption (Rouse 1991). UCD specialists aspire to design systems that accommodate users' characteristics, limits, tasks and workflows (Johnson et al. 2005). Rather than strictly relying on input from system designers, UCD enlists users as participants to help inform their design solutions. Additionally, UCD encompasses the philosophies and methodologies whereby design is guided by observing, working with and studying users and their requirements (Karat 1997). Methods of user involvement can vary from consulting with end users to analyzing their interactions with systems and information needs (Damodaran 1996). Gould and Lewis (1985) proposed three principles for UCD: (1) focus early on users and their tasks; (2) conduct empirical evaluation and measurement; and (3) apply iterative design processes. Thus, UCD involves collection of data from users and its transformation to design solutions for improving the usefulness and usability of products.

Traditionally, system designers expected users to align with how a system operated. In contrast, system development guided by user input increases the likelihood that the resulting systems will be easy to learn, minimize errors, and will also increase user productivity, acceptance and satisfaction. In contrast, failing to incorporate iterative and ongoing user feedback in the design process can result in a lack of alignment between user needs and system capabilities. There are a number of advantages to involving users during system development.

Identifying user needs early in the design phase is imperative to designing systems that meet user specifications and to keep project costs to a minimum (Johnson et al. 2005). The costs associated with making system changes escalate as system development progresses. Moreover, failing to consider users in the design process often requires system redesign, which is both costly and time-consuming (Johnson et al. 2005). The financial benefits of user involvement include increased sales and user productivity, and decreased training and user support costs. In considering aggregated evidence from user involvement in ethnographic, qualitative and quantitative studies, the following benefits have been reported: (1) more accurate user requirements, (2) minimization of superfluous functionality, and (3) improved user acceptance of systems (Kujala 2003). Thus, it has been argued that it is financially prudent to adopt good design principles and incorporate user exemplars to identify any design and usability issues early on in the development process.

Several challenges offset the benefits of user involvement. For one, methods that include users in an integral way can be more time consuming and expensive than developing a system with limited user input (Kujala 2003). Recruiting participants may be a more time consuming process in itself. It can be difficult to select the ideal users to participate in system development. Users need to be representative of the prospective user group(s); this may require a number of participants with different disciplinary backgrounds (e.g., medicine, nursing, or pharmacy) and specialties (e.g., general medicine, cardiology, or surgery) (Kushniruk and Turner 2012). Ideally, users selected for participation should be able to articulate the needs and requirements of representative end users, not just themselves. That is, there may be considerable individual variability in user needs, and this should be reflected in the resultant system. In addition, it may be difficult to attain consensus amongst the users (Kujala 2003).

There are a variety of approaches for increasing user involvement during system design (e.g., ethnography, contextual design, user-centered design, participatory design) (see Kujala 2003 for comparison among methods). The emphasis of UCD is on usability; and UCD methods include task analysis, prototyping and usability

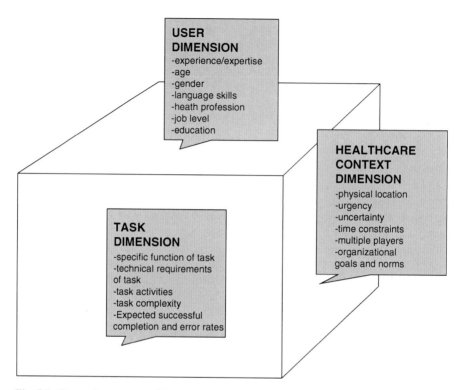

Fig. 7.1 User-task-context model (Adapted from Kushniruk and Turner 2012)

evaluations (Kujala 2003). UCD is inherently guided by user goals; that is, the emergent system should be developed driven by what users need to accomplish (Saffer 2007). Assessing user needs and obtaining feedback from users for the design of clinical information systems is challenging in clinical settings for a number of reasons: (1) healthcare is a complex domain, (2) there may be many classes of users for a particular clinical information system, (3) users may have varied healthcare and IT backgrounds, (4) clinical workflow must be carefully considered in addition to more static elements of system user interfaces, and (5) the context of use of clinical systems varies considerably. In 2012, Kushniruk and Turner proposed a three-dimensional model to aid in the modeling of end user involvement in designing and testing clinical information systems. The model can be used to both capture design requirements and also provide a basis for setting up specific usability tests to ensure a partially or fully completed system meets clinical user needs (see Fig. 7.1).

The model in Fig. 7.1 can be used to drive both the development of use case scenarios for use in scenario-based design of healthcare information systems, as well as for summative testing of systems once they are implemented (Carroll 1995; Kushniruk and Turner 2012). For example, along the User Dimension, the different classes of users of a system being developed (e.g., physicians, pharmacists, nurses) are delineated along with their attributes (e.g., level of experience/expertise, age range). Along the Task Dimension, the various tasks and the attributes of those tasks are defined for each class of user (e.g., tasks such as entry of patient data, decision support, etc.). In the past, the combination of User and Task dimensions made up a model known in the software industry as the User-Task Matrix (Hackos and Redish 1998). In our work in clinical contexts, it became apparent that a third dimension, that of "Context" also needs to be considered when designing healthcare information systems. This perspective is consistent with work from the socio-technical design literature for healthcare IT development (where the role of social context is emphasized), but differs in that it provides an explicit model of context in relation to user types and users' tasks. Context refers to the healthcare setting or environment into which healthcare IT will be deployed. As an illustration, the User-Task-Context model can be used to consider under what conditions a new speech recognition component would likely be effective for physicians dictating reports while using an electronic health record system (i.e., the Task dimension). The effectiveness of the component can be shown to vary considerably even when considering the same class of users (i.e., the User dimension), depending on whether the speech recognition component is deployed in a quiet office setting or in a noisy clinic (i.e., the Context dimension). Thus, the success or failure of health information systems and technologies is related to consideration of all 3 dimensions.

In our work developing requirements, application of this model has proven useful for activities ranging from creation of system requirements during early requirements analysis, to generation of use cases (which describe in detail the scenarios involved in specific uses of the system) and generation of scenarios that can be used to test the user model of a prototype once a system has been deployed. The system development life cycle (SDLC) provides a useful formal framework for considering where this type of user modeling can be applied and consists of the following phases: (1) the Planning Phase, where the initial planning of the system development is initiated, (2) the Analysis Phase, where there is a focus on requirements gathering, (3) the Design Phase, where detailed architectural blueprints for the system are developed, (4) the Implementation phase, where the system is programmed, and (5) the Support Phase, where the system is in use (Kushniruk 2002). In the context of the SDLC, the User-Task-Context matrix is useful at a number of stages including early in Planning and Analysis phases to specify user requirements, during the Design Phase to drive refinement of use cases, and during the Implementation Phase, to provide those testing a system with a list of users and tasks for target testing (in order to ensure the system does what it was intended for each class of user it was designed to serve).

7.3 Low-Cost Rapid Usability Engineering in Clinical Informatics

In this section, we describe methods collectively known as rapid low-cost usability engineering methods designed to be used for analyzing user interactions with a range of healthcare information systems and which can be an integral part of UCD in healthcare (Kushniruk et al. 2006; Borycki et al. 2013). As will be shown, the methods can be employed during UCD, and also upon completion of a clinical information system during its deployment phase (i.e., during the support phase of the traditional SDLC).

Usability testing involves observing representative users of a system (e.g., doctors or nurses) while they use a system or user interface to carry out representative tasks (e.g., entering medications into a clinical information system) (Nielsen 1993; Kushniruk and Patel 2004). Observing users typically involves video recording user interactions, on-screen actions and verbalizations. Such data can be transcribed and coded to identify usability problems and issues (Kushniruk and Patel 2004). Usability testing methods have been employed widely in the design and evaluation of a range of health information systems over the past several decades. Usability testing methods can be used along the entire SDLC and the focus of the testing will depend on the stage of development of the system (Borycki et al. 2011; Kushniruk 2002).

Usability engineering methods have evolved in response to advances in technology. For example, free or low-cost screen recording software and built-in microphones on laptops have enabled "low-cost rapid usability testing" to become more widely applied (Kushniruk and Borycki 2006). The goal of this method is to provide an informative usability test that is efficient and cost effective. Moreover, low-cost rapid usability testing is not limited to the confines of a laboratory setting. Rather, by employing low-cost portable methods that can be taken directly into settings like operating rooms or clinics, the approach allows for what we have referred to as "in-situ" usability testing. Such testing has the advantage of having greater fidelity than laboratory-based usability testing. Such testing can also vary in terms of whether the experimenter exerts control over the study, or allows the users' interactions to be more naturalistic, which allows for a range of study types. It also is arguably far less expensive, since if the testing can be taken into real settings after hours or when available, then the cost of the testing can be reduced (Kushniruk and Borycki 2006). Regardless of whether usability testing is conducted in a laboratory setting or in a real clinical environment, there are a number of steps that need to be considered in setting up such testing. Kushniruk and colleagues (Kushniruk and Patel 2004; Borycki and Kushniruk 2005) have previously outlined the stages of this approach:

1. Identification of testing objectives
2. Selection of participants (e.g., $n = 10$ to 20 representative users)
3. Selection of representative experimental tasks

4. Selection of an evaluation environment
5. Observation and recording of users' interaction with the health information system
6. Analysis of usability data (i.e., coding screen and/or video recordings and audio transcripts)
7. Translating findings and feedback into suggestions for system improvement

This method has been shown to drastically reduce development costs. In one study, adopting this method resulted in an estimated cost savings between 36.5 and 78.5 % (Baylis et al. 2012). Costs associated with design changes are much lower early in the SDLC. For example, identifying a usability problem or error early in the design phase may require minimal effort to fix. However, once a system is deployed, making even minimal changes may be impossible or prohibitively expensive. Further, mitigating errors before deploying the system reduces the potential of technology-induced errors (i.e., errors resulting from the use of an information system that may be caused from poor usability or from interactions with a system in a real setting) which in some cases are costly to address from a systems and human perspective in terms of patient safety (Baylis et al. 2012; Borycki and Keay 2010). As a result, this method minimizes the probability of requiring a system re-design. In addition to this, the method is appealing as it is both efficient and inexpensive to employ. Currently, experimental apparatus (i.e., the computer screen, screen recording software, and microphone) is embedded in most laptops and therefore a usability test can be conducted anywhere (Kushniruk and Borycki 2006). The low-cost rapid usability engineering approach can also be conducted remotely by employing commonly available web-conference and screen sharing software to remotely view and record the screens and audio of subjects performing tasks during usability testing remotely (Kushniruk et al. 2007, 2008; Kushniruk and Borycki 2006).

In considering at what points in the SDLC that low-cost rapid usability engineering can be applied, the literature indicates that such testing can be carried out at various stages (Kushniruk and Patel 2004). For example, in the early development of the user interface for an EHR (e.g., during the Analysis and Design phases), early prototypical designs can be analyzed by having representative users (e.g., physicians and nurses) comment on, and interact with partially functioning mock-ups and prototypes in order to determine the most effective interface. In addition, continual testing throughout the Implementation Phase is recommended as the feedback gained from end users can be used to refine the system/user interface. Finally, upon delivery of a clinical information system within an institution, the application of low-cost rapid usability engineering is highly recommended in order to ensure that systems that are beginning to be deployed are both safe and effective for end users.

An important aspect of conducting effective usability tests is the delineation of the following: (1) user classes (i.e., who are the different users or potential users of the system being designed and have they all been defined and characterized?), (2) the tasks the system will be designed to support (e.g., what tasks will the system be used for?), and (3) the context in which the system will be deployed (where will the system be implemented?). The User-Task-Context model described in the previous section can be used to decide what scenarios and use cases should be used for setting up usability testing.

7.4 Using Low-Cost Rapid Usability Engineering in Conjunction with Rapid Prototyping in UCD

Rapid prototyping uses models (ranging from paper mock-ups to wireframe models to partially functioning systems) to illustrate/simulate system functionality (Kushniruk 2002). Thus, these models depict different options about how the system *could* operate in order to gain insight and feedback from users without investing substantial time and resources in system design. For example, Axure (www.axure.com) software can be used to develop interactive wireframe mock-ups without writing any code. Similarly, Usaura (www.usaura.com) allows designers to upload screenshots or sketches and then asks users to do a task, pick from a selection or give feedback. Usaura collects a variety of data on how the users interacted with the screen (e.g., "heat maps" of user clicks, accuracy of user clicks, how long users took to click). Usaura also allows users to select their preference between display options and respond to multiple-choice questions. This software can be used to evaluate a variety of research questions (e.g., Where should a design element be placed? Which design iteration is better?). Thus, software can facilitate the development of prototypes quickly and these potential design solutions can be compared and evaluated by users.

Rapid prototyping focuses on key system functionality, and thus minimizes the time invested in system design prior to gaining user feedback about critical aspects of the system or user interface design. Moreover, rapid prototyping can be used to investigate specific system components independently. Developing components in parallel allows for the progression of other components to continue despite barriers impeding the development of specific components. Furthermore, several different solutions can be evaluated to discern the best solution before considerable investment in designing the actual system. Additionally, different ways of integrating components can be explored to determine which combinations are most successful. Thus, rapid prototyping integrates users' choice and feedback about how a system will operate with minimal expenses. Kushniruk (2002) outlines the process of incorporating rapid prototyping into system design (see Fig. 7.2). This flowchart depicts the iterative nature of rapid prototyping to refine the solution and ensure that user requirements are met by subjecting the prototypes to usability evaluations before a final solution is implemented. In Fig. 7.2, the box in the flowchart corresponding to "Prototype Testing (Usability Testing)" is the point where low-cost rapid usability testing methods can be applied.

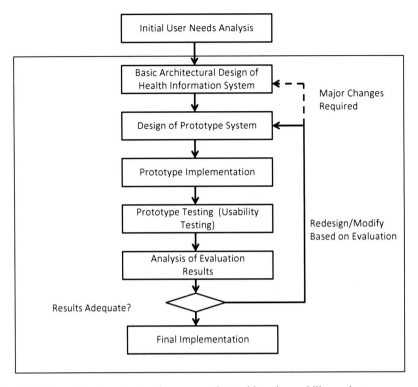

Fig. 7.2 Systems development based on prototyping and iterative usability testing

In addition, application of usability inspection methods, such as heuristic evaluation (Nielsen 1993; Nielsen and Mack 1994; Zhang et al. 2003; Carvalho et al. 2009) and cognitive walkthroughs (Kushniruk et al. 1996) are potential techniques for evaluating the usability of prototypes (a detailed description of the evaluation methods can be found in Chap. 5 in this volume). These methods do not involve observing users but rather having one or more expert analysts "stepping through" and methodically comparing the interface design against design guidelines in the case of heuristic evaluation (Nielsen 1993), and in the case of cognitive walkthrough "inspecting" areas where users might be expected to have problems by identifying user goals, actions, and system responses (Wharton et al. 1994). However, it should be noted that during rapid prototyping there is no replacement to actually observing users' interactions in terms of gaining an in-depth understanding (rather than predicting alone) of both usability and workflow problems and issues that need to be corrected on subsequent iterative cycles.

The adoption of rapid prototyping techniques in health information system design (in conjunction with usability testing) have been shown to improve the usability and usefulness of these systems while simultaneously minimizing development costs. Rapid prototyping fosters inexpensive exploration and refinement of models before a system is developed. Thus, more options are available for users to assess. In addition to *what* users are testing during system development, advancements in *how* usability tests are conducted have been made. For example, rapid approaches are now being used that can practically be incorporated within iterative prototyping cycles to feed information back into design based on analysis of user interactions with systems.

7.5 Use of Clinical Simulations in System Design and Evaluation

Clinical simulations represent a development that follows logically from usability testing methods and can be practically employed during UCD. As described above, usability testing can be characterized as involving observation of *representative users* of a system being observed/recorded while they carry out *representative tasks* (using a system being evaluated). Clinical simulations extend the realism of testing by also carrying out the evaluation in *representative environments* (i.e. settings, environments or contexts that are representative of where the system being designed or developed will ultimately be deployed in). Examples of clinical simulations include work conducted in the evaluation of medication administration systems in order to assess the impact of different system designs on usability and patient safety (Borycki et al. 2013). In a series of studies conducted "in-situ" in a hospital in Japan, realistic clinical situations were set up by using hospital rooms "after hours", where the system was to be deployed (Kushniruk et al. 2006, 2008). This approach included using mannequins (i.e. life size physical representations of the human body used in health professional education) in place of patients, as the simulations were to include not only use of computer systems in the room, but also physical interactions such as hanging intravenous bags and ergonomic aspects of the room layout (i.e. where the computer is located). This reduced the cost of setting up the in-situ testing, as the hospital room was already in place along with integration with other hospital systems and technologies. The advantages include not only reduction in cost, but also the fidelity or realism of the study was increased as the setting mirrored the actual location where the medication administration would be implemented. It also included testing the human-computer interaction involving integration with other technologies already in the hospital such as the bar code scanning technology. For this study, a User-Task-Context model was used to brainstorm a set of representative tasks that ranged from using the system to administer routine medications to medications that varied in their complexity of administration. In addition, scenarios were also created that included physical interruptions and unexpected emergency conditions. Representative users included sixteen health professionals (physicians and nurses) that were recruited to participate in 1-h sessions where they interacted with the new system to carry out the set of representative medication administration tasks. Recording of the tasks involved installing screen recording software (e.g. hypercam®) on the computer the

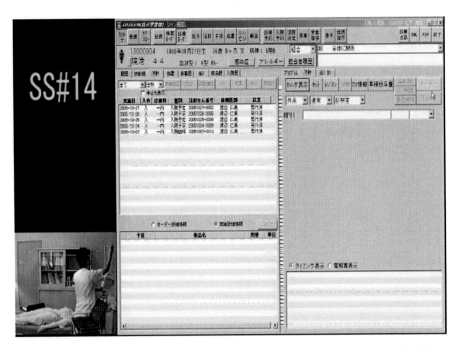

Fig. 7.3 External video view and screen view of user interactions with a medication administration system

participants accessed the medication administration system from. This allowed for recording of all user interactions with the medication administration system. In addition, a camcorder was used to obtain a wide-angle view of the physical interactions of the participants with the system and other technologies in the room (see Fig. 7.3).

Video analysis of the screen recordings in conjunction with audio recordings of users interacting in the task and external video views were integrated using Adobe® Premiere video editing software. During the analysis of the data, users' interactions were coded for: (a) usability problems in using the medication administration system, (b) ergonomic issues, and (c) issues in the integration of differing technologies (e.g. medication administration system with bar coding). The coding methodology used was modified and adapted from that described by Kushniruk and Patel (2004) and involved first transcribing all audio recordings and then observing the video and screen recordings, in order to create an annotated log file of verbalizations and actions for each participant. The interactions were coded for time taken to complete tasks and subtasks (e.g. verifying patients, reviewing medication orders, entering administration information) as well as for problems and issues encountered using the system. In addition, a post-task audio-recorded semi-structured interview was conducted to ask each participant about his or her experience in using the system. The results indicated that for routine medication administration, the system operated safely and was deemed to be usable when simple and short lists of medications were to be administered. However, as the complexity of the tasks increased it was found that the rigidity of the system locked the user into a workflow sequence, which although it supported safety (in not allowing for any deviation from a specified workflow) did pose potential safety risks when emergencies were simulated. Specifically, when a simulated emergency occurred there was not enough time for all steps to be completed in sequence (as guided by the system) and there was a need for emergency override capability. As a result of this study, such an override was included in the system design prior to widespread release (Kushniruk et al. 2006).

Carrying out system evaluation in-situ can increase the fidelity of testing while at the same time reduce costs. Another cost-effective approach involves integrating clinical simulations into the operations of simulation laboratories that are becoming increasingly commonly used for medical and nursing education purposes. An example of this is the IDX laboratory (Kushniruk et al. 2013a) that was established in Copenhagen. The laboratory was initially used for medical and nursing education purposes (i.e. computer controlled mannequins are used for training students), but has since been expanded for use in testing the usability and safety of clinical information systems. Recently, it has been used for installing candidate clinical information systems for testing those systems during a regional procurement process having the objective of selecting a system that matched the needs of users in the Copenhagen region.

Clinical simulations have fewer potential risks, offer more experimental control and are often more cost effective than testing a health information system with real patients once a system goes live. In conducting such simulations, it is valuable to build unexpected events into the simulations that emulate uncommon circumstances that occur in the real world during UCD (Kushniruk et al. 2013a). For example:

- How does the health information system react if the user is called for an emergency and there is a delayed period of non-interaction?
- What happens in the event of a power failure?
- How does the system behave if two users are trying to modify the same patient chart at the same time?

In-situ testing can be undertaken prior to implementation to minimize the potential risks of the introduction of healthcare IT. This is also a prudent approach for deployment of new electronic systems in healthcare. Specifically, a gradual roll-out of new healthcare IT enables it to be tested and limits the potential impact of technology-induced errors, whereas a "big bang" deployment of HIT has an increased potential to compromise patient safety. Further, testing should be done on a regular basis, not just at the time of deployment. Users may only find issues with the IT after months of use when they become familiar with it. Alternatively, the healthcare environment itself may evolve and may need adjustments in the HIT to accommodate these changes (Kushniruk et al. 2013a).

Clinical simulations have a number of limitations and may involve some logistical challenges. For example, although clinical simulations conducted in-situ can be cost-effective (as they do not require trying to recreate real environments) they do require permission and access to real local environments (e.g. hospital rooms) in order to carry out simulation studies (typically when such environments are not being used for patient care, such as after hours). On the other hand, conducting clinical simulations in fixed laboratories does not require such permission. However, such fixed laboratories can be expensive to build and require expertise in running the equipment. The cost may be leveraged by developing facilities for testing information systems within simulation laboratories that may already be in place for training healthcare professionals (e.g. medical and nursing students).

7.6 A Layered Approach to Evaluating Clinical Information Systems for Ensuring Usability and Safety

Thorough testing is a critical component for revealing the possible usability and system safety issues. As such, the Institute of Medicine (2012) argued "it is critical to test HIT during *all stages* of development to determine whether user requirements have been translated into software that actually does what the user wants" (p. 96). An effective approach to improving patient safety requires continuous testing (Borycki and Keay 2010). In addition, it is recommended that the fidelity of the testing environment should be gradually increased from low fidelity (e.g., an office laboratory), to medium fidelity (e.g., clinical simulation), to high fidelity (e.g., in-situ) (Kushniruk 2002; Kushniruk et al. 2013a). It is important to investigate the system in a variety of settings to reveal as many potential problems and shortcomings as possible.

In applying usability engineering in clinical informatics, system testing can (and ideally should) include a focus on the examination of the user and system (Level 1 in Fig. 7.4). From a theoretical perspective, this level can be seen as corresponding to the Human Information Processor model, which views user interactions with information systems as involving two "information processors": the human end user and the computer system (Newell and Simon 1972). At this level of testing, surface level usability problems (e.g., navigational problems, user interface consistency problems) can be readily detected. This can be followed by evaluation of use of the system in carrying out work tasks (Level 2). At this level, issues involving workflow inefficiencies and potential safety problems when using the system to carry out work tasks can often be detected. Finally, consideration of use of the system within the complex organizational setting is needed (Level 3). From a theoretical perspective, these last two levels can be construed as being at the level of distributed cognition – that is, cognition that is distributed amongst multiple intelligent agents, including various computer systems, people and representations (Patel and Kaufman 2006). This multi-layered approach to considering testing for usability and safety borrows from the three layers of human-computer interaction as

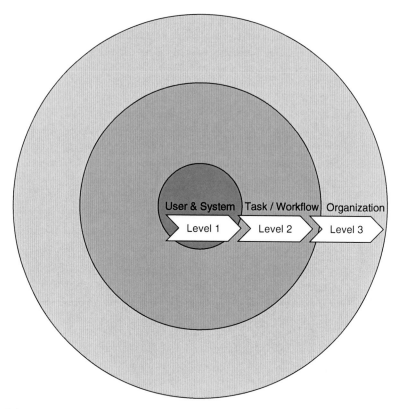

Fig. 7.4 Depiction of a layered approach to clinical information system evaluation

described by Eason (1991) and expanded on by Kushniruk et al. (2008) in the context of healthcare IT.

In our work, we have applied such a layered approach to organizing and conducting evaluations and analyses of clinical information systems. For example, in recent work conducted by Li and colleagues (2012), clinical guidelines designed for incorporation into a commercial electronic health record (EHR) system were tested using this multi-layered approach prior to being released within a large American healthcare organization. In the first phase of testing, physicians interacted with the initial prototype of the guideline design in isolation using a "traditional" laboratory-style usability testing approach that involved asking subjects to "think aloud". Based on this analysis, a variety of surface level usability problems were identified (with this level of analysis corresponding to Level 1 of Fig. 7.4). After a phase of refining the guidelines and their integration into the underlying EHR, a second phase of testing was subsequently conducted which involved observing physicians interacting with the guidelines embedded in the EHR while interviewing a "digital" patient (a video clip of a patient designed to elicit the physician's preferred way of interacting with the guidelines). This phase represented a clinical simulation, and corresponds to Level 2 of the layers described above (i.e., using the

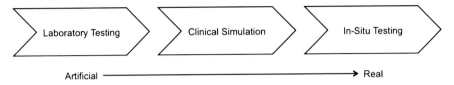

Laboratory Testing   Clinical Simulation   In-Situ Testing

Artificial ──────────────────────────────────────→ Real

Fig. 7.5 Continuum of studies to ensure system safety prior to release

system to carry out a work task involving not only the computer, but one or more other active participants). Based on results from this layer of testing it was found that the guidelines often triggered at an inappropriate point during user interaction, requiring refinement of the guidelines. In a final layer of testing, corresponding to Level 3 (i.e., testing in a socially complex setting or environment), physicians' interaction with the guidelines were recorded for a limited number of live patient interactions before deploying the system more widely. After optimizing their design, once released on a large scale, the guidelines were readily adopted by end users throughout the institution. In summary, the approach essentially moves from the artificial to the more realistic, naturalistic setting in sequence (see Fig. 7.5).

7.7   Implications of User-Centered Design for Both Improved Usability and System Safety

A major concern with serious usability problems or issues is that they may lead to medical error (Kushniruk et al. 2005). For example, if the layout of information on the screens of an electronic health record make it difficult for users to locate key information (e.g., a patient's drug allergies), then it becomes more likely that such information might not be accounted for when prescribing new medications. Furthermore, healthcare can be characterized by conditions that might cause errors, including high workloads, poor interface designs, stressful and fast-paced environments, and fatigue (Reason 1995). Thus, it is important to employ UCD coupled with usability engineering methods as a means to improve system usability and patient safety in healthcare. However, healthcare systems pose unique challenges for UCD because situations are dynamic and tasks fluctuate according to circumstances (Carayon 2012; Carvalho et al. 2009). That is, not all patients can be treated the same way or will have the same outcomes for any given treatment. Furthermore, human error in healthcare (that could be a result of poor user interface design) can result in serious medical error (Borycki et al. 2012). Recent research has indicated that the deployment of new health information systems actually has the potential to introduce technology-induced errors (Borycki and Kushniuk 2008; Borycki et al. 2009). Having increased input from healthcare providers during design and development improves the likelihood that new systems will maximize efficiency, minimize errors, and be compatible with their workflow. Further, given that healthcare is always in flux, it is imperative that systems are flexible so they can adapt to the needs and challenges of any situation.

Recently, the Institute of Medicine's (2012) report entitled *Health IT and Patient Safety: Building Safer Systems for Better Care* has indicated the need for greater emphasis on testing with end users in the design process (i.e., a user-centered design). Improved usability (e.g., easy navigation, simple intuitive data displays) was identified as being important for improving HIT safety (IOM 2012). However, successful and safe system development rests on the realization that UCD and application of user testing is a continuous process and not just a singular event at a particular stage of HIT development. UCD methods in conjunction with usability engineering should be applied throughout system development, and may involve not only usability testing but also use of in-situ clinical simulations and observation of naturalistic use of system to ensure system usability and safety (Kushniruk et al. 2013a).

In order to increase safety of systems, a number of standards have also emerged for design of user interfaces, including some that are general, and others that are specific to HIT. For example, the National Institute of Standards and Technology in the United States has developed the Common Industry Specification for Usability (NISTIR 2007), which can be used to guide system development. Other guidelines have been developed around the area of designing more usable user interfaces for web accessible systems (Usability.gov 2014). In health informatics, examples of user interface guidelines include work towards developing a common user interface for EHR systems (MCUI 2014). In addition, this has led to more specific guidelines to help in designing and assessing user interfaces involving medications or devices, such as the United Kingdom's National Health Services design for patient safety guidelines (NHS 2014). By providing more standards and well thought out guidelines to aid in design and evaluation of clinical information systems, it is expected that the potential for technology-induced error will be reduced and the learning time for mastering the use of systems will also be reduced (Kushniruk et al. 2013b).

7.8   Discussion and Future Trends

There are a number of new directions and trends in usability engineering for supporting improved design of clinical information systems. One trend involves conducting usability data collection remotely. Along these lines, the term "televaluation" has been used to describe "virtual" usability engineering (Kushniruk et al. 2001). Using this approach, system users and experimenters can be located anywhere in the world, making it readily feasible and reducing costs associated with transporting users or testers to fixed locations to carry out usability evaluations. This may involve remotely recording users interacting with systems by using remote screen monitoring and Web conferencing tools with screen sharing capabilities. Such remote testing can be carried out simply and inexpensively using remote screen sharing where the user's screens and audio (from the remote location) are seen by the experimenter on their computer (and recorded from the experimenter's computer). Moreover, variations in televaluation can also now allow for remote automated and simultaneous testing of a system in an array of different environments. Thus, usability issues that may only arise in specific environments can be identified early in the design phase. Furthermore, by removing the presence of a researcher, and any external equipment, it is less likely that participants will be affected by their participation in an experiment (Heppner et al. 2008). Televaluations typically entail "recording all human–computer inter-action (i.e., video recording all computer screens) and audio-recording all subject verbalizations as they interact with system prototypes" (Kushniruk et al. 2001). The findings from virtual usability testing can include: (1) suggestions by users for improvements to both the user interface and system functionality, (2) identification of usability problems such as lack of consistency in interface operations, and (3) quantitative measurements including time for task completion and system response times. This data can be used to create suggestions to improve health information systems' design to enhance the interface and functionality, ameliorate usability issues and reduce the time to complete tasks.

An approach known as the "Virtual Usability Laboratory" (VuLab) has been piloted to allow for both remote data collection and collation of large amounts of user tracking data, subjective questionnaire and automated interview data and other forms of both quantitative and qualitative data that can be automatically collected from any number of users of a system remotely. To aid researchers and developers in analyzing this type of data the VuLab also contains automated tools for data analysis and summarization of usability data collected remotely. The approach has been used to evaluate use of clinical guidelines in Canada, and feedback from this study has been used to refine both content and sequencing of clinical guidelines as well as health related content targeted to patients (Kushniruk et al. 2007, 2008; Wideman et al. 2007).

Another area of future research from a practical perspective includes develop-ment of rapid and automated or semi-automated methods to speed up analyses of usability data to fit in rapid prototyping and agile approaches to UCD. In order for the methods to be employed more widely, this is perhaps one of the greatest challenges. Methodological approaches such as low-cost rapid usability engineer-ing (Kushniruk et al. 2006) and IDA (Instant Data Analysis) (Kjeldskov et al. 2004) are attempts at reducing schedule and cost barriers to application of usability testing in system design and deployment. Other approaches to increasing the speed of usability analyses for incorporation into rapid prototyping include the work of Dumas and Salzman (2006) in the development of the Rapid Iterative Test and Evaluation (RITE) method. The RITE method argues for continually repeating the same evaluation tasks and redesigning until the problems have been fixed or until there are no more resources. The RUE (Rapid Usability Evaluation) method also attempts to reduce the time required to complete the appropriate sections of the testing method (Russ et al. 2010). Although these approaches attempt to speed up time and lessen resources needed for user testing, rapid and agile application of usability testing in the design and deployment of many health information systems has not yet become the norm. However, with methodological advances including potential for automation of testing processes, the situation may gradually improve. In addition, critical comparison of methodological approaches (Jaspers 2009) is essential for determination of the most appropriate and practical methods for carrying out usability engineering in healthcare.

7.9 Conclusion

The usability and safety of healthcare information systems depend on improved input from users in design. In this chapter, we have discussed approaches to UCD that incorporate key elements from usability engineering. The application of these approaches is necessary for not only ensuring the usability of clinical information systems, but also their safety. It should be noted that the approaches described in this chapter have also begun to be used in the selection and procurement of clinical information systems that better match user needs in clinical settings, in addition to their use during the design and implementation processes (Kushniruk et al. 2010). In addition, the extension of usability testing to clinical simulations is leading to new ways of testing systems in order to identify and prevent both usability errors and safety hazards. A key aspect of more widely introducing these methods into HIT and health informatics is that of reducing the cost and effort required to apply usability engineering in healthcare. Along these lines, research has already begun to indicate that the effort in terms of cost and manpower to apply the methods described in this chapter is well worth the effort (Baylis et al. 2012).

Discussion Questions
1. What are the essential characteristics of user-centered design (UCD)?
2. What are the issues and challenges in applying UCD in healthcare IT design?
3. What are some of the main issues in understanding and representing user needs as a basis of UCD in healthcare?
4. How can usability testing methods be practically applied in UCD and rapid prototyping?
5. How do clinical simulations extend usability testing approaches?

Additional Readings

Kushniruk, A. (2002). Evaluation in the design of health information systems: Application of approaches emerging from usability engineering. *Computers in Biology and Medicine, 32*(3), 141–149.

Kushniruk, A. W., & Borycki, E. M. (2006). Low-cost rapid usability engineering: Designing and customizing usable healthcare information systems. *Healthcare Quarterly, 9*(4), 98–100.

Kushniruk, A. W., & Patel, V. L. (2004). Cognitive and usability engineering approaches to the evaluation of clinical information systems. *Journal of Biomedical Informatics, 37*(1), 56–76.

Kushniruk, A., Nohr, C., Jensen, S., & Borycki, E. M. (2013). From usability testing to clinical simulations: Bringing context into the design and evaluation of usable and safe health information technologies. *Yearbook of Medical Informatics, 8*(1), 78–85.

Preece, J., Rogers, Y., & Sharp, H. (2011). *Interaction design: Beyond human-computer interaction* (3rd ed.). New York: Wiley.

References

Baylis, T., Kushniruk, A. W., & Borycki, E. M. (2012). Low-cost usability for health information systems: Is it worth the effort? *Studies in Health Technology and Informatics, 180*, 363–367.

Beuscart-Zéphir, M. C., Pelayo, S., Ancequx, F., Meaux, J., Degroisse, M., & Degoulet, P. (2005). Impact of CPOE on doctor–nurse cooperation for the medication ordering and administration process. *International Journal of Medical Informatics, 74*(7), 629–641.

Borycki, E., & Keay, E. (2010). Methods to assess the safety of health information systems. *Healthcare Quarterly, 13*, 49–54.

Borycki, E., & Kushniruk, A. W. (2005). Identifying and preventing technology-induced error using simulations: Application of usability engineering techniques. *Healthcare Quarterly, 8*, 99–105.

Borycki, E. M., & Kushniuk, A. W. (2008). Where do technology-induced errors come from? Towards a model for conceptualizing and diagnosing errors caused by technology. In A. W. Kushniruk & E. M. Borycki (Eds.), *Human, social and organizational aspects of health information systems* (pp. 148–166). Hershey: IGI Global.

Borycki, E. M., Kushniruk, A., Keay, E., Nicoll, J., Anderson, J., & Anderson, M. (2009). Toward an integrated simulation approach for predicting and preventing technology-induced errors in healthcare: Implications for healthcare decision-makers. *Healthcare Quarterly, 12*, 90–96.

Borycki, E. M., Kushniruk, A. W., Kuwata, S., & Kannry, J. (2011). Engineering the electronic health record for safety: A multi-level video-based approach to diagnosing and preventing technology-induced error arising from usability problems. *Studies in Health Technology and Informatics, 164*, 197–205.

Borycki, E. M., Kushniruk, A. W., Bellwood, P., & Brender, J. (2012). Technology-induced errors: The current use of frameworks and models from the biomedical and life sciences literatures. *Methods of Information Medicine, 51*(2), 95–103.

Borycki, E., Kushniruk, A., Nohr, C., Takeda, H., Kuwata, S., Carvalho, C., Bainbridge, M., & Kannry, J. (2013). Usability methods for ensuring health information technology safety. *Yearbook of Medical Informatics, 8*(1), 20–27.

Carayon, P. (2012). *Handbook of human factors and ergonomics in health care and patient safety* (2nd ed.). Boca Raton: CRC Press.

Carroll, J. M. (1995). *Scenario-based design: Envisioning work and technology in system development*. New York: Wiley.

Carvalho, C. J., Borycki, E. M., & Kushniruk, A. W. (2009). Ensuring the safety of health information systems: Using heuristics for patient safety. *Healthcare Quarterly, 12*, 49–54.

Damodaran, L. (1996). User involvement in the systems design process – A practical guide for users. *Behaviour & Information Technology, 15*(6), 363–377.

Dumas, J. S., & Salzman, M. C. (2006). Usability assessment methods. *Reviews of Human Factors and Ergonomics, 2*(1), 109–140.

Eason, K. D. (1991). Ergonomics perspective on advances in human-computer interaction. *Ergonomics, 34*(6), 721–741.

Gould, J. D., & Lewis, C. (1985). Designing for usability: Key principles and what designers think. *Communications of the ACM, 28*(3), 300–311.

Hackos, J. T., & Redish, J. C. (1998). *User and task analysis for interface design*. New York: Wiley.

Heppner, P. P., Wampold, B. E., & Kivlighan, D. M. (2008). *Research design in counseling* (3rd ed.). New York: Thomson.

Institute of Medicine (U.S.). Committee on Patient Safety and Health Information Technology. (2012). *Health IT and patient safety: Building safer systems for better care*. Washington, DC: National Academies Press.

Jaspers, M. W. (2009). A comparison of usability methods for testing interactive health technologies: Methodological aspects and empirical evidence. *International Journal of Medical Informatics, 78*, 340–353.

Johnson, T. R., Johnson, C. M., & Zhang, J. (2005). A user-centered framework for redesigning health care interfaces. *Journal of Biomedical Informatics, 38*(1), 75–87.

Karat, J. (1997). Evolving the scope of user-centered design. *Association for Computing Machinery. Communications of the ACM, 40*(7), 33.

Kaufman, D. R., Patel, V. L., Hilliman, C., Morin, P. C., Pevzner, J., Weinstock, R. S., & Starren, J. (2003). Usability in the real world: Assessing medical information technologies in patients' homes. *Journal of Biomedical Informatics, 36*(1), 45–60.

Kjeldskov, J., Skov, M. B., & Stage, J. (2004). Instant data analysis: Conducting usability evaluations in a day. In *NordiCHI '04* (pp. 233–240). ACM.

Koppel, R., Metlay, J., Cohen, A., Abaluck, B., Localio, A., Kimmel, S., & Strom, B. (2005). Role of CPOE in facilitating medication errors. *Journal of the American Medical Association, 293* (10), 1197–1203.

Kujala, S. (2003). User involvement: A review of the benefits and challenges. *Behaviour & Information Technology, 22*(1), 1–16.

Kushniruk, A. W., & Borycki, E. M. (2006). Low-cost rapid usability engineering: Designing and customizing usable healthcare information systems. *Healthcare Quarterly, 9*(4), 98–102.

Kushniruk, A., & Turner, P. (2012). A framework for user involvement and context in the design and development of safe e-Health systems. *Studies in Health Technology and Informatics, 180*, 353–357.

Kushniruk, A. W., Kaufman, D. R., Patel, V. L., Levesque, Y., & Lottin, P. (1996). Assessment of a computerized patient record system: A cognitive approach to evaluating an emerging medical technology. *M.D. Computing, 13*(5), 406–415.

Kushniruk, A. W., Patel, C., Patel, V. L., & Cimino, J. J. (2001). 'Televaluation' of clinical information systems: An integrative approach to assessing web-based systems. *International Journal of Medical Informatics, 61*(1), 45–70.

Kushniruk, A. W., Triola, M., Borycki, E. M., Stein, B., & Kannry, J. (2005). Technology induced error and usability: The relationship between usability problems and prescription errors when using a handheld application. *International Journal of Medical Informatics, 74*(7–8), 519–526.

Kushniruk, A., Owston, R., Ho, F., Pitts, K., Wideman, H., Brown, C., & Chu, S. (2007, February). Design of the VULab: A quantitative and qualitative tool for analyzing use of on-line health information resources. In *Proceedings of ITCH 2007*, Victoria, BC, Canada.

Kushniruk, A. W., Borycki, E. M., Kuwata, S., & Watanabe, H. (2008). Using a low-cost simulation for assessing the impact of a medication administration system on workflow. *Studies in Health Technology and Informatics, 136*, 567–572.

Kushniruk, A. W., Beuscart-Zephir, M. C., Grzes, A., Borycki, E., Watbled, L., & Kannry, J. (2010, September). Increasing the safety of healthcare information systems through improved procurement: Toward a framework for selection of safe healthcare systems. *Healthcare Quarterly, 13*, 53–58.

Kushniruk, A. W., Bates, D. W., Bainbridge, M., Househ, M., & Borycki, E. (2013). National efforts to improve health information system safety in Canada, the United States of America and England. *International Journal of Medical Informatics, 82*(5), e149–e160.

Li, A. C., Kannry, J. L., Kushniruk, A., Chrimes, D., McGinn, T. G., Edonyabo, D., & Mann, D. M. (2012). Integrating usability testing and think-aloud protocol analysis with "near live" clinical simulations in evaluating clinical decision support. *International Journal of Medical Informatics, 81*(11), 761–772.

Mao, J. Y., Vrendenburg, K., Smith, P. W., & Carey, T. (2005). The state of user-centered design practice. *IEEE Engineering Management Review, 33*(2), 51.

MCUI. (2014). *Microsoft common user interface.* Accessed from http://www.mscui.net/

Newell, A., & Simon, H. A. (1972). *Human problem solving.* Englewood Cliffs: Prentice-Hall.

NHS. (2014). *National health service – Design for patient safety guidelines.* Accessed from http://www.nrls.npsa.nhs.uk/resources/collections/design-for-patient-safety/

Nielsen, J. (1993). *Usability engineering.* San Diego: Academic.

Nielsen, J., & Mack, R. L. (1994). *Usability inspection methods.* New York: Wiley.

NISTR. (2007). *Common industry specification for usability requirments – NISTIR 7432.* Accessed from http://zing.ncsl.nist.gov/iusr/documents/CISU-R-IR7432.pdf

Patel, V. L., & Kaufman, D. (2006). Cognitive science and biomedical informatics. In E. Shortliffe & J. Cimino (Eds.), *Biomedical informatics: Computer applications in health care and biomedicine.* London: Springer.

Patel, V. L., & Kushniruk, A. W. (1998). Interface design for health care environments: The role of cognitive science. In *Proceedings of the AMIA symposium* (p. 29). In C. Chute (Ed.), Philadelphia: Hanley & Belfus, Inc.

Reason, J. (1995). Understanding adverse events: Human factors. *Quality in Health Care, 4*, 80–89.

Rouse, W. B. (1991). *Design for success: A human-centered approach to designing successful products and systems.* New York: Wiley.

Russ, A. L., Baker, D. A., Fahner, W. J., Milligan, B. S., Cox, L., Hagg, H. K., & Salleem, J. J. (2010). A rapid usability evaluation method (RUE) method for health information technology. In *AMIA 2010 symposium proceedings* (pp. 702–706). Bethusda, MD: American Medical Informatics Association.

Saffer, D. (2007). *Designing for interaction: Creating smart applications and clever devices.* Berkeley: New Riders.

Usabilility.gov. (2014). *Usabilility.gove – Improving the user experience.* Accessed from http://guidelines.usability.gov/

Wharton, C., Rieman, J., Lewis, C., & Polson, P. (1994). The cognitive walkthrough method: A practitioner's guide. In J. Nielsen & R. Mack (Eds.), *Usability inspection methods.* New York: Wiley.

Wideman, H., Owston, R., Brown, C., Kushniruk, A., Ho, F., & Pitts, K. (2007, March). Unpacking the potential of educational gaming: A new tool for gaming research. *Simulation & Gaming, 38*(1), 1–21.

Zhang, J., Johnson, T. R., Patel, V. L., Paige, D. L., & Kubose, T. (2003). Using usability heuristics to evaluate patient safety of medical devices. *Journal of Biomedical Informatics, 36*(1), 23–30.

Chapter 8
Human Computer Interaction in Medical Devices

Todd R. Johnson, Harold Thimbleby, Peter Killoran, and J. Franck Diaz-Garelli

8.1 Introduction

Intuitively, we might think of a medical device as any tool that is specifically designed for health or for promoting health. Although this intuitive notion is sufficient for everyday purposes, it is not sufficient for medical device designers. What counts as a medical device, and the requirements for testing, using, and selling a device, are defined through regulations and standards that are designed to protect the safety of patients and caregivers. These regulations are one of several factors that affect the user interface design and evaluation of medical devices. Others include the safety-critical nature of medical devices, the diversity of users, extreme and noisy use environments, the lack of user interface standards for medical devices, and the small physical space often available for the user interface.

This chapter provides an introduction to medical device HCI regulations and the challenges that result from the regulatory requirements and the complexity and variation within healthcare. We demonstrate these challenges using specific examples along with two case studies: one showing how HCI and broader human factors engineering played a major role in reducing deaths related to the use of anesthesia machines, and another showing how simple changes to number entry interfaces can decrease the chance of serious medical errors.

T.R. Johnson, Ph.D. (✉) • P. Killoran, M.S., M.D. • J.F. Diaz-Garelli, M.S.
School of Biomedical Informatics, University of Texas Health Science Center at Houston, Houston, TX, USA
e-mail: todd.r.johnson@uth.tmc.edu

H. Thimbleby, FRCPE, HonFRCP, Ph.D.
Department of Computer Science, Swansea University, Swansea, Wales, UK

© Springer International Publishing Switzerland 2015
V.L. Patel et al. (eds.), *Cognitive Informatics for Biomedicine*, Health Informatics,
DOI 10.1007/978-3-319-17272-9_8

8.2   Human Computer Interaction and Related Fields

The field of human computer interaction is intimately concerned with medical devices because medical devices are used by humans (usually caregivers, but increasingly patients) and they often include computers. HCI is not concerned so much with whether a device performs within technical specifications, but with other important matters like whether it is usable, helps reduce error, and is enjoyable to use (Carroll 2003). HCI helps make informed trade-offs, for example, how to make a device smaller without making it too small for people to use (for instance because the screen is illegible), or how to make a system secure, but not so secure that nobody can use it or so secure that everybody reverts to sticking password reminders up, and thus circumventing the security features. HCI thus covers a very broad range of important topics that help improve the safety, ease of use and user satisfaction of medical devices. Different emphases on analytic foci and different types of methods emerge from different areas of inquiry concerned with devices:

- **HF**, Human Factors (sometimes called **ergonomics**)—the study of how humans perform and behave, particularly while operating complex systems or working in complex environments, often with tough working conditions such as interruptions, fatigue, vibration and so forth.
- **HFE**, Human Factors Engineering—human factors specifically used to help engineer or design improved working environments and systems.
- **HCI**, Human Computer Interaction (sometimes CHI, which is more pronounceable)—many complex systems involve computers; hence, HCI is HF and HFE in the context of complex, computer-based systems.
- **UCD**, User Centered Design—a key slogan of HCI and HFE; to design a system for human use, one must focus, or center, design efforts on the user and their tasks.
- **UX**, User Experience—originally, HFE focused on work environments and performance of work-related goals; in contrast, UX emphasizes the experience of the user rather than the organization. Do they enjoy their work? Of course, if users have a good experience, their work will improve too!

8.3   Why Should We Be Concerned About HCI?

We all know what we like and what we find easy to use. Some companies, like Apple, are adept at capitalizing on this and designing devices we enjoy using. However, what we enjoy using and what makes for a safe and reliable experience for professionals to use to perform demanding clinical tasks can be very different. In particular, user errors occur primarily because the errors are not noticed; and if we do not notice our own errors, how can we possibly know what is best in environments where errors may have disastrous consequences? In addition, people are very different and our own skills and preferences—with which we are very familiar—are not a good indicator of anyone else's skills and preferences. In short, to design or procure safe and usable systems for other people to use requires an understanding of scientific principles and methods that underlie user-centered design (UCD), which is aimed at ensuring we do not misunderstand what or who we are designing for.

8.4   What Is a Medical Device?

The U.S. Federal Food, Drug, and Cosmetic Act (Office of the Commissioner 2002) defines a medical device as "an instrument, apparatus, implement, machine, contrivance, implant, *in vitro* reagent, or other similar or related article, including a component part, or accessory that is:

- Recognized in the official National Formulary, or the US Pharmacopoeia, or any supplement to them,
- Intended for use in the diagnosis of disease or other conditions, or in the cure, mitigation, treatment, or prevention of disease, in man or other animals, or
- Intended to affect the structure or any function of the body of man or other animals, and which does not achieve any of its primary intended purposes through chemical action within or on the body of man or other animals and which is not dependent upon being metabolized for the achievement of any of its primary intended purposes."

This definition offers an initial starting point for device manufacturers. In practice, whether a device is considered a "medical device" and the legal requirements to market a medical device are complex. In 2011, the FDA issued draft guidance indicating that they intend to apply regulatory oversight to mobile medical applications that meet the above definition of a medical device and "whose functionality could pose a risk to a patient's safety if the mobile application were to not function as intended" (U.S. Department of Health and Human Services, Food and Drug Administration 2013). There is also considerable controversy over Electronic Health Records (EHRs) and other forms of HIT, with some arguing that EHRs should be classified and regulated as high risk medical devices (Institute of Medicine 2012).

The European Union (EU) uses a similar, but not identical, definition of medical devices (The Council of the European Communities 2007). Specific details and differences of the definitions and regulations around the world are beyond the scope of this chapter. In the rest of this chapter, we will use the FDA framework as an example of how regulations affect HCI. Since regulations vary by region and change over time, HCI designers must be aware of current regulations for their target market early in the design process. When a medical device is marketed in different countries, HCI expertise is also needed to balance international issues, cultural differences, and so on to ensure devices are usable where they are needed.

8.5 Regulatory History and Human Factors Engineering Requirements

The Federal Food, Drug, and Cosmetic Act (FFDCA) of 1938 contributed to the formal definition of a medical device and its status in law. The Food and Drug Administration's (FDA) mission was to determine whether a device was safe and effective as opposed to defective, unsafe, filthy, or produced in unsanitary conditions (adulterated), or against statements, designs, or labeling that was false or misleading (misbranded). Enforcement was predominantly based on post-market inspection and complaints, until the 1960s when the FDA shifted to more proactive oversight of life-saving devices and medical equipment as opposed to screening for fraudulent and dangerous products.

In 1976, new legislation defined devices and divided them into three classes based on potential risks, with varying regulatory control for each class (*Medical Device Amendments of* 1976). Class I devices are those that have minimal potential for harm, such as dental floss and elastic bandages. Many Class I devices are exempt from the regulatory process. Class II devices have greater potential for harm, such as powered wheelchairs. Class III devices are those with the highest potential risks, such as replacement heart valves, breast implants, and implantable pacemakers.

The Medical Device Amendments Act of 1976 also established the provisions for pre-market notifications (the so-called 510 k) (U.S. Food and Drug Administration, Center for Devices and Radiological Health 2014), and inspection and enforcement of good manufacturing practices (U.S. Food and Drug Administration 2008).

In 1995, the Association for the Advancement of Medical Instrumentation (AAMI) and the FDA held a joint conference in Washington D.C. to discuss human factors and medical devices (Association for the Advancement of Medical Instrumentation 1996). This was the first large scale attempt to include human factors in FDA regulations. Two publications were key to the evolution of manufacturing standards and made human factors an active part of the design process for the first time. *Quality System – Design Controls Regulations* were published under 21 CFR part 820 in 1996 (61 FR 52602) and went into effect in 1997, harmonizing requirements to international standards, primarily, the International Organization for Standards (ISO) 9001:1994 series of quality standards (International Organization for Standardization 1994). From an HCI perspective, the most important clause in the Design Controls Regulations states "Design validation shall ensure that devices conform to defined user needs and intended uses and shall include testing of production units under actual or simulated use conditions." The second important publication, *Do it by design: An introduction to human factors in medical devices,* was issued in 1996 as guidance to help medical device manufacturers take human factors into account during product design phases (Sawyer 1996).

In 2000, the FDA's Center for Devices and Radiological Health (CDRH) released human factors guidance including that "human error" should be considered in risk analysis (Kaye and Crowley 2000). In 2001, the American National Standards Institutes (ANSI) and the AAMI released standard HE74 *Human Factors Design Process for Medical Devices* (Association for the Advancement of Medical Instrumentation 2001). In 2006, the International Electrical Commission (IEC) released standard 60601-1-6 on medical electrical equipment, which included human factors of alarm systems (Part 1–6: *General requirements for basic safety and essential performance – Collateral standard: Usability*) (International Electrochemical Commission 2006). In 2007, the IEC released standard 62366, *Application of usability engineering to medical devices* (International Electrochemical Commission 2007), and ANSI/AAMI/ISO released 14971:2007, detailing how human factors engineering can be used as part of risk analysis (International Organization for Standardization 2007). In 2009, the ANSI and the AAMI released standard HE75:2009 *Human Factors Engineering – Design of Medical Devices* (Association for the Advancement of Medical Instrumentation 2009).

In addition to pre-market requirements, regulations also cover post-market surveillance of medical devices. Manufacturers, importers, and device user facilities are required to report all device-related adverse events and product problems, which includes reporting of "use errors": outcomes that are different than intended due to the way a device was used, but not caused by malfunctions. In addition, the FDA encourages healthcare professionals, patients, caregivers, and consumers to voluntarily submit reports. Reports going back to 1991 are publicly available online through a web-based search engine called MAUDE (Manufacturer and User Facility Device Experience) ("MAUDE – Manufacturer and User Facility Device Experience" n.d.). MAUDE can be used for downloading data for importing into databases. These reports are an important source of information regarding possible human factors issues with medical devices; however, they must be used with caution because there is often insufficient data to determine whether a use error was due to a design problem or to a user problem. In addition, the data cannot be used to evaluate rates of adverse events or compare rates across devices, due to the incomplete nature of the reports and lack of availability of the number of devices in use at the time of the report.

At present, the regulatory environment continues to evolve. For example, the Institute of Medicine recently issued a report, at the FDA's request, of the 510 (k) clearance process (Council 2011). This refers to Section 510(k) of the FFDCA, which outlines a streamlined pre-market approval process for medical devices that are "substantially equivalent" to an existing device that was cleared through the same process. The IOM report finds that the 510(k) process is flawed because many existing devices were never assessed for safety and effectiveness. As a result, 510 (k) clearance is not a determination that a device is safe and effective. They recommend that the FDA develop a new integrated pre-market and post-market regulatory system, instead of continuing to modify the existing system.

Taken together, the regulations, guidance documents and recognized standards offer both general and specific guidelines and recommendations for applying human factors engineering to medical device design including documentation requirements for devices that require FDA approval. Many of the standards include extensive background material and references for further reading. Before beginning any medical device interface design project, it is essential for HCI designers to have a thorough understanding of these documents.

8.6 Impact of Medical Device Design on Patient Safety

Many studies have examined the role and extent of human factors issues on errors involving medical devices. Overall, these reports indicate that more problems are caused by device-use errors than device failures. An early study showed that 82 % of all preventable medical errors involving anesthesia devices were due to human error (Cooper et al. 1984). Another suggested that patients may be 3–10 times more at risk due to user error than to device failure (Grant 1998). A study of errors involving infusion pumps found that the most frequent cause of patient harm was user error and inadequate device education (McConnell et al. 1996). It is important to note that use error does not mean the user is at fault; many use errors have multiple causes, including poor training, poor device design, overwork, fatigue and interruptions, poor operating procedures and even poor handwriting. In fact, FDA data collected between 1985 and 1989 demonstrated that 45–50 % of device recalls stemmed from poor product design (O'Connel n.d.). More recent studies suggest that, despite efforts to improve device user interfaces and safety, device use errors continue to be a substantial source of adverse events. For example, studies of "smart" infusion pumps (which contain dose error reduction systems sensitive to drugs and safe dosing ranges) have found that they have had only limited effects on patient safety (Brannon 2006; Cummings and McGowan 2011; Rothschild et al. 2005; Trbovich et al. 2010).

The limited impact of efforts to improve device safety mirrors the generally limited results of more than a decade of effort to improve patient safety in the US, despite demonstrated success in controlled studies of specific interventions (Wachter et al. 2013).

8.7 Unique Challenges of Medical Device Design

Usability is ultimately a product of the interplay of a device (including its user interface), its use environment, its user(s), the characteristics of the patients who are being treated, and the tasks being performed with the device. Although device manufacturers must consider all of these elements, the diversity, complexity, and ever-changing nature of healthcare poses design problems that common methods of user-centered design do not adequately address. Below we review each of these areas in the context of medical device design.

8.7.1 Medical Device Users

Users of medical devices range from healthcare professionals to patients and their family members. Professionals are more likely to understand the medical role of devices, have experience using the devices, and may be familiar with similar devices. However, professionals often must use a number of similar devices of different models by the same or multiple manufacturers. For example, the same hospital may use different models of infusion pumps, each with user interfaces that may be very or just slightly different. This diversity in design may be for historical reasons (older and newer devices in the same setting), clinical reasons (some models are better for certain areas of care or tasks), or because the user works in multiple healthcare settings. Although familiarity with a family of devices can have positive transfer of skill effects, it can also lead to negative transfer where the user's knowledge of one device leads to use errors on a different device (Gosbee 2002; Woltz et al. 2000). Healthcare professionals also tend to be extremely busy, which can result in limited time for formal training on new devices. This increases their need to rely on their mental models and operating knowledge of previous devices— knowledge that may not correctly transfer to the new device.

An increasing number of devices are being used outside traditional healthcare settings by patients or lay-caregivers. In some cases, these devices are specifically designed for non-professional users and settings. One common example are glucose meters, which had significant problems in early designs (Rogers et al. 2001). In other cases, patients and lay-caregivers must use devices that were designed for healthcare professionals operating in a clinical setting.

Designing medical devices for non-professional users is challenging because these users exhibit much more variation in abilities and knowledge than healthcare professionals. They may have a wide range of physical, cognitive or perceptual disabilities, and their educational background and understanding of the clinical context can vary greatly. Although non-professional users may need to go through training prior to device use, their actual use is much harder to monitor than in more controlled, professional settings.

In April 2010, the FDA issued the Medical Device Home Use Initiative guidance document (U.S. Food and Drug Administration Center for Devices and Radiological Health 2010). It lists caregiver knowledge, device usability, and environmental unpredictability as three unique challenges. A companion draft guidance document, issued in 2012, provides design considerations for medical devices intended for home use (U.S. Food and Drug Administration, Center for Devices and Radiological Health 2012). Many of the recommendations address the differences between professional and non-professional users. For instance, the guidance specifically recommends that designers take literacy level and emotional issues into consideration, and design the interface so that it is "inherently apparent to users how to use the device."

There is considerable need for additional research on designing medical devices to accommodate a wide variety of user characteristics. More accessible medical devices could benefit both non-professional and professional users, because as the workforce ages, professional users will face some of the same challenges as non-professional users. Existing medical devices designed for professionals rarely consider even common disabilities, making it difficult for caregivers with disabilities to use, or even access, the devices (Winters and Story 2007).

8.7.2   Variability in Patients

Even when a patient is not a direct user of a device, characteristics of the patient being treated, tested, or monitored can still affect device use, and thus must be considered during device design. For example, adults, young children, and neonates (premature and newborn infants) have very different dosing limits for medications. As a result, vendors have designed infusion pumps that the user can place in different operating modes, depending on the patient being treated. This has caused mode confusion errors when a pump is inadvertently placed in the wrong mode, but operated as if it is in the correct mode (Obradovich and Woods 1996). Patients with several comorbidities increase task complexity and often the number of devices involved in their care. Device designers must also consider patient disabilities. For instance, patients who cannot stand on their own, such as those who use wheelchairs, may have difficulty getting a mammogram because most mammography equipment requires that the patient stand and remain still (Todd and Stuifbergen 2011).

8.7.3   Use Environments

The diversity and complexity of medical device use environments present a number of design challenges. There are roughly four different environments: in-patient facilities (such as hospitals and nursing homes), pre-hospital emergency settings, outpatient clinics, and homes. Although variation is more extreme across these settings, there is also considerable variation within each. Here we highlight some of the major differences among these environments.

The hospital setting is the most controlled of all healthcare settings. Equipment, staffing, room and unit layout, and room assignments may all be managed to optimize care. However, patients in hospitals tend to be those who require immediate medical monitoring and intervention, ranging from nearly constant monitoring and therapy (such as in an intensive care unit) to relatively infrequent observation. Multiple devices are often in use for a single patient, which can lead to connector and alarm confusion, as well as equipment placement that is less than ideal for optimal use. For instance, many medical devices have digital displays that are inset in a bezel, such that if viewed from an angle above the device, the bezel will obscure the top or sides of the numbers, perhaps making a 7 appear as a 1 (Thimbleby 2007).

In this and other healthcare environments, many safety-critical devices are in constant operation even when a trained provider is not present. Although medical devices include visual and audible alerts, these may not be heard outside a patient's room. Some devices also have high rates of false alarms, so the alarms tend to be ignored, or patients ask providers to lower the alarm volume so that they are not woken at night. There is considerable body of research on medical device alarm design; for a review see (U.S. Food and Drug Administration Center for Devices and Radiological Health 2011).

The in-patient environment is also subject to numerous interruptions, and it may be noisy, have non-optimal lighting and limited space for equipment placement. Multiple devices are often mounted on a single wheeled pole, which can become unstable and pose a hazard to patients and providers. Providers are typically time-constrained due either to workload or emergent clinical situations. This has design implications for speed and ease of use that we explore below.

Pre-hospital emergency settings include injury scenes and ground or air ambulances. Ambulances present unique design challenges due to the available space and vehicle motion, vibration, and noise. A user interface that works well at the hospital bedside may not be suited for use in ambulances. For example, during an observational session of paramedics who were operating in an ambulance equipped with an early telemedicine system, one of the authors (TRJ) observed that the paramedics used a raised bezel around a wall-mounted computer touchscreen to anchor their fingers so they could successfully use the telemedicine interface: the bezel allowed the user's hand to rise and fall with the movement of the vehicle and the touchscreen. To access menus on the top half of the screen, the paramedics hooked their fingers on top of the bezel and used their thumb to touch the screen. To access menus on the lower half, the paramedics hooked their thumb on the bezel at the bottom of the screen and used a finger to touch the screen. The bezel was not intentionally designed for this purpose—it was simply an artifact of the method used to mount the screen. Without the bezel, the paramedics would have had trouble using the touchscreen interface while the ambulance was moving.

Outpatient clinics are perhaps the simplest environment with respect to medical devices; however, efforts to reduce the number of emergency department visits and in-patient stays are increasing the complexity of care in outpatient clinics. With increased complexity of care comes an increase in the number and complexity of medical devices. Similar economic pressures are demanding faster and faster visits, meaning that common outpatient medical devices that are easier and faster to use can play a role in assisting the shift to "better care for less." For example, medical devices that directly send patient vital signs to the electronic medical records can offer significant efficiency gains, but also pose design challenges in terms of patient identification and preventing errors that result from removing the user from overseeing the data entry process.

The home care environment, which may also include work and recreational sites, is a growing but challenging environment for medical device design. An aging population, patient preference, and economic pressures, along with constantly wired mobile technology, are leading to new ways to monitor and care for patients who would normally require care in a traditional healthcare setting. However, the home setting is one of the most diverse and uncontrolled environments. The FDA's draft guidance on home-use medical devices lists a number of environmental considerations, including contaminants, childproofing, resistance to tampering, and possible implications of security screenings while traveling with medical devices (U.S. Food and Drug Administration, Center for Devices and Radiological Health 2012).

8.7.4 Tasks

The safety-critical nature and complexity of tasks in which medical devices play a role, greatly affect device usability and safety. In HCI the notion of task is broadly defined. It may be used to refer to something very general that a person wants or needs to do, such as diagnosing or monitoring a patient, or to something very specific, such as turning off an infusion pump. When designing and evaluating a medical device interface, it is important for designers to consider both device-specific tasks and broader tasks in which the device plays a role. For example, clinicians sometimes manage a patient's pain by using a patient-controlled anal-gesia pump. This is a type of infusion pump that is loaded with pain control medication, then programmed to allow the patient to deliver the medication as needed—up to a programmed dose and rate limit. Device-specific tasks include programming the pump (typically done by a nurse) and signaling the need for more pain medication (typically done by the patient). However, these tasks are just subtasks of the broader pain management task. Likewise, pain management is just one subtask of treating a patient. While a single device-specific task might seem relatively simple when analyzed in isolation, designers need to consider that that task is being done in the context of a complex suite of tasks involving multiple agents and multiple devices, often over extended periods of time.

As medicine has progressed, the complexity of clinical tasks has increased. As with other areas of technology, the introduction of computer-controlled medical devices has supported and enabled more and more complex interventions, further raising task complexity. To support more complex interventions, designers have added additional functionality to medical devices, in much the same way that mobile phones have continued to gain functionality. For example, some infusion pumps can deliver several medications, each with their own rate and total doses. Infusions may also be programmed to change over time. Medical devices are increasingly connected to other devices and clinical information systems. They may be operated or reconfigured remotely or even automatically. Many can be customized at the institutional level to provide default values and modes designed to ensure efficiency of care and safe dose limits.

When devices are designed to perform more and more functions, their user interfaces necessarily increase in complexity. At the same time, designers are pressured to keep device size as small as possible to maximize space utilization and the ability to transport the device (and to reduce manufacturing and storage costs). The pressure to keep devices as small as possible can lead to serious compromises in display and control design. For example, multi-channel infusion pumps may only display the program for a single channel, requiring user interaction to view other channels. Physical controls may be placed too close together with each control serving multiple functions. On some devices controls are placed at the back of the device where they are hard to see and may be inadvertently changed when moving or holding the device. Small screen and font sizes may also make it difficult for users to accurately read the display, particularly when not standing directly in front of the screen, such as when a provider is on the opposite side of a patient's bed. A user may not realize a screen is difficult to use; they may just misread it and not know they have misread the display.

Infection control is a major concern in nearly all healthcare settings. It is an overarching task in which almost all device tasks are embedded. To prevent infection, providers often use medical devices while gloved, so traditional consumer-oriented interaction technology and user interfaces may not work or work reliably. Devices must also be easy to disinfect, and must work under extreme conditions, such as when splashed with fluids.

Because users are often time-constrained, they must be able to quickly and accurately assess and change the state of the device, or use the device to get an accurate assessment of the patient's clinical state. Small displays, confusing icons and information displays, and the need to change modes to access critical information, all raise the probability of adverse events. When used in the context of multiple medical devices, the time element increases the chance of alarm, connector, and device confusion. For instance, nurses have correctly programmed the wrong infusion channel, because they had difficulty tracking down which tube was connected to which pump and which channel on the pump.

Many devices must continue to operate when removed from a main power source, such as during a power outage or during patient transport. Devices typically have built-in batteries in addition to a power cord. The design of power source and battery status displays is critical for the safe operation of these devices. Since the devices continue to operate while unplugged, and since operators are not always present, patients have been harmed when devices have run out of battery power because they were either inadvertently unplugged or were not plugged in after transportation or setup. In some cases, these errors were the result of poorly designed power status displays.

8.7.5   *Devices*

Unlike consumer applications that have user interfaces based on mature operating systems with standardized user interface elements and interaction guidelines, medical devices are often completely custom-designed user interface projects involving blends of custom hardware, software, displays, and interaction devices. Although this gives designers tremendous flexibility to develop innovative devices, it also means that designers do not benefit from the years of user interface development and research experience embedded in modern consumer products. In particular, users familiar with everyday devices may be caught up by medical device idiosyncrasies. The small form-factor of many medical devices adds additional challenges to user interface design, both in terms of the amount of information that can be displayed at once and the design of physical controls.

With the advent of more powerful mobile technology, such as smartphones and tablets, the number and importance of mobile medical applications are expected to increase. As noted above, the FDA intends to regulate mobile medical applications that meet the definition of device, pose more than minimal risk to patients, and either transform a mobile device into a medical device or are an accessory to a regulated mobile device. Mobile medical applications can offer additional HCI challenges (Poole 2013). Unlike dedicated medical devices, they share the device with several other applications that could affect the functioning of the mobile health application. For example, a mobile health alert may be lost among a number of other, non-health related application alerts. Mobile app developers and users vary more than for traditional medical devices. Because users typically have their mobile devices on or near them at all times, the same user may use the mobile health app under a wide range of environmental and social conditions. In addition to standard usability factors, such as the design of visual and audible feedback, designers must also address battery issues, Internet connectivity, security, and privacy. There is also a need to integrate information from a number of health-related devices and display it in a way that permits a user to understand relationships. For example, a person might want to view weight, blood pressure, sleep, and exercise in an integrated display by date, despite the fact that each is collected by different devices and applications.

8.8   Methods for Medical Device Interface Design and Evaluation

The FDA provides comprehensive draft guidance on the human factors engineering process for medical device design along with recommended methods (U.S. Food and Drug Administration Center for Devices and Radiological Health 2011). The main goal of the process is to understand and mitigate use-related hazards so that device use is safe and effective. The process has four main steps: identifying and investigating anticipated and unanticipated use-related hazards, prioritizing risks associated with use-related hazards, developing and implementing risk mitigation and control strategies, and validation testing. The steps must be carried out in the context of an analysis of the intended users, tasks, use environments, and (once designed or prototyped) the device user interface.

It is never possible to design a good device without doing user testing. How users will use a device is unknown until they try it in a realistic environment; even in the lab, user behavior can be misleading. Crucially, if designers modify a design to improve user performance, it becomes necessary to do more user testing in case new problems have been accidentally introduced. Hence all devices should be tested *iteratively* until they meet the design criteria appropriate for their intended use. International standards such as ISO 9241 (International Organization for Standardization 2006) and 14971 (International Organization for Standardization 2007) should be referred to for more details on design processes.

Since medical devices are used in safety-critical settings where even infrequent errors can result in major harm, user tests are not sufficient for ensuring safety. Testing with humans gets harder and harder as user interface design improves. For example, if only 1 % of user actions are errors, user tests have to be performed 100 times longer to get reliable results. As a result, user tests must be supplemented by two further approaches. The first is to use computer models of users to "stress test" devices. These simulated users try to get the device to do everything it is intended to do, while making key-press slips. Using this approach, it is easy to perform billions of tests, and to cover all of a device's features (Thimbleby 2007).

Secondly, devices should be designed using formal methods—modern software engineering—so that it can be proved they satisfy their design requirements (Dix 2013). Programming medical devices without proof today is irresponsible, but as we have emphasized it is always essential to perform user tests—a device might be "correct" but correctly implementing a poorly-conceived design!

Our own experiments, discussed in Case Study 2 (Cauchi et al. 2012), show that user interfaces can be made from 2 times to 20 times safer, and that the improvements to the user interface do not need to affect error-free behavior, so users need no retraining to benefit from the improved safety.

Since medical device user interface design challenges stem from the interplay of a number of factors as we described in the previous section, it is also important to use a human factors framework that takes a systems-based approach to design. Contextual Design offers a systematic set of methods and tools to help designers analyze the context in which devices are used and then to use this information to inform user interface design (Holtzblatt and Beyer 2013). Universal Design (Story et al. 1998) and Inclusive Design (Clarkson 2003) are two design frameworks that provide design guidelines and methods for producing devices and applications for a broader range of user abilities and disabilities.

The moral of the story is that Human Factors and HCI can help make better and safer medical devices, and that current devices unfortunately leave much to be desired in terms of their quality, but this is primarily because manufacturers are not using HCI well enough given the complexity of healthcare.

8.9 Case Study 1: Human Factors in the Evolution of Anesthesia Machines

The progressive improvement in anesthesia machine safety over the last century is a striking example of how risks associated with increased complexity have been mitigated through improvements in design. More than 50 years after the first public demonstration of ether in 1846 (Viets 1949), anesthesia machines at the start of the twentieth century looked more like industrial equipment than a medical device (Drägerwerk 2012). Early development had focused on increasing the efficiency of drug delivery and to control cost, so that the benefits of anesthesia during dental and surgical procedures could reach as many patients as possible. Techniques for accurately measuring gas flow rates were still decades away and patient monitoring was limited to "keeping a finger on the pulse". Interaction with the device was limited to adjusting valves that regulated the flow of anesthetic gasses and oxygen to the patient without the assistance of safety features that might prevent overdose or alert the anesthetist to an interruption in gas delivery.

Over the subsequent decades, advances in technology led to gradual design enhancements. For example, as the ability to accurately measure flow rates and drug concentration became available, these components were incorporated into the design. Engineering approaches to improving machine safety were also developed in this period. In response to patient deaths involving delivery of hypoxic gas mixtures due to incorrect attachment of gas supply tanks to the machine, the pin-index safety system was introduced in 1948 which made it virtually impossible to connect a nitrous oxygen cylinder to an oxygen intake valve. While introduction of this technology undoubtedly reduced errors and saved lives, deaths associated with incorrect gas connections continued for decades. In short, although technological solutions to specific safety issues improved anesthesia practice and mitigated the potential for errors, a paradigmatic shift in perspective by taking into account the "human factor" was ostensibly missing.

By the 1950s, anesthesia machines began to resemble contemporary designs. One of the most striking changes in appearance during this period was driven by the desire to integrate the device into the clinical workflow. Early machines, which had appeared like collections of tubes, valves, and tanks assembled on a wheeled platform, had evolved into a workstation that included a flat surface where documentation could be completed or drugs and procedural equipment placed for immediate access. In addition, storage drawers were also integrated into the design where additional emergency equipment could be available in easy reach. The appearance of these enhancements signaled a shift in design priorities away from purely technological enhancements to a design that addressed the global needs of the anesthetist using the machine in a clinical setting, where regulating gas flow is only one of the many tasks to be completed.

By modern standards, anesthesia was still a hazardous business in the 1950s, with one study of nearly 600,000 patients reporting anesthetic related mortality in 1 in 1,560 patients (Beecher and Todd 1954). However, the pace of innovation in machine design continued to advance utilizing both engineering and human factors approaches. Innovations in engineering included development of fail-safe components to detect and alert clinicians to the presence of hypoxic gas mixtures, enhancing safety beyond what the pin-index system had been able to achieve. Human factors approaches included efforts to standardize equipment and machine design across manufacturers. For example, the variation between manufacturers in tubing diameter used to connect patient endotracheal tubes to the anesthesia circuit was widely recognized as a hazard, because incompatibility could have disastrous implications. Standardization of equipment to ensure compatibility regardless of manufacturer would improve safety by reducing the number of variables a clinician needed to consider while preparing for a case or in response to an unexpected circumstance. Broad design issues were addressed by the American National Standards Association Committee z79, which further advocated for safety standards in anesthesia machine design that would reduce the potential for human error (Betcher 1982). For example, the relative ordering of gas flow control knobs was specified, so that the oxygen control valve would be located in the same relative position on every machine regardless of manufacturer. Similarly, the texture of the oxygen control valve was specified so that it would always have a ridged feel, while nitrous oxide and air would be smooth, giving the anesthetist a tactile cue for the valve being adjusted. While earlier approaches to improving safety had emphasized enhanced mechanical engineering, these enhancements were more directed at improving cognitive performance. Standard positioning of gas control valves could eliminate the clinician's need to remember the specific model of the machine in use during a crisis, while the standard "feel" of the oxygen control knob could enhance cognitive performance by engaging other senses.

By the 1970s, enhanced designs had started to make their way into clinical use as older equipment was retired. However, adverse events due to poor equipment design continued to be reported. In a 1976 report Dr. Rendell-Baker expressed his concerns about the role of poor design and inadequate consideration of human factors in anesthetic gas delivery systems (Rendell-Baker 1976). He noted numerous examples where safe operation of the machine required strict compliance with specific operating instructions by the anesthetist that were not necessarily explicit. In one instance, he described a design where oxygen delivery could be entirely routed through the vaporizer. If the breathing circuit needed to be flushed with fresh oxygen, as might be required after induction of anesthesia, all gas flow (including oxygen) would be vented to the atmosphere rather than to the patient. If the clinician then neglected to re-open the vaporizer, no gas would flow to the patient. The only acknowledgement of this risk from the manufacturer was in an informational brochure, described by Dr. Rendell-Baker:

> "should the anesthesiologist turn the Shunt Valve to the OFF position, he will automatically isolate the vaporizer, and the O_2, previously passing through the vaporizer will be vented to atmosphere. It will then be necessary to maintain a flow of metabolic O_2, from a direct O_2

flowmeter to the patient circuit. By thus acknowledging the performance characteristics of the apparatus, the operator can fully appreciate its efficiency with complete safety." This final sentence must rate as a masterpiece of Orwellian "1984" logic! Rendell-Baker 1976, p. 28

As a result of this design, the patient's well-being under anesthesia was critically dependent on the cognitive performance of the anesthetist to compensate for the design flaws of the equipment. Dr. Rendell-Baker went on to advocate for a fail-safe gas delivery system that incorporated continuous delivery of oxygen to the patient, an approach that would allow the anesthetist to recover from an operational error with much less risk of harm to the patient. While acknowledging the role of human error in anesthesia mishaps, there clearly were many areas where safety could be improved with engineering approaches that limited the potential for human error. Dr. Rendell-Baker recommended that "The aim of the design engineer should be to eliminate as many mechanical hazards as possible. Safety should not depend upon the user's memory and ability to carry out the correct procedure."

At the same time, rigorous analysis of anesthetic mishaps using formal human factors techniques was also underway. Cooper et al. (1978) used a modified critical-incident analysis technique to examine the characteristics of human error and equipment failure in anesthetic practice. In most cases, they found that preventable incidents were related to human error (82 %), rather than overt equipment failure (14 %), but poor design was often contributory in cases of human error and inadequate experience in cases of equipment failure. The complexity of both gaining an initial understanding of machine safety and then designing a mitigation strategy is illustrated by one of their findings. At some point prior to the start of the study, the hospital had changed the shape of the oxygen control valve to a large, protruding, square knob, presumably in response to recommendations previously discussed. This change in equipment design was intended to improve the cognitive performance of the anesthetist, but as an unintended consequence, the impact of an object on the work surface could cause unintentional rotation of the knob and result in decreased oxygen flow. Clearly, improved safety would depend on deep understanding of the clinical environment, engineering requirements, and human factors. Recognizing that improvements in machine design had largely progressed in an ad hoc manner for nearly 50 years, Cooper et al. later noted "Improvements and developments have been individual and narrow, arising in response to each specific safety problem as discovered and designed" (Cooper et al. 1978). In response to the existing machine design where "new concepts, as they have emerged, have been added to the system in the form of new and separate boxes and gadgets that further complicate the maze of wires, cords, and objects which currently clutters the operating room and the anesthetist's visual field", he proposed a complete redesign. His proposed machine would explicitly "eliminate human-factors problems... and lay a suitable technological foundation for the development of new techniques in anesthesia management". The importance of man-machine communication links that operated with a minimum of attention and effort was emphasized, and the anesthetist was conceived of as a controller, processing both patient physiologic sensors and machine effectors that would support decision-making and action-taking by the anesthetist.

The innovations advocated by Cooper et al. would take years to reach routine clinical practice. So, despite these technological innovations and awareness of human factors, anesthesia in the early 1980s was still considered risky. Anesthetic related mortality had improved, but was still estimated to be 1–2 per 10,000 anesthetics (Keenan and Boyan 1985; Lunn and Mushin 1982). Malpractice insurance was very expensive for anesthesiologists, and a disproportionate amount of payments were related to anesthesia (Pierce 1996).

The issue of patient safety was brought to public attention in 1982 when a documentary entitled "The Deep Sleep" aired on television. The program asserted that more than 6,000 patients would die or suffer brain damage from preventable causes associated with anesthesia that year. Its broadcast was followed by an immediate public outcry (Pierce 2007). The American Society of Anesthesiologists (ASA) responded, and by dedicating significant resources to making anesthesia safer, was able to make a big difference in a short period of time.

The ASA started by gathering consensus and studying the issues, both technological and human. In 1985, the Anesthesia Patient Safety Foundation (APSF) was created with a mission that "no patient shall be harmed by anesthesia," (Cooper and Pierce 1986) and a year later the Anesthesia Closed Claims project was launched as a collaborative effort between anesthesiologists, hospitals, lawyers, and insurance carriers to develop a standardized method of analyzing and learning from anesthesia related mishaps (Cheney 1999).

Closed claims data have been used extensively to analyze anesthesia related risks and improve outcomes. While incidents related to equipment have been analyzed repeatedly since its inception, claims related to gas delivery systems have decreased to 1 % since 1990, with a similar decline in the severity of harm (Mehta et al. 2013).

Anesthesia today is safer than it has ever been. Some estimates of mortality are now as low as 1–2 per 250,000 (Haller et al. 2011) and malpractice premiums and payouts are now similar to other specialties. Such rapid, dramatic declines in mortality are rare in medicine, and have been achieved in part by improved fail-safe engineering, but also by addressing human factors that inherently pose error risks. As we celebrate the decline of equipment related injury in the Closed Claims Database, it is important to remember that the majority of the claims involving gas delivery (85 %) are still related to human error without equipment failure (Mehta et al. 2013). Clearly, Human Factors will play a central role in future advancements in anesthesia machines related patient safety.

8.10   Case Study 2: User Interface Details—Illustrating the Value of HCI

HCI is a broad topic, but its impact can be seen even in small details. Take numbers. You press buttons and a number appears in the medical device, perhaps the infusion rate in mL per hour. On the Baxter Colleague 3 infusion pump, you can type 1.5 and that's what you will get, but if you type 100.5 the Baxter ignores the decimal point and you will get 1,005, which is ten times larger. The designers obviously decided that large numbers do not need decimal points; no number needs to be given to four digits of precision. So the Baxter ignores decimals, which sort of makes sense, but a rule of HCI is to provide useful feedback to the user. On the Baxter, when you press keys, they click, confirming that you pressed them hard enough. This is good feedback. Unfortunately, when you press a decimal point you get a click whether or not the Baxter ignores it. This is a design defect. In fact, the whole idea is an HCI defect: we know from eye tracking experiments (Oladimeji et al. 2011) that users do not look at displays as much as they look at keyboards, so a user will not notice the display shows 1005 instead of 100.5, which is what they expect. We know this and HCI dictates we should design to accommodate what users expect.

The BBraun Infusomat infusion pump handles numbers differently; instead of a numeric keypad there are 4 arrow keys and a cursor. The user can move the cursor left or right by using the left and right arrow keys, and can increase or decrease the digit the cursor is over by using the up and down arrow keys (see Fig. 8.1). The behavior of the Infusomat depends on its mode. In VTBI (Volume To Be Infused) if the display shows 0.0 with the cursor on the tenths position and the user presses the right arrow key (to move the cursor to the right from the tenths to the hundredths position) and then presses 'up' to increase the 0 to a 1, the display will change to 0.1, not to 0.01. The designers have made a decision to change what the users do to mean something else, and (worse) the keystroke feedback (click sounds) seem to confirm the device is obeying the keystrokes. The design is likely to cause problems. The solution would be to make an alarm sound so as to draw the user's attention to the divergence of what the pump is doing and what it was told to do. Moreover, the alarm should stay activated until the user acknowledges it, for instance by pressing [CLEAR].

Caregivers must often make calculations while using medical devices, such as to convert between different units. However, calculators vary greatly in how they detect and flag use errors. The Apple iPhone calculator detects some use errors. For example, keying 1/0. = instead of 1/0.7 = will give Error rather than 2.04. Unfortunately, continuing the calculation after an error, for instance 1/0. + 2 × 3 will give the wrong answer—here 6 rather than Error. The calculator spots an error and reports it, but the Error message is not persistent; in fact, the user is allowed to enter an erroneous calculation, and the iPhone defectively just does the last part of the calculation. The user may take 6 as the answer, and if so it would be tempting to say they would be wrong—in fact, the calculator is wrong, and its design induced the user to make this error.

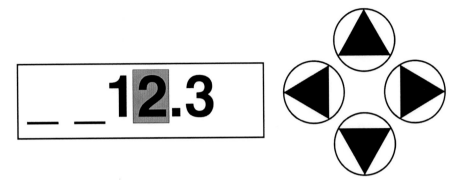

Fig. 8.1 A 4-key number entry design. The *left/right "arrows"* move the cursor left and right, and the *up/down arrows* increase or decrease the digit the cursor is over. The cursor is shown here as a *gray box*, but on many designs it will flash, and perhaps invert video as well. Some defective designs allow *left/right arrows* to wraparound the cursor position: e.g., pressing too many rights will bring the cursor round to the far left, so a user trying to enter a fractional digit could accidentally enter a 1000s digit. Some designs adjust digits independently, and others have "carry" so incrementing a digit goes −8–9–10, rather than −8–9–0. The four-key design has a low user error rate but it is complex to ensure it handles boundary cases correctly and in the best way for the user. For example, an easy way of changing 10–100 goes via 0, which may be a prohibited value and automatically set a minimum value like 1, which the user will find counter-productive!

Many devices keep a log, and the log may be used as legal evidence after an incident. If the log says the infusion pump delivered 15 mL, then it is tempting to think the user told it to deliver 15 mL, and if this is the cause of the incident, then it would seem the user is to blame. But it is not so simple. On some devices, the delete key does not work as expected. For example, keying 1. [DEL] 5 may result in 5 rather than the intended 1.5, an error that is 3.33 times out yet the log will say the user keyed 5, not 1.5 (or even 1. [DEL] 5). Thus the log in this case probably correctly describes what the infusion pump did, but not what the user asked it to do. Logs are also susceptible to key bounce errors, where the user presses a key once but the device treats it as two or more presses; again the log will say what the device does, but is a misleading account of what the user did.

Reducing the number of keys to enter numbers makes using a device easier, and also reduces the amount of time a user needs to look at the keyboard. Some devices use up/down arrows to increase and decrease numbers (see Fig. 8.2). Not only are there fewer keys, but the user model is that the displayed number has to be changed to be correct; like the 4-key style mentioned above, therefore, 2-key number entry has lower error rates. Instead of the design being "the user keys a number" the design is "the number displayed is wrong; the user corrects it" and therefore they are forced to look at the display and to expect errors they will correct. Such interfaces are much more reliable, yet they are slower and therefore some might claim they are "less usable." However, to say they are less usable is to confuse speed with ease of use; but in a healthcare environment, ease of use is not as important as whether a device can be used reliably. Obviously it is an advantage

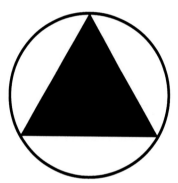
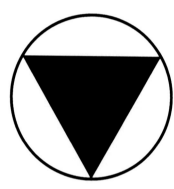

Fig. 8.2 2-key number entry. Pressing the "*up*" *triangle* (on the *left*) increases the number and pressing the "*down*" *triangle* decreases the number. Typically, holding a button down repeatedly increments or decrements the number, and holding it down for several seconds speeds up the rate of change. Some devices swap the up/down keys, and some additionally have "fast" keys (e.g., which increment and decrement in 10s or 100 s rather than 1 s)

that people like a design, but it should not be the top criterion. A better way to understand the trade-off is that cars with brakes are slower (in fact, that is the point of brakes) but they are much safer and arguably also much easier to drive than cars without brakes. Likewise, slowing down a user may improve their performance overall.

Feedback is important—users cannot always pay full attention to a device (they have distracting jobs) so devices must make clear whether user actions "work" or not. In all the designs discussed, keys normally change the display, but in boundary cases (e.g., when too many digits have been pressed) the display cannot change or possibly changes in a non-standard way (e.g., not going above a preset maximum value). Hence buttons should make two sorts of noise: that they have been pressed successfully, and possibly that they have been pressed but nothing can happen. Many designs beep once for success and twice for failure, as of course a double beep for a single key press is an error in any case. Some buttons (such as [cancel] or buttons that cause confirmatory displays to appear) should make distinctive sounds.

8.11   Conclusions

The HCI of medical devices is an important but complex topic due to their safety-critical nature, regulatory requirements, and the complexity and heterogeneity of their users and use environments. This chapter provided only a brief overview of these issues. The key messages are:

1. Humans make errors sooner or later and designers should design for error. The key point in medical device design is that use error should be managed and so far as possible not lead to patient harm. For example, correctly implemented UNDO or DELETE keys allows users to make errors and to correct them.
2. Designers, too, are human and can never know enough about the context of use of a device. Medical devices help highly trained professionals in complex, stressful environments, and they do not understand complex issues of engineering design. It is *inevitable* that design requirements are going to have oversights. Devices have to be user-tested in realistic environments and improved in light of experimental results, in a repeating process called *iterative design*.
3. To fully assess device usability, designers should augment user tests with simulation and formal software engineering approaches. Simulated users that make keystroke errors can exercise the full range of device operations. Formal methods, such as model checking, can prove that the device works as intended.
4. There are numerous relevant international standards, and these are both a regulatory framework of minimum standards as well as an excellent resource of authoritative literature.

There is considerable need for research that addresses common issues across medical devices; more so, there is considerable need for the research to be applied! Research on medical device alarms and data entry interfaces are good examples of such work, but additional work is needed in other areas, such as improving situational awareness when using one or more devices.

This chapter gives only a basic introduction to the challenges of designing interfaces for medical devices. A comprehensive review can be found in the *Handbook of Human Factors in Medical Device Design* (Weinger et al. 2011) and in the FDA guidance documents and regulatory standards.

Discussion Questions
1. What are the similarities and differences between HCI for medical devices vs. non-medical devices?
2. Pick a type of medical device, such as an insulin pump, and then search MAUDE for related reports. Can you separate use-related errors from other types of problems, such as malfunctions or unrelated issues? Are they consistent kinds of use errors? Do they vary based on the model? What kinds of data would you like to gather to further clarify possible use-related errors?
3. Discuss the definition of a medical device with respect to sample mobile apps. Can you find examples of apps that meet and do not meet the definition?

4. Pick a simple mobile device, such as a blood pressure monitor, and consider how well it meets the needs of a diverse set of users and use environments.
5. Based on the definition of a medical device, do you think electronic health record systems (EHRs) are medical devices? If EHRs were regulated as medical devices, how might this affect the stakeholders, including EHR vendors, doctors, and patients?

Acknowledgments This work was partly funded by EPSRC grant [EP/L019272/1].

Additional Readings

Kaye, R., & Crowley, J. (2000). *Medical device use-safety: Incorporating human factors engineering into risk management.* Silver Spring: U.S. Food and Drug Administration, Center for Devices and Radiological Health. Retrieved from http://www.fda.gov/downloads/MedicalDevices/DeviceRegulationandGuidance/GuidanceDocuments/UCM094461.pdf

Sawyer, D. (1996). *Do it by design – An introduction to human factors in medical devices.* Rockville: U.S. Food and Drug Administration, Center for Devices and Radiological Health. Retrieved from http://www.fda.gov/medicaldevices/deviceregulationandguidance/guidancedocuments/ucm094957.htm

Weinger, M. B., Wiklund, M. E., & Gardner-Bonneau, D. J. (2011). *Handbook of human factors in medical device design.* Boca Raton: CRC Press.

References

Association for the Advancement of Medical Instrumentation. (1996). *Human factors in medical devices: Design, regulation, and patient safety* (Conference report). Arlington: Author. Retrieved from http://www.fda.gov/MedicalDevices/DeviceRegulationandGuidance/HumanFactors/ucm126018.htm

Association for the Advancement of Medical Instrumentation. (2001). *Human factors design process for medical devices.* Arlington: Author.

Association for the Advancement of Medical Instrumentation. (2009). *Human factors engineering – Design of medical devices.* Arlington: Author.

Beecher, H. K., & Todd, D. P. (1954). A study of the deaths associated with anesthesia and surgery: Based on a study of 599, 548 anesthesias in ten institutions 1948–1952, inclusive. *Annals of Surgery, 140*(1), 2–35.

Betcher, A. M. (1982). Historical development of the American Society of Anesthesiologists, Inc. In P. Volpitto & L. Vandam (Eds.), *The genesis of contemporary American Anesthesiology* (Vol. 134, pp. 185–211). Springfield: Charles C. Thomas. Retrieved from http://www.woodlibrarymuseum.org/Finding_Aid/ASA/ASA/Betcher%20Historical%20Development%20of%20The%20American%20Society%20of%20Anesthesiologists,%20Inc..pdf

Brannon, T. S. (2006). Ad hoc versus standardized admixtures for continuous infusion drugs in neonatal intensive care: Cognitive task analysis of safety at the bedside. *AMIA Annual Symposium Proceedings, 862.*

Carroll, J. M. (2003). *HCI models, theories, and frameworks: Toward a multidisciplinary science* (1st ed.). Amsterdam/Boston: Morgan Kaufmann.

Cauchi, A., Gimblett, A., Thimbleby, H., Curzon, P., & Masci, P. (2012). Safer "5-key" number entry user interfaces using differential formal analysis. In *Proceedings of the 26th annual BCS interaction specialist group conference on people and computers* (pp. 29–38). Swinton: British Computer Society. Retrieved from http://dl.acm.org/citation.cfm?id=2377916.2377921

Cheney, F. W. (1999). The American Society of anesthesiologists closed claims proj ...: Anesthesiology. *Anesthesiology, 91*(2), 552–556.

Clarkson, J. (2003). *Inclusive design: Design for the whole population.* London/New York: Springer Science & Business Media.

Cooper, J. B., & Pierce, E. C. (1986). Safety foundation organized. *Anesthesia Patient Safety Foundation Newsletter, 1*(1), 1–8.

Cooper, J. B., Newbower, R. S., Long, C. D., & McPeek, B. (1978a). Preventable anesthesia mishaps: A study of human factors. *Anesthesiology, 49*(6), 399–406.

Cooper, J. B., Newbower, R. S., Moore, J. W., & Trautman, E. D. (1978b). A new anesthesia delivery system. *Anesthesiology, 49*(5), 310–318.

Cooper, J. B., Newbower, R. S., & Kitz, R. J. (1984). An analysis of major errors and equipment failures in anesthesia management: Considerations for prevention and detection. *Anesthesiology, 60*(1), 34–42.

Cummings, K., & McGowan, R. (2011). "Smart" infusion pumps are selectively intelligent: Nursing 2013. *Nursing, 41*(3), 58–59.

Dix, A. J. (2013). Formal methods. In M. Soegaard & R. F. Dam (Eds.), *The encyclopedia of human-computer interaction* (2nd ed.). Aarhus: The Interaction Design Foundation. Retrieved from http://www.interaction-design.org/encyclopedia/formal_methods.html

Drägerwerk, A. G. (2012). *The history of Anaesthesia at Dräger 1898–1966* (2nd Rev.). Author. Retrieved from http://www.draeger.com/sites/assets/PublishingImages/Generic/UK/Booklets/4212-Br-History-of-Anaesthesia_A5_en_191212-LR.pdf

Gosbee, J. (2002). Human factors engineering and patient safety. *Quality & Safety in Health Care, 11*(4), 352–354. doi:10.1136/qhc.11.4.352.

Grant, L. (1998). Medical equipment. Devices and desires. *The Health Service Journal, 108* (5603), 34–35.

Haller, G., Laroche, T., & Clergue, F. (2011). Morbidity in anaesthesia: Today and tomorrow. *Best Practice & Research. Clinical Anaesthesiology, 25*(2), 123–132.

Holtzblatt, K., & Beyer, H. R. (2013). Contextual design. In *The encyclopedia of human-computer interaction* (2nd ed.). Retrieved from http://www.interaction-design.org/encyclopedia/contextual_design.html

Institute of Medicine. (2012). *Health IT and patient safety: Building safer systems for better care.* Washington, DC: The National Academies Press. Retrieved from http://www.nap.edu/catalog.php?record_id=13269

International Electrochemical Commission. (2006). *IEC 60601-1-6: Medical electrical equipment – Part 1–6 general requirements for basic safety and essential performance – Colateral standard: Usability.* Geneva: Author.

International Electrochemical Commission. (2007). *IEC 62366 – Medical devices – Application of usability engineering to medical devices.* Geneva: Author.

International Organization for Standardization. (1994). *ISO 9001:1994 – Quality systems – Model for quality assurance in design, development, production, installation and servicing.* Geneva: Author. Retrieved from http://www.iso.org/iso/iso_catalogue/catalogue_tc/catalogue_detail.htm?csnumber=38193

International Organization for Standardization. (2006). *ISO 9241 – Ergonomics of human-system interaction.* Geneva: Author. Retrieved from http://www.iso.org/iso/iso_catalogue/catalogue_tc/catalogue_detail.htm?csnumber=38193

International Organization for Standardization. (2007). *ISO 14971:2007 – Medical devices – Application of risk management to medical devices.* Geneva: Author. Retrieved from http://www.iso.org/iso/iso_catalogue/catalogue_tc/catalogue_detail.htm?csnumber=38193

Keenan, R. L., & Boyan, C. P. (1985). Cardiac arrest due to anesthesia: A study of incidence and causes. *The Journal of the American Medical Association, 253*(16), 2373–2377.

Lunn, J. N., & Mushin, W. W. (1982). Mortality associated with anaesthesia. *Anaesthesia, 37*(8), 856.

MAUDE – Manufacturer and User Facility Device Experience. (n.d.). Retrieved May 30, 2014, from http://www.accessdata.fda.gov/scripts/cdrh/cfdocs/cfMAUDE/search.CFM

McConnell, E. A., Cattonar, M., & Manning, J. (1996). Australian registered nurse medical device education: A comparison of simple vs. complex devices. *Journal of Advanced Nursing, 23*(2), 322–328.

Medical Device Amendments of 1976. Pub. L. No. 94–295 (1976).

Mehta, S. P., Eisenkraft, J. B., Posner, K. L., & Domino, K. B. (2013). Patient injuries from anesthesia gas delivery equipment: A closed claims update. *Anesthesiology, 119*(4), 788–795.

National Council. (2011). *Medical devices and the public's health: The FDA 510 (k) clearance process at 35 years [Internet].* Washington, DC: The National Academies Press [cited 2015 May 26]. Available from: http://216.230.117.100/~/media/Files/Report%20Files/2011/Medical-Devices-and-the-Publics-Health-The-FDA-510k-Clearance-Process-at-35-Years/Testimony-Challoner.pdf

O'Connel, G. W. (n.d.). *Human factors in the GMP inspection process.* Retrieved May 30, 2014, from http://www.fda.gov/MedicalDevices/DeviceRegulationandGuidance/HumanFactors/ucm128186.htm

Obradovich, J. H., & Woods, D. D. (1996). Special section: Users as designers: How people cope with poor HCI design in computer-based medical devices. *Human Factors: The Journal of the Human Factors and Ergonomics Society, 38*(4), 574–592. doi:10.1518/001872096778827251.

Office of the Commissioner. Federal Food, Drug, and Cosmetic Act FD&C Act 21 CFR 201 (H) [21 U.S.C. 321], § 21 CFR 201(h). (2002). Retrieved from http://www.fda.gov/regulatoryinformation/legislation/federalfooddrugandcosmeticactfdcact/fdcactchaptersiandiishorttitleanddefinitions/ucm086297.htm

Oladimeji, P., Thimbleby, H., & Cox, A. (2011). Number entry interfaces and their effects on errors and number perception. In *Proceedings IFIP conference on human-computer interaction, interact 2011* (Vol. IV, pp. 178–185). Heidelberg/New York: Springer.

Pierce, E. C. (1996). The 34th Rovenstine Lecture: 40 years behind the mask: Safety revisited. *Anesthesiology, 84*(4), 965–975.

Pierce, Jr., E. C. (2007). Looking back: Doctor pierce reflects. *Anesthesia Patient Safety Foundation Newsletter, 22*(1). Retrieved from http://www.apsf.org/newsletters/html/2007/spring/02_looking_back.htm

Poole, E. S. (2013). HCI and mobile health interventions. *Translational Behavioral Medicine, 3*(4), 402–405. doi:10.1007/s13142-013-0214-3.

Rendell-Baker, L. (1976). Some gas machine hazards and their elimination. *Anesthesia & Analgesia, 55*(1). Retrieved from http://journals.lww.com/anesthesia-analgesia/Fulltext/1976/01000/Some_Gas_Machine_Hazards_and_Their_Elimination_.6.aspx

Rogers, W. A., Mykityshyn, A. L., Campbell, R. H., & Fisk, A. D. (2001). Analysis of a "simple" medical device. *Ergonomics in Design, 9*(1), 6–14.

Rothschild, J. M., Keohane, C. A., Cook, E. F., Orav, E. J., Burdick, E., Thompson, S., . . . Bates, D. W. (2005). A controlled trial of smart infusion pumps to improve medication safety in critically ill patients. *Critical Care Medicine, 33*(3), 533–540.

Story, M. F., Mueller, J. L., & Mace, R. L. (1998). *The universal design file: Designing for people of all ages and abilities* (Rev. ed.). Retrieved from http://eric.ed.gov/?id=ED460554

The Council of the European Communities. (2007). *EU medical devices directive – MDD 93/42/EEC and 2007/47/EC.* Author. Retrieved from http://www.emergogroup.com/resources/regulations-europe/regulations-EU-MDD93-42-EEC#1

Thimbleby, H. (2007). *Press on: Principles of interaction programming.* Cambridge, MA: The MIT Press.

Todd, A., & Stuifbergen, A. (2011). Barriers and facilitators related to breast cancer screening. *International Journal of MS Care, 13*(2), 49–56. doi:10.7224/1537-2073-13.2.49.

Trbovich, P. L., Pinkney, S., Cafazzo, J. A., & Easty, A. C. (2010). The impact of traditional and smart pump infusion technology on nurse medication administration performance in a simulated inpatient unit. *Quality & Safety in Health Care, 19*(5), 430–434. doi:10.1136/qshc.2009. 032839.

U.S. Department of Health and Human Services, Food and Drug Administration. (2013, September 25). *Mobile medical applications: Guidance for industry and food and drug administration staff.* Retrieved from http://www.fda.gov/downloads/MedicalDevices/ DeviceRegulationandGuidance/GuidanceDocuments/UCM263366.pdf

U.S. Food and Drug Administration. (2008). *Good manufacturing practice (GMP) guidelines/ inspection checklist.* Author. Retrieved from http://www.fda.gov/cosmetics/guidance regulation/guidancedocuments/ucm2005190.htm

U.S. Food and Drug Administration Center for Devices and Radiological Health. (2010). *Medical device home use initiative.* Silver Spring. Retrieved from http://www.fda.gov/downloads/ medicaldevices/productsandmedicalprocedures/homehealthandconsumer/homeusedevices/ ucm209056.pdf

U.S. Food and Drug Administration Center for Devices and Radiological Health. (2011, June 22). *Draft guidance: Applying human factors and usability engineering to optimize medical device design.* Author. Retrieved from http://www.fda.gov/medicaldevices/deviceregulationand guidance/guidancedocuments/ucm259748.htm

U.S. Food and Drug Administration, Center for Devices and Radiological Health. (2012). *Draft guidance for industry and FDA staff – Design considerations for devices intended for home use.* Silver Spring: Author. Retrieved from http://www.fda.gov/medicaldevices/ deviceregulationandguidance/guidancedocuments/ucm331675.htm

U.S. Food and Drug Administration, Center for Devices and Radiological Health. (2014). *Premarket notification (510k).* Retrieved May 30, 2014, from http://www.fda.gov/ medicaldevices/deviceregulationandguidance/howtomarketyourdevice/ premarketsubmissions/premarketnotification510k/default.htm

Viets, H. R. (1949). The earliest printed references in newspapers and journals to the first public demonstration of ether anesthesia in 1846. *Journal of the History of Medicine and Allied Sciences, IV*(2), 149–169. doi:10.1093/jhmas/IV.2.149.

Wachter, R. M., Pronovost, P., & Shekelle, P. (2013). Strategies to improve patient safety: The evidence base matures. *Annals of Internal Medicine, 158*(5_Part_1), 350–352. doi:10.7326/ 0003-4819-158-5-201303050-00010.

Winters, J. M., & Story, M. F. (2007). *Medical instrumentation: Accessibility and usability considerations.* Boca Raton: CRC Press.

Woltz, D. J., Gardner, M. K., & Bell, B. G. (2000). Negative transfer errors in sequential cognitive skills: Strong-but-wrong sequence application. *Journal of Experimental Psychology: Learning, Memory, and Cognition, 26*(3), 601–625. doi:10.1037/0278-7393.26.3.601.

Chapter 9
Applying HCI Principles in Designing Usable Systems for Dentistry

Elsbeth Kalenderian, Muhammad Walji, and Rachel Ramoni

9.1 Introduction

In 2012, close to 650 million patient visits were conducted in dental offices throughout the United States. Dentists, like physicians, routinely perform highly technical procedures in complex environments, work in teams, (Taichman et al. 2010) and have rapidly begun to adopt electronic health records (EHRs). Unfortunately, there is another parallel to medical practice: the usability of dental EHRs is a growing concern. Data stored in dental EHRs are not only used to coordinate care for an individual patient, but also can be aggregated and mined to determine the efficacy of treatments or adherence to standards of care. One of the biggest limitations of data stored in dental EHRs has been the lack of adoption of a standardized terminology to document dental diagnoses. As a structured diagnosis code is not required as part of dental billing, there has been little to no emphasis on the importance of accurately documenting a diagnosis as part of a patient's health record. In this chapter, we review our previously published research in developing and disseminating the Dental Diagnostic System (DDS) Dental Diagnostic Terminology (formerly called the EZCodes) amongst dental school clinics. In order to

E. Kalenderian, DDS, MPH, Ph.D. (✉)
Department of Oral Health Policy and Epidemiology, Harvard School of Dental Medicine, Boston, MA, USA
e-mail: Elsbeth_kalenderian@hsdm.harvard.edu

M. Walji, Ph.D.
Department of Diagnostic and Biomedical Sciences, School of Dentistry, University of Texas Health Science Center at Houston, Houston, TX, USA
e-mail: Muhammad.F.Walji@uth.tmc.edu

R. Ramoni, DMD, ScD
Oral Health Policy and Epidemiology, Harvard School of Dental Medicine, Boston, MA, USA

Center for Biomedical Informatics, Harvard Medical School, Boston, MA, USA
e-mail: Rachel_ramoni@hms.harvard.edu

© Springer International Publishing Switzerland 2015
V.L. Patel et al. (eds.), *Cognitive Informatics for Biomedicine*, Health Informatics,
DOI 10.1007/978-3-319-17272-9_9

bring DDS into the clinic, we applied human computer interaction (HCI) principles to re-designing a treatment-planning module in a widely used dental EHR called axiUm (Exan Corp., Vancouver, Canada) in close collaboration with the vendor. American academic dentistry is well positioned to leverage on the promise of the EHR to advance scientific knowledge and improve health care quality, as 51 of the 65 U.S. dental schools use AxiUm as their EHR. To contextualize this undertaking, we begin by describing the dental profession and practice, with a major focus on the United States. We then describe our human-computer interaction studies, highlighting the relevance of the work to usability studies, secondary use of data, and inter-professional practice.

9.1.1 Characteristics of the Dental Team

The dental practitioner will rarely perform care without a dental assistant present chair-side as "fourhanded" dentistry significantly improves productivity, (Finkbeiner 2000) efficiency, (University of Alabama at Birmingham Four-Handed Dentistry 2011) as well as ergonomics (Finkbeiner 2001). Hygienists and sometimes a nurse further round out the clinical dental team. Front and back office personnel are responsible for patient scheduling, billing and other administrative duties.

The majority of the 195,000 dentists in the U.S. work in small practices, although ownership declined from 91 to 86 % between 1991 and 2010. During the same period, solo practitioners declined from 67 to 59 % (Guay et al. 2012) and as one might imagine, group practices increased in number: between 2008 and 2010, the number of dentists joining a company-owned practice grew from 5.4 to 6.4 % (Guay et al. 2012). By contrast, in the medical profession physicians started to integrate in large group practices as early as the 1990s, associated with the rise of managed care in medicine (Anderson and Grey 2013). This is in contrast to our Canadian colleagues where 98.3 % of the 19,563 (Canadian Dental Association Dental Health Services in Canada 2010). Canadian licensed dentists work in private practice, of whom 79 % are owners (Service Canada Dentists. Government of Canada 2014).

In the teaching practices within dental schools, the workflow is different than in private practices. Students provide care under the supervision of full-time or adjunct faculty members. In most dental schools, students frequently practice without a dedicated dental assistant or are assisted by a fellow dental student. Thus, the students themselves are responsible for data entry into the EHR and might also schedule appointments for their patients.

9.1.2 Workflow in the Dental Operatory

Even before the introduction of computers, a lot was happening in a small space within the modern dental operatory, the space in which the dental team performs its clinical work. Dentists may have two to three operatories occupied at the same time; on average, the operatory turnover occurs every 30 min.

The EHR-endowed dental operatory is typically set up in one of two ways: either with the EHR at the 12 o'clock position, essentially behind the dentist, or attached to the dental chair. The latter more readily allows the patient to be included in treatment planning and education as documents, instructional videos and digital radiographs can easily be displayed by swiveling the EHR within eyesight of the patient. Most often, the dental assistant enters data into the EHR via a wireless keyboard chair-side. The most intensive data entry occurs during the intra-oral exam, when the dentist calls out findings that the dental assistant documents in the EHR. Figure 9.1.

Dentistry has a unique clinical workflow, (Button et al. 1999) yet only a few studies have been conducted on workflow and the role of technology in the dental clinic (Button et al. 1999; Wotman et al. 2001). Nevertheless, previous studies have demonstrated that limited consideration of HCI related issues often interferes with the dental clinic workflow. For example, Irwin et al. showed that over 60 % of the 27 "breakdowns" during initial examination and treatment planning using EHRs in general dentist practices were associated with technology (Irwin et al. 2009). Usability issues and unfamiliarity with chair-side use of clinically relevant electronic data were major barriers to EHR adoption for dental practitioners, (Schleyer

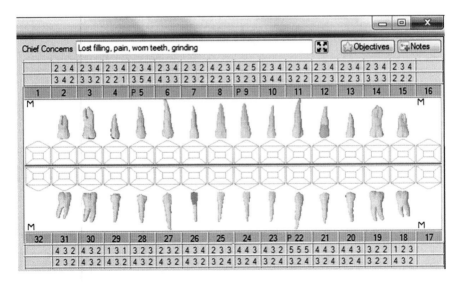

Fig. 9.1 Recording of pocket depth (numbers in mm in *red*), bleeding points (P), missing teeth (M) and existing restorations (*colored areas* on teeth) in the EHR

et al. 2006, 2007; John et al. 2003; Thyvalikakath et al. 2007, 2008) not unlike the barriers associated with medical provider encounters (Miller and Sim 2004; Fitzpatrick and Koh 2005; Simon et al. 2007). In the U.S., the axiUm EHR has achieved near ubiquity in dental academic settings. This is not to say that the axiUm EHR has surmounted the usability challenges of the private practice dental EHRs; indeed, a survey and interview study conducted during the implementation of axiUm at the University of Texas Health Science Center at Houston Dental Branch identified usability as a major concern (Walji et al. 2009).

9.1.3   Development of a Standardized Dental Diagnostic Terminology

A complete list of patient problems and diagnoses is a cornerstone of the medico-legal document that is the patient record. It serves as a valuable tool for providers assessing a patient's clinical status, succinctly communicates this information between providers and to front desk and administrative personnel, and serves as a fulcrum around which research and quality improvement levers pivot.

Early efforts to standardize dental diagnostic terms have fallen short with respect to comprehensiveness and availability (World Health Organization 1973; Ettelbrick et al. 2000). Subsequently, the ICD-DA (application of the International Classification of Diseases to Dentistry and Stomatology) was added to ICD-8 in 1965 (World Health Organization 1973). However, the oral health coverage of the ICD terminology continues to call for improvement (Ettelbrick et al. 2000). Over the years, some groups independently generated dental diagnostic terminologies (Orlowsky and Glusman 1969; Gregg and Boyd 1996; Bader et al. 1999). Of these, the Toronto Codes (Leake et al. 1999) have been systematically evaluated, (Leake 2002) while we do not know to what extent the other terminologies have met dental teams' diagnostic documentation needs (Sabbah 1999). In the early 1990s, the American Dental Association (ADA) started the development of SNODENT, a Systematized Nomenclature for Dentistry. In 1998, the ADA entered into an agreement to incorporate SNODENT Version I into SNOMED (SNODENT Update 2004). SNODENT is composed of diagnoses, signs, symptoms and complaints, and currently includes over 7700 terms (Goldberg et al. 2005; Torres-Urquidy and Schleyer 2006). In 2012, SNODENT Version II was incorporated into the SNOMED CT. Until its recent inclusion into SNOMED CT, SNODENT was only available by license and was maintained by the ADA. As a result, SNODENT is currently not widely implemented. In 2007, our research team developed the EZCodes, (Kalenderian et al. 2011) renamed Dental Diagnostic System or DDS for short, to enhance the proper and consistent registration of diagnostic findings. The DDS has been mapped to SNOMED, ICD 9, ICD 10, ICD 9-CM and ICD 10-CM

(CM is the American version of ICD 9 and 10). With 1518 terms, the DDS is developed as an interface terminology (a set of terms designed to be compatible with the natural language of the user, used to mediate between a user's colloquial conceptualizations of concept descriptions and an underlying reference terminology (Clinical Information Modeling Initiative (CIMI) Category: Interface terminology 2012)) to be used in the dental clinic with SNOMED CT as its back-end reference terminology (a terminology where each term has a codable, computerusable definition to support retrieval and data aggregation (Reference Terminology)). The few DDS terms that did not have adequate coverage with SNOMED terms were submitted for integration with SNOMED, of which the majority has been accepted. As such, SNOMED truly functions as the reference terminology for the DDS terminology. Similarly, we have submitted terms to ICD in an effort to enhance the ICD oral health classification and improve the mapping between DDS and ICD oral health terms. The DDS terminology is also in its last phase of becoming a norm in The Netherlands, meaning that it will be the standardized diagnostic terminology that all Dutch dentists are expected to use (Nederlands Tandartsenblad Nederlandse Norm voor diagnostische termen).

However, prior analyses of the EZCodes (DDS) terminology in use in an EHR demonstrated both low utilization and frequent errors (Kalenderian et al. 2011). Between July 2010 and June 2011, the EZCodes were utilized 12 % of the time in three dental schools. More than 1,000 terms of the available 1,321 terms were never chosen. Caries and periodontics were the most frequently used categories. 60.5 % of the EZCodes entries were found to be valid (Blumenthal and Glaser 2007). The low utilization rate reiterated findings from an earlier study, (White et al. 2011) but also suggested the need to conduct more training, improve the EHR interface, and add descriptions and synonyms to the terms.

In Sect. 9.2, we describe our approach in using HCI principles to systematically identify usability problems, and to drive the re-design of an existing EHR to enhance the effective and efficient entry of dental diagnostic terms.

To put this work in context, we first review some of the recent and relevant literature regarding usability, dental EHRs and interface terminologies. A number of researchers have established that dental EHRs have some distance to go to be usable. Reynolds and colleagues provide a brief overview of dental informatics, reiterating that usability challenges represent a primary hurdle to the adoption of dental EHRs (Reynolds et al. 2008). In 2008, Hill, Stewart, and Ash explored the impact of EHRs on dental faculty and students in the dental academic setting. Newly developed clinical processes were considered more time consuming than previous paper processes. The end users' needs appeared to be intense, immediate and significant. Here too, the authors reported significant usability problems standing in the way of smooth implementation. Additionally, changes in workflow were significant and often cumbersome (Hill et al. 2010a). Juvé-Udina reported on the evaluation of the usability of the diagnosis axis in a nursing interface terminology. Utilization of the diagnostic terms was high at 92.3 % where some of the concepts were used rarely and others as often as 51.4 % (Juve-Udina 2013). Thyvalikakath et al. similarly concluded that using a combination of heuristic evaluation and user tests methods showed that the four major commercial dental EHRs had significant usability problems (Thyvalikakath et al. 2009). Despite the fact that dental EHR usability is an established problem, little has been published on the use of cognitive engineering approaches, like think-aloud protocols, workflow observations and semi-structured interviews, to remedy the issues (Thyvalikakath et al. 2014).

9.1.4 Challenges of Dental EHR Use and Usability

Although healthcare providers, including dental providers, increasingly adopt EHRs, in part driven by current significant governmental incentives (Marcotte et al. 2012) and the hope for increased efficiency and quality (Blumenthal and Glaser 2007; Chaudhry et al. 2006), usability issues remain a major barrier to adoption (Patel et al. 2008; Zhang 2005a, b). As with medical EHRs, a user-centered designed dental EHR facilitates good usability, assuring that the user can efficiently and effectively complete work tasks satisfactorily and successfully (Walji et al. 2014). It is also understood that, on the contrary, a poorly designed EHR with poor usability can lead to potential patient safety issues (Horsky et al. 2005a, b; Ash et al. 2004).

There is a plethora of challenges of dental EHR use and usability concerns. Usability challenges include visual as well as functional interface design problems (Thyvalikakath et al. 2009). Illogical button placement, unanticipated button functionality, difficulty switching between the odontogram and periodontal chart, inability to easily delete a mistaken entry on the odontogram, the need for better visual representation of dental findings and the fact that many icons resemble each other in shape and color are just some specific examples of interface design problems detected in the dental EHR (Reynolds et al. 2008; Thyvalikakath et al. 2009; Walji et al. 2013; Song et al. 2010).

Low chair-side adoption rate of dental EHRs is also thought to be, in part, due to the unsuitability of the conventional EHR set-up in the dental operatory (Reynolds et al. 2008). Keyboards and mice are potential sources of infection and need protective covers (D'Antonio et al. 2013). Electronic clinical data entry is often believed to take longer than entering this information in the paper chart or is thought to be impractical because the dental assistant is needed to perform other duties (Reynolds et al. 2008). Additionally, the inability to effectively use clinical decision support within the dental EHR to positively influence dental patient care outcomes (Schleyer and Thyvalikakath 2012) and the lack of integration of evidence based guidelines (Song et al. 2010) into the EHR have limited adoption by dental practitioners.

9.2 Applying Theory to Practice: Redesigning a Treatment Planning Module in a Dental EHR

9.2.1 Design Challenge

Because the axiUm EHR is widely used amongst dental school clinics to document patient care, it was possible to work in close collaboration with the vendor to redevelop one of its existing modules, using a participatory, work-centered design approach with an aim to better support the diagnostic-centric treatment planning process for dental students. Specifically, the existing treatment planning module within the EHR was deemed too complicated and difficult to use. Several dental institutions had also recently adopted the DDS Dental Diagnostic Terminology (formerly called the EZCodes), which drove the diagnostic entry functionality of the Treatment Planning module.

The work of treatment planning in dentistry is the process of using information obtained from the patient history, clinical examination and diagnostic tests to formulate a sequence of treatment steps designed to eliminate disease and restore efficient, comfortable aesthetic and masticatory function to a patient. When developing a treatment plan, the provider should follow a general phasing and sequencing format designed to solve the patient's dental problems in a way that first manages the patient's emergent concerns (e.g., pain and infection). The next step is disease (e.g., caries) removal and tooth restoration; then, tooth replacement and reconstruction. Once these priorities have been met, aesthetic and cosmetic concerns are addressed, and lastly, preventive and maintenance measures are ensured. Any given phase may contain several individual procedures, some of which may be sequenced in a specific order (Stefanac and Nesbit 2007).

The Treatment Planning module in the axiUm EHR was originally developed with input from dental educators and thought leaders, and follows the treatment planning philosophy of Stefanac (Stefanac and Nesbit 2007). In order to develop a treatment plan within axiUm, a user (i) enters the patient's problems/complaints; (ii) selects the appropriate diagnoses from a comprehensive list; (iii) enters the treatment objectives, which represent the intent or rationale for the final treatment plan, usually expressed as short statements and clear goals from both the student's and patient's perspectives; and (iv) enters a detailed plan for treating each of the selected diagnoses (Fig. 9.2). Following treatment planning, the student obtains instructor approval and patient consent before beginning treatment.

9.2.2 Design Approach

A participatory design process to systematically identify challenges in the use of the existing Treatment Planning Module was used to inform an improved user interface that effectively supports the underlying needs of the end users. As summarized in

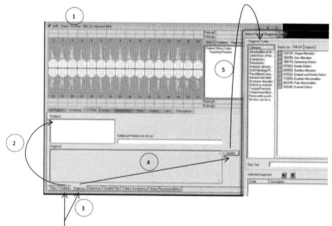

In the (1) 'treatment planning' module, the student (2) enters the problems and (3) moves to the 'Diagnosis' tab. Here, the appropriate diagnoses may be selected by (4) clicking on the 'update' button and working through (5) the list of the 'Clinical Diagnosis Codes'.

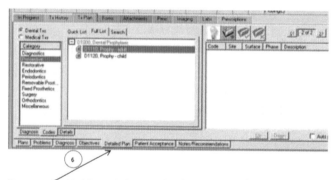

Treatment is added for each diagnosis by clicking on the (6) 'Detailed Plan' tab, selecting the appropriate treatment category and subsequently, the suitable treatment from the full list.

Fig. 9.2 Original treatment planning process in axiUm (Reprinted from Tokede et al. permission required)

Fig. 9.3, usability challenges were first identified and prioritized. New mockups were then developed, tested, refined and implemented in the EHR by the vendor. After further usability assessments, the new module was released to customers. Post-implementation usability assessments were conducted to determine the impact of the re-design in comparison to the original version.

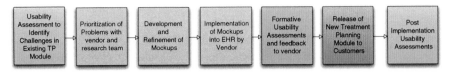

Fig. 9.3 Overall process for assessing, improving and implementing the Treatment Planning (TP) Module in axiUm

9.2.2.1 Usability Assessment to Identify Challenges in Existing Treatment Planning Module

In general, a terminology is evaluated in terms of its ability to represent relevant concepts, and user interfaces are evaluated in terms of their usability. As Patel and Cimino noted, a combined approach towards evaluating both the terminology and the user interface offers a more holistic perspective on how the task is carried out and where it can be improved (Cimino et al. 2001). Consider when a user would like to enter a diagnosis into the Treatment Planning module but faces significant hurdles or fails. The reason for the failure might be any one or a combination of the following: inadequate completeness of the terminology (e.g., the terminology does not represent the diagnosis), poor usability (e.g., the interface does not provide adequate access to the diagnostic terminology), or insufficient representation within the terminology (e.g., poor organization of the terminology). The same problems could underpin the selection of a term that does not capture the intended meaning. By attending to both the terminology and the user interface, we can begin to characterize the breadth of the causes of failure. Thus, we analyzed the following when considering this human computer interaction challenge: (1) use of the DDS terminology itself, (2) use of the existing Treatment Planning interface and (3) use of the DDS terminology as part of clinic workflow.

We conducted usability assessments of EHRs at two dental schools: Harvard School of Dental Medicine (HSDM) and University of California, San Francisco (UCSF). Both institutions have university-owned clinics to train dental students as well as residents (post graduate students). Both dental schools also have a private faculty practice, use the axiUm EHR system, and were early adopters of the DDS dental diagnostic terminology. Study participants included a sample of third and fourth year dental students (who were actively involved with delivering patient care), residents, and faculty. These groups represent the primary users of the DDS dental diagnostic terminology. As mentioned previously, dental students are responsible for updating the dental patient record under the supervision of attending faculty. Because one does not get many opportunities to overhaul a major module within the EHR, we conducted three complementary usability assessments in order to maximize our ability to capture challenges. We will summarize that work here; we have published full details in the International Journal of Medical Informatics (Walji et al. 2013, 2014).

Think-Aloud User Testing We created two pre-defined scenarios to assess users' interactions with DDS in the axiUm Treatment Planning module: a simple task of entering one diagnosis and a more complex treatment-planning task. Participants were asked to think aloud (Ericsson and Simon 1993) and verbalize their thoughts as they worked through each scenario. As part of user testing, quantitative data was captured to assess if tasks were completed successfully (a measure of effectiveness) and the amount of time spent in accomplishing the task (a measure of efficiency). To evaluate whether a user successfully completed the tasks, we had to define the correct path to complete the tasks. We did this using Hierarchical Task Analysis (HTA) (Diaper and Stanton 2004) after gathering input from expert dentists at each site. After determining the appropriate path to complete the tasks, we calculated the expert performance time, which is the time it would take an expert (who makes no errors) to complete the tasks. We did this using CogTool, (John et al. 2004) an open source software that predicts performance time on the basis of application screenshots and the specification of a path to complete a specific task. After completing the exercises, participants were asked to provide additional feedback on the use of the module, and complete a user satisfaction survey using the validated and widely used System Usability Scale (Brooke 1996).

Observations Using Ethnography Observational data were collected over a 3-day period by a trained researcher in order to provide insight into the clinical workflow, information gathering and diagnostic decision-making process in the clinical environment where the dentists and dental students worked. To minimize any impact on patient care, a non-participatory observational technique was used. The researcher engaged with the dental team members only if there was a need for any clarification or during downtime such as when a patient did not show for an appointment. Observational data were captured using paper-based field notes. Each set of observations occurred for approximately 4 h, in two separate shifts (morning and afternoon). The primary purpose of the observations was to capture overall clinical workflow and to identify how diagnoses were made and captured in the EHR using the DDS dental diagnostic terminology, and to identify any associated challenges. Actual clinical work was not part of the observation.

Semi-structured Interviews The third approach we took for evaluating the terminology and interface was to conduct semi-structured interviews with open-ended questions. The semi-structured format ensured uniformity of questions asked, while the open-ended format allowed the interviewees to express themselves. New questions were allowed to arise as a result of the discussion. The prepared questions focused on two broad themes: (1) the perception and internal representation of the clinic, patient care and role of dentists/students within the clinic; and (2) the nature of the workflow and environment of care within this dental clinic with the use of EHR. The questions were influenced by the knowledge gained from the observations. Interviews lasted approximately 30 min each. The interview data were collected in order to assess information on the role, situational awareness and general work philosophy of the subjects in the dental clinic. The sample was representative of those who are usually present in the clinical environment and as such included dental third and fourth year students, residents and faculty.

Findings User testing revealed that only 22 % of users were able to successfully complete all of the steps in the simple task of entering one diagnosis, while no user was able to complete the more complex treatment-planning task. Table 9.1 provides an overview of the 24 high-level usability problems that were found through the use of the three methods. The methods together identified a total of 187 usability violations: 54 % via user testing, 28 % via the semi-structured interview and 18 % from the survey method, with modest overlap (Walji et al. 2014). Interface-related problems included unexpected approaches for displaying diagnosis, lack of visibility, and inconsistent use of user interface widgets. User interface widgets are elements of the interface with which a user interacts. Terminology related issues included missing and mis-categorized concepts. Work domain issues involved both absent and superfluous functions. In collaboration with the vendor, each usability problem was prioritized and a timeline set to resolve the concerns.

9.2.2.2   Participatory Prioritization of Problems with the Vendor and Broad-Based Research Team

Based on the findings from the usability studies, a diverse group comprising of clinicians, secondary data users, usability experts, terminology developers/ researchers, and the vendor design team assessed each of the 24 findings and prioritized each issue, and how it may be addressed in future versions of the EHR. Involvement of the vendor was critical at this stage. Several problems had solutions or workarounds that could be implemented immediately by re-configuration or customization in the existing version of the Treatment Planning module. For example, the ability to enter free text could be disabled for end users. The research team also gained greater appreciation of the vendor's development schedule and rationale for some of their earlier design decisions. The vendor's development team, for the first time, had empirical evidence of specific usability problems faced by users. The prioritization process, which occurred during a face-to-face meeting with the CEO as well as several follow-up phone calls, provided a common understanding of the major usability problems and a process by which they could be addressed.

9.2.2.3   Development and Refinement of Mockups

Over 2–3 months, the usability team developed low fidelity mockups and made presentations of this work to the larger, broad-based team in weekly conference calls. After several iterations, a consensus design was developed. As shown in

Table 9.1 Summary of usability problems, priorities and timeframe to address and implement solutions

	Usability problem (PRIORITY)	
	Description/example	Timeframe to implement solutions
Interface	**1. Illogical ordering of terms(HIGH)**	**Immediate**: Reorder alphabeti-
	Terms are ordered based on numeric code rather than alphabetically	cally; **≤1 year**: Users to customize ordering
	2. Term names not fully visible(HIGH)	**≤6 months**
	Users select incorrect diagnosis as they are unable to read the full name	
	3. Time consuming to enter a diagnosis(HIGH)	**≤1 year**
	User must navigate several screens and scroll through a long list to find and select a diagnosis	
	4. Inconsistent naming and placement of user interface widgets(HIGH)	**≤6 months**
	To add a new diagnosis, a user must click a button labeled "Update"	
	5. Ineffective feedback to confirm diagnosis entry(HIGH)	**≤1 year**
	User only sees the numeric code for the diagnosis and not the name of the term.	
	6. Search results do not match users expectations(MEDIUM)	**≤1 year**
	A search for "pericornitis" retrieves 3 concepts with the same name but a different numerical code	
	7. Users unaware of important functions to help find a diagnosis(MEDIUM)	**≤1 year**
	System defaults to "quick list", so some users do not navigate the "full list" or discover the use of the search feature	
	8. Limited flexibility in user interface(MEDIUM)	**≤1 year**
	User unable to modify an entered diagnosis on the "details" page and must go back to previous screens to edit diagnosis	
	9. Distinction between Category Name and Concept unclear(MEDIUM)	**Immediate**
	Users attempt to select a category name.	
Terminology	**10. Inappropriate granularity/specificity of concepts(MEDIUM)**	**≤1 year**
	Some sub-categories have a large number of concepts making it very difficult for users to find an appropriate term	

(continued)

Table 9.1 (continued)

	Usability problem ^(PRIORITY) Description/example	Timeframe to implement solutions
	11. Some concepts appear missing/not included^(HIGH)	≤6 months
	Examples of missing concepts according to users include: missing tooth, arrested caries, and attritional teeth	
	12. Some concepts not classified in appropriate categories/sub categories^(HIGH)	≤6 months
	Example: aesthetic concerns	
	13. Abbreviations not recognized by users^(HIGH)	≤6 months
	Example: F/U, NOS, VDO	
	14. Visibility of the numeric code for a diagnostic term^(HIGH)	**Immediate**: Use Quicklist to hide code ≤**1 year**: Remove numeric code in UI
	Although the numeric code is a meaningless identifier, users had an expectation that the identifier should provide some meaning	
	15. Users not clear about the meaning of some concepts^(MEDIUM)	≤1 year
	Novice users (students) had difficulty distinguishing between similar terms, and definitions and synonyms were not provided	
Work domain	**16. Free text option can be used circumvent structured data entry**^(HIGH)	**Immediate**: Disable option ≤**1 year**: Remove option altogether
	Instead of selecting a structured term, some users free text the name of the diagnosis.	
	17. Synonyms not displayed^(HIGH)	≤1 year
	Users must search by preferred term name	
	18. Knowledge level of diagnostic term concepts and how to enter in EHR limited^(HIGH)	≤1 year
	Users appear to have had little concerted education and training either by institution or vendor	
	19. Only one diagnosis can be entered for each treatment^(HIGH)	≤1 year
	Endodontic discipline require that treatments are justified using both a pulpal and periapical diagnosis	
	20. Diagnosis cannot be charted using the Odontogram or Periogram^(HIGH)	≤2 year
	Users chart findings using	

(continued)

Table 9.1 (continued)

Usability problem [(PRIORITY)]	
Description/example	Timeframe to implement solutions
21. No historical view of when a diagnosis has been added or modified[(HIGH)]	≤1 year
22. No decision support to help suggest appropriate diagnoses, or alert if inappropriate ones are selected[(MEDIUM)]	≤2 year
23. No way to indicate state of diagnosis (i.e differential, working or definitive)[(MEDIUM)]	≤1 year
24. Users forced to enter a diagnosis for treatments that may not require them.[(MEDIUM)]	≤1 year

Reproduced from Walji et al. (2013) used with permission

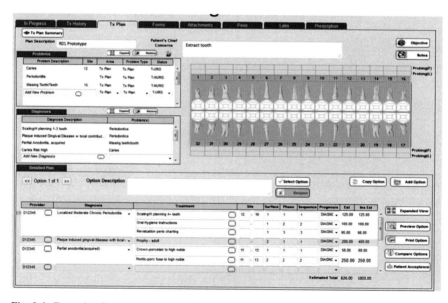

Fig. 9.4 Example of a mature mockup of a new Treatment Planning interface

Fig. 9.4, key design features included (1) one screen for entering problems, diagnoses and treatments to provide situational awareness to users, (2) autocomplete functionality to enter problems, diagnoses and treatments, and (3) ability to explicitly link problems, diagnoses and treatments.

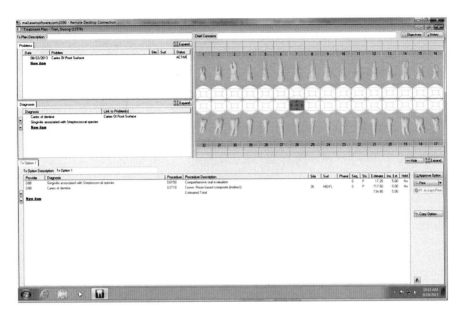

Fig. 9.5 Treatment Planning interface in axiUm after implementation by vendor

9.2.2.4 Implementation of Mockups into EHR

The vendor's design team was then responsible for determining how to implement the mockups within its EHR using their existing development tools (Microsoft Visual C++ .Net). Some of the desired functionality, such as drag and drop to reorder concepts, was not possible due to the underlying design architecture. In each case, the vendor would provide alternative solutions to meet the intent of the enhancement. Figure 9.5 shows a screenshot of the newly developed Treatment Planning module in the axiUm EHR. The approximate development time from receiving the mockups to full implementation was 6 months.

9.2.2.5 Next Steps: Assessing Impact of the New Treatment Planning Module

This design case demonstrates how a participatory, work-centered design process can be used to re-design an EHR module to support the treatment planning process in dentistry. The vendor released the new Treatment Planning module in February 2014. In ongoing work, the research team is conducting comprehensive assessments to determine the impact of the new interface on efficiency, effectiveness, and satisfaction.

9.3 Implications for Practice

9.3.1 Importance of Collaborative Teams for the Design of Usable Systems

"It takes work, and new ways of thinking, and new kinds and methods of openness, to bring substantively new voices into a conversation. Similarly, to bring users' knowledges and perspectives directly into computer specification and design, it is necessary to do more than "just add users and stir."" (Muller and Druin 2003)

Human-computer interaction has, as a field, undergone an evolution from technological solutions to complex problems of human interaction with computers, to user-centered design, (Thursky and Mahemoff 2007) to participatory design (Teixeira et al. 2011). This evolution represents shifts from designing without users to designing with users in mind to designing with users. This last approach, called participatory design, is a set of theories and practices engaging end-users as full participants in design. Rather than replacing user-centered design, participatory design has subsumed user-centered approaches, like the work-centered design approach we used, into its rich and diverse toolbox, which draws upon fields such as graphic design, architecture, psychology, anthropology, software engineering, and communications studies. Participatory design has likewise been applied to a diverse set of applications, as wide ranging as land use in Africa (d'Aquino and Bah 2014) to designing technology for children with special needs (Frauenberger et al. 2011).

In a strict user-centered design process, the researcher serves as the interface between the user and designer. The researcher collects primary data or uses secondary sources to learn about the user's needs, which are translated by the researcher into design criteria. The designer interprets these criteria, typically through mockups. The researcher and user reappear in the process for usability testing. In user-centered design, the researcher, designer, and user have distinct roles: the user is not integral to the design team, but is instead spoken for by the researcher. A key participatory design principle is to blur and bridge the distinctions among these roles through mutual learning, often through face-to-face interaction and prototyping.

The way that we have operationalized participatory design principles in the context of standardized dental diagnostic term entry into the EHR has been to bring together a broad range of stakeholders in a series of virtual and face-to-face working sessions. The breadth of the stakeholders at each meeting reflected the wide-ranging impact of building and implementing the terms and the interface to the terms. Each team member brought a different, relevant perspective; they included the CEO of the dental EHR company, the lead architect of the dental EHR company, practicing dentists, usability experts, epidemiologists, data warehouse experts, and dental clinic administrators. Through close interaction and real-time problem solving, we were able to learn from each other and to find solutions that would meet each stakeholder's needs while respecting the limitations other stakeholders faced.

Participatory design was a good fit with our goal of enhancing standardized dental diagnostic term entry in the context of an EHR. We had a committed, and funded, set of core participants who were willing to devote scores of hours to the project; we had sufficient technical latitude to accommodate end-user feedback given the close partnership with the EHR vendor; and as the developers of the diagnostic terminology, we had the ability to make necessary changes to the terms as required. In addition, as has been the case in many participatory design applications, our scope was tightly focused (Pilemalm and Timpka 2008). Were we to have considered the totality of the user experience when interacting with the EHR, the type of participatory approach we took would have been infeasible given our timeline and budget. As has been noted elsewhere, participatory design is costly (Pilemalm and Timpka 2008). A much leaner approach to usability analysis is the use of heuristics evaluation, i.e., assessing how well a given system adheres to best practices for interaction design, which is well-suited to eliminating initial design decisions that would violate a heuristic. As design progresses to implementation, though, more user engagement is needed to identify usability challenges. In a 2009 study of four dental EHRs, heuristic evaluation was found to anticipate half of the usability problems identified through empirical testing with end users (Thyvalikakath et al. 2009). User testing is not, of course, the only way to incorporate user participation. Other approaches include interviews and surveys. Though we found the survey approach to be comparatively less effective in our own work, surveys have the advantage of being inexpensive and quick to yield results, which may be the best option in some circumstances (Walji et al. 2014).

9.3.2 Impact on Secondary Use of Data

Although the discussion of whether the use of EHRs will lower costs and improve care is still open, there are fewer questions about the significance of the data generated through clinical care. Given the monetary and time expense of clinical trials, it is only sensible to use the informational and biological by-products of health care delivery to expand our knowledge and improve practice (Kohane 2013). Before being the object of a researcher's analysis, these data were entered in a variety of systems, which in turn, sit in a variety of contexts, both of which may have usability implications. Here, it is useful to draw out what is meant by the term usability, as it covers a large swath of concepts. Over the decades, the literature has surfaced a wide range of both narrow and broad definitions of usability. A frequently-referenced definition is that framed within the ISO 9241 standard, in which usability is defined as the "[e]xtent to which a product can be used by specified users to achieve specified goals with effectiveness, efficiency, and satisfaction." (International Organization for Standardization 1998) In turn, satisfaction is defined as "freedom from discomfort, and positive attitudes towards the user of the product"; efficiency is defined as the "resources expended in relation to the accuracy and completeness with which users achieve goals"; and effectiveness is defined as the "accuracy and completeness with which users achieve specified goals."

It would be tempting to surmise that effectiveness, efficiency, and satisfaction depend on one another, but alas, the field has an under-developed understanding of the relationships among usability measures (Hornbaeck 2006). Indeed, some have posited that any relationships among them depend on other factors, such as application domain, use context, user experience, and task complexity (Association for Computing Machinery CHI 2000). What this means is that distinct aspects of usability need to be measured separately, that we cannot rely upon efficiency to tell us about effectiveness, for example.

In the setting of secondary use of data, effectiveness is key: in the context of dental diagnostic terms, for instance, secondary users of data rely upon the primary users to have effectively entered valid diagnostic terms, even if such entry entailed discomfort and expenditure of resources on the part of the individual who entered the data. Indeed, part of the challenge of promoting the valid documentation of standardized diagnostic terms is that it has not been a professional norm in dentistry and thus inherently involves additional effort than does failing to enter the diagnosis. Thus, the assessments we conducted captured utilization, the proportion of times that any diagnostic term was entered when a diagnosis was appropriate, as well as valid use, the proportion of diagnostic terms entered that were an appropriate match for the treatment provided.

9.3.3 Impact on Inter-professional Practice

It is an artifact of the history of dentistry in the United States, (Centers for Medicare & Medicaid Services Medicare Dental Coverage 2013; Bebinger 2014) rather than anatomy or physiology, that oral health is perceived as separable from general health, as if there were an impenetrable firewall between the two. Unfortunately, in the case of bridging medical and dental data, there most often is such a technical and policy-based firewall, with no broadly adopted ways to communicate efficiently across the divide. In 2013, the Advisory Committee on Training in Primacy Care Medicine and Dentistry wrote, "the separation between oral health and systemic health does not serve the needs of patients. There must be a mutual interaction between oral health and systemic health using efficient inter-professional communication." Inter-professional practice is being promoted as a way to achieve the so-called Triple Aim of (1) enhanced population health, (2) reduced costs of care, and (3) optimal patient care experience (Advisory Committee on Training in Primary Care Medicine and Dentistry 2013; Berwick et al. 2008). Informatics infrastructure can pose both barriers to and opportunities for collaborative practice between medicine and dentistry; the Advisory Committee recommended that dental practices should interact and integrate more effectively with medicine and other health professions in terms of quality measure and health information systems (Advisory Committee on Training in Primary Care Medicine and Dentistry 2013).

Under the right conditions, EHRs in the dental clinic setting could serve to bridge the inter-professional information gap in a way that is not possible in a paper-based world. In the most straightforward scenario, the medical and dental records would be integrated into a single system. EHR systems with oral health modules are deployed through the Indian Health Service, the Department of Veteran's Affairs, as well as the Cattails medical and dental EHRs developed and used at the Marshfield Clinic in Marshfield, WI (Advisory Committee on Training in Primary Care Medicine and Dentistry 2013; Schleyer and Eisner 1994). Unfortunately, these cases are the rare exception rather than the rule. As noted by Powell and Din, "the essential core improvement to bring medicine and dentistry closer together is the integration of medical and dental care and data. Currently, many medical records and data exist separate and distinct from dental records and data for the same patient" (Powell and Din 2011). Even in the context of clinical care, there are no channels through which to exchange data between medical and dental EHRs. In practice, thus, the little information that is exchanged between the medical and dental settings is typically done through letters or telephone calls. Information exchanged in this way can make its way into the record only as a PDF or image or as free-text notes entered by a clinician. In 2009, the ADA announced an agreement with HL7 (Health Level 7) to enhance the coordination of patient care between medical and dental practices using a dental extension to the Continuity of Care Document (CCD), (Health Level 7 International Health Level Seven and the American Dental Association Sign Agreement to Develop Joint Healthcare IT Standard Initiatives 2009; Health Level 7 International HL7/ASTM Implementation Guide for CDA® R2 -Continuity of Care Document (CCD®) Release 1) though the routine exchange of such documents has not yet come to pass.

In addition to the technical details of how clinical information is exchanged across the professional divide, we should consider the communicative value of the information. One of the primary goals of standardizing dental diagnostic terms is to enhance communication between providers, with patients, and with third parties like payors (Kalenderian et al. 2011). Thus, ensuring that both the terminology itself as well as the EHR design, deployment, and use support effective and efficient documentation of standardized dental diagnostic terms serves inter-professional practice at its most basic level. Taking a step back, it is also worth noting that poor usability and a steep learning curve have been reported as barriers to adoption of EHRs in dentistry, as was mentioned in Sect. 9.1.4 of this chapter. Even in the dental academic setting, in which EHRs are widespread, users have expressed doubt that the systems improve efficiency and effectiveness (Thyvalikakath et al. 2014).

Improving EHR usability could not only enhance inter-professional practice but also could heal the fractured perceptions of EHRs within larger dental practices in which administrative and clinical duties are divided. In a study in a large dental teaching practice at an academic center, administrators articulated the most and broadest benefits of an EHR: in fact, the technology had so enhanced the quantity and quality of accessible information to the point that it was described as

Additional Readings

Kalenderian, E., Ramoni, R. L., White, J. M., et al. (2011). The development of a dental diagnostic terminology. *Journal of Dental Education, 75*(1), 68–76.

Muller, M., & Druin, A. (2003). *Participatory design: The third space in HCI. The human-computer interaction handbook.* Hillside: L. Erlbaum Associates Inc.

Norman, D. A. (2005). Human-centered design considered harmful. *Interactions, 12*(4), 14–19.

References

Advisory Committee on Training in Primary Care Medicine and Dentistry. (2013). *Interprofessional education.* Rockville: Health Resources and Services Administration.

Anderson, G. D., & Grey, E. B. (2013). *The MSO's prognosis after the ACA: A viable integration tool?* Phoenix: Physicians and Physician Organizations Law Institute. http://www.healthlawyers.org/Events/Programs/Materials/Documents/PHY13/B_anderson_grey.pdf. Accessed 2 May 2014.

Ash, J. S., Berg, M., & Coiera, E. (2004). Some unintended consequences of information technology in health care: The nature of patient care information system-related errors. *Journal of the American Medical Informatics Association, 11*(2), 104–112.

Association for Computing Machinery CHI. (2000). *Measuring usability: Are effectiveness, efficiency, and satisfaction really correlated?* Paper presented at Conference on human factors in computing systems, The Hague, The Netherlands.

Bader, J. D., Shugars, D. A., White, B. A., & Rindal, D. B. (1999). Development of effectiveness of care and use of services measures for dental care plans. *Journal of Public Health Dentistry, 59*(3), 142–149.

Bebinger, M. (2014). *Put back the teeth? Why we separate dental and medical care.* WBUR's CommonHealth Reform and Reality, Boston, MA.

Berwick, D. M., Nolan, T. W., & Whittington, J. (2008). The triple aim: Care, health, and cost. *Health Affairs (Millwood), 27*(3), 759–769.

Blumenthal, D., & Glaser, J. P. (2007). Information technology comes to medicine. *New England Journal of Medicine, 356*(24), 2527–2534.

Brooke, J. (1996). *A "quick and dirty" usability scale.* London: Taylor & Francis.

Button, P. S., Doyle, K., Karitis, J. W., & Selhorst, C. (1999). Automating clinical documentation in dentistry: Case study of a clinical integration model. *Journal of Healthcare Information Management, 13*(3), 31–40.

Canadian Dental Association Dental Health Services in Canada. (2010). *Fact and figures.* http://www.med.uottawa.ca/sim/data/Dental/Dental_Health_Services_in_Canada_June_2010.pdf. Accessed 6 July 2014.

Centers for Medicare & Medicaid Services Medicare Dental Coverage. Baltimore: Centers for Medicare & Medicaid Services 2013. http://cms.hhs.gov/Medicare/Coverage/MedicareDentalCoverage/index.html

Chaudhry, B., Wang, J., Wu, S., et al. (2006). Systematic review: Impact of health information technology on quality, efficiency, and costs of medical care. *Annals of Internal Medicine, 144*(10), 742–752.

Cimino, J. J., Patel, V. L., & Kushniruk, A. W. (2001). Studying the human-computer-terminology interface. *Journal of the American Medical Informatics Association, 8*(2), 163–173.

Clinical Information Modeling Initiative (CIMI) Category: Interface terminology. (2012). http://informatics.mayo.edu/CIMI/index.php/Category:Interface_Terminology. Accessed 14 July 2014.

D'Antonio, N. N., Rihs, J. D., Stout, J. E., & Yu, V. L. (2013). Computer keyboard covers impregnated with a novel antimicrobial polymer significantly reduce microbial contamination. *American Journal of Infection Control, 41*(4), 337–339.

d'Aquino, P., & Bah, A. (2014). Multi-level participatory design of land use policies in African drylands: A method to embed adaptability skills of drylands societies in a policy framework. *Journal of Environmental Management, 132,* 207–219.

Diaper, D., & Stanton, N. A. (2004). *The handbook of task analysis for human-computer interaction.* Mahwah: Lawrence Erlbaum.

Ericsson, K. A., & Simon, H. A. (1993). *Protocol analysis: Verbal reports as data* (Rev. ed.). Cambridge, MA: MIT Press.

Ettelbrick, K. L., Webb, M. D., & Seale, N. S. (2000). Hospital charges for dental caries related emergency admissions. *Pediatric Dentistry, 22*(1), 21–25.

Exan Corp., Vancouver, Canada. http://www.axiumdental.com. Accessed 29 July 2014.

Finkbeiner, B. L. (2000). Four-handed dentistry revisited. *Journal of Contemporary Dental Practice, 1*(4), 74–86.

Finkbeiner, B. L. (2001). Selecting equipment for the ergonomic four-handed dental practice. *Journal of Contemporary Dental Practice, 2*(4), 44–52.

Fitzpatrick, J., & Koh, J. S. (2005). If you build it (right), they will come: The physician-friendly CPOE. Not everything works as planned right out of the box. A Mississippi hospital customizes its electronic order entry system for maximum use by physicians. *Health Management Technology, 26*(1), 52–53.

Frauenberger, C., Good, J., & Keay-Bright, W. (2011, March). Designing technology for children with special needs: Bridging perspectives through participatory design. Available from: Ipswich. Accessed 4 July 2014. *Codesign (Serial Online), 7*(1), 1–28.

Goldberg, L. J., Ceusters, W., Eisner, J., & Smith, B. (2005). The significance of SNODENT. *Studies in Health Technology and Informatics, 116,* 737–742.

Gregg, T. A., & Boyd, D. H. (1996). A computer software package to facilitate clinical audit of outpatient paediatric dentistry. *International Journal of Paediatric Dentistry, 6*(1), 45–51.

Guay, A. H., Wall, T. P., Petersen, B. C., & Lazar, V. F. (2012). Evolving trends in size and structure of group dental practices in the United States. *Journal of Dental Education, 76*(8), 1036–1044.

Health Level 7 International Health Level Seven and the American Dental Association Sign Agreement to Develop Joint Healthcare IT Standard Initiatives. (2009). Ann Arbor.

Health Level 7 International HL7/ASTM Implementation Guide for CDA® R2 -Continuity of Care Document (CCD®) Release 1. Ann Arbor: Health Level 7 International. http://www.hl7.org/implement/standards/product_brief.cfm?product_id=6. Accessed 4 May 2014.

Hill, H. K., Stewart, D. C., & Ash, J. S. (2010a). The training and support needs of faculty and students using a health information technology system were significant: A case study in a dental school. *AMIA Annual Symposium Proceedings, 2010,* 301–305.

Hill, H. K., Stewart, D. C., & Ash, J. S. (2010b). Health Information Technology Systems profoundly impact users: A case study in a dental school. *Journal of Dental Education, 74*(4), 434–445.

Hornbaeck, K. (2006). Current practice in measuring usability: Challenges to usability studies and research. *International Journal of Human-Computer Studies, 64,* 79–102.

Horsky, J., Kuperman, G. J., & Patel, V. L. (2005a). Comprehensive analysis of a medication dosing error related to CPOE. *Journal of the American Medical Informatics Association, 12*(4), 377–382.

Horsky, J., Zhang, J., & Patel, V. L. (2005b). To err is not entirely human: Complex technology and user cognition. *Journal of Biomedical Informatics, 38*(4), 264–266.

International Organization for Standardization. (1998). *Ergonomic requirements for office work with visual display terminals. Part 11: Guidance on usability.* Geneva: International Organization for Standardization.

Irwin, J. Y., Torres-Urquidy, M. H., Schleyer, T., & Monaco, V. (2009). A preliminary model of work during initial examination and treatment planning appointments. *British Dental Journal, 206*(1), E1; discussion 24–5.

John, J. H., Thomas, D., & Richards, D. (2003). Questionnaire survey on the use of computerisation in dental practices across the Thames Valley Region. *British Dental Journal, 195*(10), 585–590; discussion 79.

John, B., Prevas, K., Salvucci, D., & Koedinger, K. (2004). *Predictive human performance modeling made easy.* Paper presented at: CHI Conference on Human Factors in Computing Systems, Vienna, Austria.

Juve-Udina, M. E. (2013). What patients' problems do nurses e-chart? Longitudinal study to evaluate the usability of an interface terminology. *International Journal of Nursing Studies, 50* (12), 1698–1710.

Kalenderian, E., Ramoni, R. L., White, J. M., et al. (2011). The development of a dental diagnostic terminology. *Journal of Dental Education, 75*(1), 68–76.

Kohane, I. S. (2013). Secondary use of health information: Are we asking the right question? *JAMA Internal Medicine, 173*(19), 1806–1807.

Leake, J. L. (2002). Diagnostic codes in dentistry – Definition, utility and developments to date. *Journal of the Canadian Dental Association, 68*(7), 403–406.

Leake, J. L., Main, P. A., & Sabbah, W. (1999). A system of diagnostic codes for dental health care. *Journal of Public Health Dentistry, 59*(3), 162–170.

Marcotte, L., Seidman, J., Trudel, K., et al. (2012). Achieving meaningful use of health information technology: A guide for physicians to the EHR incentive programs. *Archives of Internal Medicine, 172*(9), 731–736.

Miller, R. H., & Sim, I. (2004). Physicians' use of electronic medical records: Barriers and solutions. *Health Affairs (Millwood), 23*(2), 116–126.

Muller, M., & Druin, A. (2003). *Participatory design: The third space in HCI. The human-computer interaction handbook.* Hillside: L. Erlbaum Associates Inc.

Nederlands Tandartsenblad Nederlandse Norm voor diagnostische termen. Nieuwegein, Nederland: Nederlandse Maatschappij van Tandartsen 2014. http://www.ntblad.nl. Accessed 14 July 2014.

Orlowsky, W. J., & Glusman, M. (1969). Recovery of aversive thresholds following midbrain lesions in the cat. *Journal of Comparative Physiology and Psychology, 67*(2), 245–251.

Patel, V. L., Zhang, J., Yoskowitz, N. A., Green, R., & Sayan, O. R. (2008). Translational cognition for decision support in critical care environments: A review. *Journal of Biomedical Informatics, 41*(3), 413–431.

Pilemalm, S., & Timpka, T. (2008). Third generation participatory design in health informatics – Making user participation applicable to large-scale information system projects. *Journal of Biomedical Informatics, 41*(2), 327–339.

Powell, V. J. H., & Din, F. M. (2011). *Rational and need to articulate medical and dental data.* New York: Springer.

Reference Terminology. http://informatics.mayo.edu/CIMI/index.php/Category:Reference_Terminology. Accessed 1 Apr 2013.

Reynolds, P. A., Harper, J., & Dunne, S. (2008). Better informed in clinical practice – A brief overview of dental informatics. *British Dental Journal, 204*(6), 313–317.

Sabbah, W. (1999). *Assessing the validity of North York dental diagnostic codes.* Faculty of Dentistry. Toronto: University of Toronto.

Schleyer, T., & Eisner, J. (1994). The computer-based oral health record: An essential tool for cross-provider quality management. *Journal of the California Dental Association, 22*(11), 57–58; 60–61; 3–4.

Schleyer, T., & Thyvalikakath, T. P. (2012). Alert fatigue. *Journal of the American Dental Association, 143*(4), 332–333; author reply 33–4.

Schleyer, T. K., Thyvalikakath, T. P., Spallek, H., et al. (2006). Clinical computing in general dentistry. *Journal of the American Medical Informatics Association, 13*(3), 344–352.

Schleyer, T., Spallek, H., & Hernandez, P. (2007). A qualitative investigation of the content of dental paper-based and computer-based patient record formats. *Journal of the American Medical Informatics Association, 14*(4), 515–526.

Service Canada Dentists. Government of Canada 2014. http://www.servicecanada.gc.ca/eng/qc/job_futures/statistics/3113.shtml. Accessed 6 July 2014.

Simon, S. R., Kaushal, R., Cleary, P. D., et al. (2007). Correlates of electronic health record adoption in office practices: A statewide survey. *Journal of the American Medical Informatics Association, 14*(1), 110–117.

SNODENT Update. (2004). *National Committee on Vital and Health Statistics (NCVHS); Subcommittee on Standards and Security*. Chicago: American Dental Association.

Song, M., Spallek, H., Polk, D., Schleyer, T., & Wali, T. (2010). How information systems should support the information needs of general dentists in clinical settings: Suggestions from a qualitative study. *BMC Medical Informatics and Decision Making, 10*, 7.

Stefanac, S. J., & Nesbit, S. P. (2007). *Treatment planning in dentistry* (2nd ed.). St. Louis: Mosby.

Taichman, R., Pinsky, H., & Sarment, D. (2010). *Pilot safety protocol could help dentists reduce errors*. Ann Arbor: University of Michigan. http://ns.umich.edu/htdocs/releases/story.php?id=7906. Accessed 25 Apr 2011.

Teixeira, L., Saavedra, V., Ferreira, C., & Santos, B. S. (2011). Using participatory design in a health information system. *Conference Proceedings IEEE Engineering in Medical Biology Society, 2011*, 5339–5342.

Thursky, K. A., & Mahemoff, M. (2007). User-centered design techniques for a computerised antibiotic decision support system in an intensive care unit. *International Journal of Medical Informatics, 76*(10), 760–768.

Thyvalikakath, T. P., Schleyer, T. K., & Monaco, V. (2007). Heuristic evaluation of clinical functions in four practice management systems: A pilot study. *Journal of the American Dental Association, 138*(2), 209–210, 12–8.

Thyvalikakath, T. P., Monaco, V., Thambuganipalle, H. B., & Schleyer, T. (2008). A usability evaluation of four commercial dental computer-based patient record systems. *Journal of the American Dental Association, 139*(12), 1632–1642.

Thyvalikakath, T. P., Monaco, V., Thambuganipalle, H., & Schleyer, T. (2009). Comparative study of heuristic evaluation and usability testing methods. *Studies in Health Technology and Informatics, 143*, 322–327.

Thyvalikakath, T. P., Dziabiak, M. P., Johnson, R., et al. (2014). Advancing cognitive engineering methods to support user interface design for electronic health records. *International Journal of Medical Informatics, 83*(4), 292–302.

Torres-Urquidy, M. H., & Schleyer, T. (2006). Evaluation of the systematized nomenclature of dentistry using case reports: Preliminary results. *AMIA Annual Symposium Proceedings, 2006*, 1124.

University of Alabama at Birmingham Four-Handed Dentistry. (2011). Birmingham. https://www.uab.edu/uabmagazine/breakthroughs/healthcare/four-handed-dentistry. Accessed 2 May 2014.

Uretz, M. (2014a). 10 reasons why your dental practice will soon be using Electronic Health Records (EHRs). http://practicemanagement.dentalproductsreport.com/technology-ehr/10-reasons-why-your-dental-practice-will-soon-be-using-electronic-health-records-ehrs. Accessed 14 July 2014.

Uretz, M. (2014b). *ADA Professional Product Review, 9*(2). http://www.dentalsoftwareadvisor.com/wp-content/uploads/2014/05/PPR_Vol_9_Iss_2_April_2014_PDF.25-29.pdf

Walji, M. F., Taylor, D., Langabeer, J. R., 2nd, & Valenza, J. A. (2009). Factors influencing implementation and outcomes of a dental electronic patient record system. *Journal of Dental Education, 73*(5), 589–600.

Walji, M. F., Kalenderian, E., Tran, D., et al. (2013). Detection and characterization of usability problems in structured data entry interfaces in dentistry. *International Journal of Medical Informatics, 82*(2), 128–138.

Walji, M. F., Kalenderian, E., Piotrowski, M., et al. (2014). Are three methods better than one? A comparative assessment of usability evaluation methods in an EHR. *International Journal of Medical Informatics, 83*(5), 361–367.

White, J. M., Kalenderian, E., Stark, P. C., et al. (2011). Evaluating a dental diagnostic terminology in an electronic health record. *Journal of Dental Education, 75*(5), 605–615.

World Health Organization. (1973). *Application of the international classification of diseases to dentistry and stomatology* (1st ed.). Geneva: World Health Organization.

Wotman, S., Lalumandier, J., Nelson, S., & Stange, K. (2001). Implications for dental education of a dental school-initiated practice research network. *Journal of Dental Education, 65*(8), 751–759.

Zhang, J. (2005a). Human-centered computing in health information systems. Part 2: Evaluation. *Journal of Biomedical Informatics, 38*(3), 173–175.

Zhang, J. (2005b). Human-centered computing in health information systems. Part 1: Analysis and design. *Journal of Biomedical Informatics, 38*(1), 1–3.

Chapter 10
Design for Supporting Healthcare Teams

Charlotte Tang, Yan Xiao, Yunan Chen, and Paul N. Gorman

10.1   Introduction

Healthcare today is a team sport, no longer dominated by the vision of a single nurse or doctor interacting with a patient. Rather, modern healthcare occurs through a coordinated action of many individuals, possessing diverse skills and expertise, sometimes collocated but often distributed in time and space. Obvious examples of healthcare teams include a surgical team performing an operation, emergency department (ED) personnel stabilizing a trauma patient, a "code team" responding to in-hospital cardiac arrest, and daily bedside rounds by multi-disciplinary teams in an intensive care unit. Less obvious are examples of health professional communication and collaboration that do not occur face-to-face. For example, a nurse may notice unexpected symptoms in her patient during night-shift, contact a pharmacist to learn that this is a medication side effect, pass this information on verbally at shift report so other nurses can monitor the effects, record the information in the medical record for all clinicians to be aware of, and perhaps add a paper or electronic "post-it" note for the physician, suggesting a change of the medication order at morning rounds.

In these contexts, electronic health records (EHR) and other health information technologies (HIT) can function in ways that support healthcare teams, becoming a

C. Tang (✉)
Department of Computer Science, Engineering and Physics, University of Michigan-Flint, Flint, MI, USA
e-mail: tcharlot@umflint.edu

Y. Xiao
Human Factors & Patient Safety Science, Baylor Scott & White Health, Dallas, TX, USA

Y. Chen
Department of Informatics, University of California, Irvine, Irvine, CA, USA

P.N. Gorman
Department of Medical Informatics and Clinical Epidemiology, Oregon Health & Science University, Portland, OR, USA

© Springer International Publishing Switzerland 2015   215
V.L. Patel et al. (eds.), *Cognitive Informatics for Biomedicine*, Health Informatics,
DOI 10.1007/978-3-319-17272-9_10

routine part of healthcare delivery and changing the ways teams work, communicate and collaborate. Outside the hospital, consumer-centered HIT such as patient portals and personal health records (PHR) can enable individuals to become more effectively engaged in their care, sharing information and communicating with multiple members of the healthcare team. In this chapter, we review healthcare teams, key concepts and theories of teamwork, and present two case studies on teamwork in healthcare.

10.1.1 Diversity of Healthcare Teams

In team research literature, an often adopted definition of a team is "*a distinguishable set of two or more people who interact dynamically, interdependently, and adaptively toward a common and valued goal/object/mission, who have each been assigned specific roles or functions to perform, and who have a limited life span of membership*" (Salas et al. 1992, p. 4). This definition goes beyond mere affiliation, emphasizing common goals and specific role assignments. In healthcare, role assignments may be perceived differently by different parties or may at times be unclear. For example, a surgeon, a nurse, and a patient may identify team membership or roles and responsibilities differently, and changing conditions and personnel in attendance may make assignments less clear and require re-negotiation. Table 10.1 lists several key characteristics of healthcare teams with examples.

It is important to recognize that a great variety of teams exist in healthcare, with varying degrees of shared objectives, clarity of role specifications, and interdependencies. For example, ED care is characterized by unpredictable and changing

Table 10.1 Key characteristics of healthcare teams

Healthcare team characteristics	Examples
Multidisciplinary	Multidisciplinary rounds in pediatric intensive care unit (Fig. 10.3)
Dynamic team formation, composition, and role assignment, blurry role differentiation	Ad hoc medical teams formed in ED to stabilize trauma patients
Distributed or collocated teams, or a combination	Multidisciplinary Medical Team (MMT) meetings with remote consultation with specialists; telemedicine
Coordination needed for continuous coverage	Shift handovers in inpatient care; patient transfer to ICU for close monitoring
May be defined by profession, discipline, physical location, temporal shift, patient needs, etc.	Pharmacists vs. radiologists; outpatient unit vs. ICU; day nurses vs. night nurses
Communication mediated through cognitive artifacts	EHR for physicians and nurses to communicate; whiteboard for residents' patient assignment; intercom for broadcasting within a medical unit

combinations of patient care needs, sometimes shifting abruptly from low-demand to highly complex and urgent. In response, ED teams tend to be highly adaptive and ephemeral, changing in composition, roles, and assignments based on shifting requirements of a fluctuating group of patients and care issues. Intensive care units (ICUs) also exhibit such ad hoc, self-assembling teams, which then dissolve once conditions have stabilized. For ICU teamwork, strategy and goal formulation was the most common team tasks, and the level of teamwork was significantly associated with ICU patient outcomes, as found in a recent systematic review (Dietz et al. 2014). By contrast, other healthcare contexts are characterized by stable, well defined teams, for example, a cardiac surgery suite where a small and select group of surgeons, nurses, surgical technicians, perfusionists, and anesthesiologists work together frequently, developing well defined roles and responsibilities, and familiar communication patterns.

A recent review of teamwork in healthcare (Xiao et al. 2013) used the concept of "organizational shell" to understand various types of teams in healthcare in terms of how an organization provides a structural context for the functioning of a team. A team may find a strong infrastructure ("organizational shell") with explicit requirements on personnel with respect to training, skills, knowledge, certification, and privileges; well thought-out structures for team tasks such as protocols, standardized operating procedures; and well-designed technology support. Such a strong organizational shell reduces coordination needs (Ginnett 1993). In many healthcare settings, work demands may be less predictable or work systems less well designed. In these cases, team membership and task assignments may be less clear, work practices become adaptive, and workarounds become common. Such fluid behavioral norms and authority arrangements render it difficult to make general statements about healthcare teams independent of the care context and the degree to which an "organizational shell" exists.

In addition to the role that an "organizational shell" may provide, multiple factors contribute to effective team functioning in healthcare, including prior education, training, and experience, professional group influences, regulatory policies, and cultural norms (Ginnett 1993). As a result, team roles, expectations, and lines of authority are sustained across contexts and organizations, exhibiting what amounts to interoperability of health professionals as they move across organizational contexts.

10.1.2 Characteristics of Healthcare Teams

Xiao et al. (2013) highlight several features commonly found in healthcare teams, two of which are very relevant to the design of HIT. First, team composition changes, depending on settings and needs, or simply over time. A family physician may work with different supporting staff in her clinic to address varying issues and patient care needs. A nurse often must contact different physicians at different times of the day when making referral appointments for a patient so that her routine practices are not impacted. Hospital staff such as interns and residents in training, hospitalist physicians, or surgical specialists may rotate on and off duty over a short cycle time, resulting in fluctuating configurations of staff and a high degree of adaptability by team members. Moreover, team composition can change as a function of a patient's illness and treatment trajectory, when the needs of a patient change. HIT can thus play important roles in enabling team members to see which clinicians have participated in the care of a patient and in providing up-to-date information on the roles of each team member in relation to a patient.

Second, the delineation of responsibility and the communication structure in healthcare teams may become unclear across temporal or functional boundaries. Individual patients, particularly in hospital settings, require participation by changing groups of health professionals, with cross-coverage responsibilities over nights or weekends and other changes to work and personnel arrangements. In military settings, a designated and clear structure for communication and role differentiation can reduce the overhead of communication and negotiation (MacMillan et al. 2002), a principle that may be applied in healthcare settings as well.

Definition of teams can have profound implications for how HIT should be designed to enhance team communication and collaboration. For example, teams may be defined by profession and discipline, by physical or temporal context, or by emerging patient needs. Examples of professional or disciplinary teams include (a) surgeons who share the care of patients who have had surgery, (b) nurses who share responsibility for care of patients on a nursing unit, or (c) physical therapists who share responsibility for therapy needs of patients distributed throughout the hospital. Examples of contextually defined teams include the multidisciplinary team responsible for patients in a specific location such as an operating room or emergency department, or those responsible for care over a specific period of time such as the night shift. Examples of teams defined by emerging care needs include the ad hoc, self-assembling teams that form and dissolve in response to emergent needs in an intensive care unit or delivery room.

These forms of team definition and composition have implications for the processes and artifacts or tools used for communication and collaboration. To illustrate, a surgical resident may consider the attending surgeons and surgical residents on his/her surgical service as his/her team, sharing responsibility for the preoperative and postoperative care of patients receiving surgery from a member of their group. Such a group will typically have routines for group discussion to share patient information and care plans (during "rounds"), as well as shared cognitive artifacts (either paper or electronic) for recording and transferring this information within the group. These routines and artifacts support transfer of information, division of responsibility, and shared situation awareness that enable them to achieve the shared goal of caring for all the patients on their service throughout the day, ideally with processes that are robust to disruptions in availability and responsibility, such as when members of the team are unexpectedly called to or are delayed in the operating room, requiring others on the team to shift roles and responsibilities.

In contrast, multidisciplinary teams that are defined by context often have distinct routines or work processes for working together such as multidisciplinary rounds, and informal rules for turn-taking in discourse, as well as separate artifacts, such as whiteboards or printed lists, that support the somewhat different work that is accomplished in a multidisciplinary context.

Team composition and function may not be perceived in the same way by all members. As an example, the clinicians and staff who provide care to a patient often have defined roles and common goals, even though the patient may never think of them as comprising a team. At the same time, the patient's family and loved ones may play significant roles in the determination and delivery of care, even though the clinician may be unaware of this. In designing HIT, it may thus be constructive to consider the entire group of healthcare professionals and family members as a team.

When healthcare teams working together to care for an individual patient are not located together in the same place at the same time, the need for technologies to support their interaction is especially great. In these cases, communication among team members in healthcare must be mediated by appropriate technologies, such as fax machines and increasingly through the EHR, whether by use of a common EHR system or through development of mechanisms for interoperability. As such, the design of HIT has direct impact on how team members "*interact dynamically, interdependently, and adaptively*" (Salas et al. 1992, p. 4). Inadequate understanding of how teams coordinate has resulted in suboptimal patient care (e.g., Abraham and Reddy 2008; Ash et al. 2004). Two examples are communication of medication orders and use of bar code medication administration systems (BCMA). With communication of medication orders, a physician may assume an order, once entered, will be acted upon immediately by the pharmacist or nurse, when in fact, many EHR implementations require the nurse to log in and specifically look for new orders. With BCMA systems, a nurse may assume the system checks the identity of the medication and of the patient, when in fact some systems do not confirm the identity of the patient (Henneman et al. 2012). Similar "illusion of communication" leads to many incidences of communication breakdowns (Ash et al. 2004). Therefore, some hospitals have developed policies, for example, for physicians to talk directly with nurses when time-sensitive orders are placed on EHR, so that harmful delays can be avoided.

10.1.3 Teamwork in Healthcare Practices

Healthcare work can be highly dynamic, requiring intense, often multidisciplinary, collaboration. Patient care teams often consist of a large number of personnel ranging from clinicians, e.g., doctors, nurses, and pharmacists, to non-clinical members, e.g., unit coordinators, administrative staff, and those responsible for equipment supply and maintenance (Lee et al. 2012; Strauss et al. 1985). These team members may be collocated, such as those in emergency care or during a routine family doctor visit (Aronsky et al. 2007; Benham-Hutchins and Effken 2010), but more often, they are distributed over different spatial locations (Bardram and Bossen 2005; Abraham and Reddy 2008). This is particularly the case for patients with complex or multiple illnesses, who require coordinated care from different specialists, each contributing to the treatment plan. Although HIT such as the EHR can help facilitate communication between distributed collaborators, the need for clinicians to move between distributed locations while conducting medical work has been found to be indispensible (Bardram and Bossen 2003, 2005). In addition, hospital work is typically under "continuous coverage" (Zerubavel 1979) in order to offer around-the-clock patient care. Thus, temporal coordination of work among team members must be carefully maintained (Reddy et al. 2002, 2006). Taken together, these collaboration challenges increase the risk of communication breakdowns and can negatively impact the quality of patient care if they are not properly considered and addressed (Chen 2010; Ebright et al. 2004; Gandhi 2006; Horwitz et al. 2009; Patterson et al. 2004; Riesenberg et al. 2010).

Healthcare is often considered information work as collaboration relies on a variety of information media, such as verbal exchange, paper, and display media (Bardram 2000; Cabitza et al. 2005; Kovalainen et al. 1998; Luff et al. 1992; Randell et al. 2010; Xiao et al. 2001). In particular, paper artifacts are often used to record and track a work plan, as a bedside information source, opportune notepad, and tool for information transfer within and across shifts (Tang and Carpendale 2007, 2008). In addition, patients' medical records are instrumental in supporting collaborative practices, acting as a "collection and distributing device" (Berg 1996) that constitutes and mediates social relations and interrelated patient care tasks. The medical records also serve as a communication vehicle, linking heterogeneous health professionals and mediating much of the healthcare system (Berg and Bowker 1997).

10.2 Key Concepts and Theories for Team Performance

10.2.1 Sociotechnical Aspects of Teamwork

Previous studies on healthcare teamwork investigated a variety of sociotechnical issues, e.g., mobility (Bardram and Bossen 2003, 2005; Morán et al. 2007), temporality (Bardram 2000; Reddy and Dourish 2002; Reddy et al. 2006), coordinating artifacts (Bardram and Bossen 2005; Cabitza et al. 2005), communication channels (Coiera and Tombs 1998; Gurses et al. 2006; Patterson et al. 2004), and richness of information (Baldwin and McGinnis 1994; Bates et al. 2003; Currie 2002; Kerr 2002). From these studies, we have gained considerable insights into the processes and challenges for achieving effective collaboration in healthcare.

10.2.1.1 Dynamic Communication Behaviors

Effective communication is essential for successful teamwork. In medical settings, communication is ubiquitous and accounts for a substantial portion of daily routines, including interactions and information sharing in varying contexts, across temporal and spatial dimensions (Bardram and Bossen 2005; Bossen 2002; Schmidt and Bannon 1992). Communication failure among clinicians, however, has been frequently found to contribute to preventable adverse events (Gurses et al. 2006).

Face-to-face communication offers a richer communication experience, providing paralinguistic and nonverbal information in addition to the words themselves, and likely offers the best quality and spectrum of communication (Kraut et al. 1988; Orlikowski and Hofman 1997; Hatten-Masterson and Griffiths 2009; Xiao et al. 2001). Furthermore, colocation of healthcare work permits indirect and informal communication (Vuckovic et al. 2004), enhancing situational awareness among members of the group in a manner similar to more formalized coordination mechanisms such as "voice loops" (Patterson et al. 1999). The mobile and dynamic nature of medical work presents challenges to effective communication. Artifacts such as whiteboards and bulletin boards, used both synchronously and asynchronously, provide a flexible shared workspace that facilitates joint discussion and provide shared and persistent information display (Wilson et al. 2006; Xiao et al. 2001, 2007), promoting awareness and coordination of ongoing activities (Bardram 2000; Xiao et al. 2001).

In hospitals especially, healthcare work is peripatetic: it is necessary for patients, health professionals, and equipment to move among spatially distributed "work centers" (e.g. emergency department, imaging suite, operating room, intensive care unit), each with specialized personnel and equipment. Mobility is therefore crucial, for people, equipment, and the HIT that connects them. Thus, Bardram and Bossen (2005) regarded medical work as *mobility work* because mobility is often required to bring together *"the right configuration of people, resources, knowledge and place in order to carry out tasks"*. Although mobility itself does not usually accomplish any concrete tasks, without mobility, many tasks cannot be fulfilled. In particular, mobility enables distributed collaborators to conduct rich face-to-face communication, and to access information artifacts such as large whiteboards located in different units in order to achieve effective patient care.

Meanwhile, communication across temporal boundaries such as work shifts is essential to ensure continuity of monitoring, diagnosis, and treatment regimes. Staggers and Jennings (2009) investigated nursing shift report in seven medical and surgical units to identify the content and context of information exchange across nursing shifts. Their findings aligned with the results of a systematic review of studies on nursing and physician handovers (Collins et al. 2011), which revealed that there were many types and situational varieties of handovers and shift handovers and concluded that these could be better supported by an EHR system if a standardized set of key information was exchanged in a structured manner.

In addition, medical team members such as physicians, nurses, and pharmacists typically have different temporal work routines and shift cycles, increasing the challenges of coordinating team activities Reddy and Dourish (2002). Breakdowns in communication between teams have been found to contribute to many adverse events. For example, Horwitz et al. (2009), examining adverse events at the transition from ED to in-hospital care, found that "communication failure at some point of care was central to most" reported errors. As an example, an investigation into the amputation of a patient's wrong leg revealed an inadvertent communication error during shift report (Strople and Ottani 2006). More recent research on patient handover between medical units in the same hospital revealed a variety of communication challenges that involved competing departmental goals, resources, and teams. This sometimes led to limited information sharing between departments. For example, a department may conceal bed availability information from other departments so that they can make their own decisions on bed assignments, which not only affected the inter-departmental coordination but also reduced the organizational efficiency (Abraham and Reddy 2008; Abraham 2013).

10.2.1.2 Medical Records for Supporting Collaborative Work

Amongst the diversity of coordination artifacts and mechanisms used in healthcare work, patient medical records are the fundamental information infrastructure enabling collaboration across time and space. Medical records are not merely a documentation tool for patient's health conditions (Berg 1996), but also an information collection and distribution device that connects interrelated patient care tasks and social relations in a clinical environment. For instance, while a surgical team interacts face-to-face inside an operating room, team members also communicate through clinical notes in the patient's medical record when working independently on different threads of patient care activities.

In recent years, EHR systems have been widely implemented to replace paper medical records in clinical settings. The benefits of EHR systems include improvements in accessibility, patient safety, accountability, and cost-savings (Bates et al. 2001, 2003). However, the design of these systems has largely focused on EHR systems as an information storage and retrieval tool for administrative, research, and legal usage (Paul et al. 2003), with little attention to how the EHR can support communication, coordination, and collaboration of healthcare teams (Ackerman et al. 2008; Berg et al. 2006). Many prior studies reported cases in which poorly designed HIT systems have led to unintended negative consequences after deployment, including dissatisfaction, adoption failures, inefficiencies, and even increased medical errors (Campbell et al. 2006; Edinger et al. 2012; Handel and Poltrock 2011; Hardstone et al. 2004). These studies suggest that HIT systems do not properly support communication and coordination activities in team-based healthcare.

In contrast, properly designed and implemented HIT solutions have the potential to support collaboration among a variety of stakeholders, from patients to clinicians, individuals to institutions, and policymakers at all levels. In recent years, through government programs and incentives, the EHR and other HIT have become virtually universal, making it critically important and timely to address these issues resulting from the complex interplay among human, organizational, and technological systems in healthcare.

Relational Coordination and Social Interaction in Teamwork

The dynamic and often urgent nature of healthcare work amplifies the need for effective coordination of interdependent work tasks. In this respect, interpersonal communication and relationships have been found to facilitate work coordination (Gittel 2002), as evidenced in the reduction of adverse events such as hospital-acquired infections and medication errors (Havens et al. 2010). Specifically, work coordination in healthcare settings requires frequent communication of accurate and timely information, and can be enhanced through relationships via shared goals, shared knowledge, and mutual respect. Such relational coordination is particularly instrumental in healthcare settings as patients' illness trajectories are often associated with a high degree of uncertainty. For example, when a patient's condition unexpectedly becomes unstable, effective communication and efficient work coordination among relevant healthcare team members would be critical for addressing the unexpected emergency. Coordination among team members can be more effective if positive interpersonal relationships exist (Grudin 1988; Orlikowski and Scott 2008; Whittaker et al. 1994; Kraut et al. 1988; Nardi et al. 2000; Gittel 2002).

Interpersonal relationships are often achieved through informal social interactions, which are generally characterized by being impromptu, brief and context-rich, and often involve small groups of people triggered by their proximity (Whittaker et al. 1994; Nardi et al. 2000). These informal social interactions are important for articulating work among team members and coordinating shared resources for collaboration (Bannon and Schmidt 1992; Berg 1999). Yet, as healthcare work becomes more fragmented and time-pressured, clinicians less frequently find time to interact socially with their colleagues during their shift (Tang and Carpendale 2008). This may be made worse by HIT because systems may hinder articulation work and social interactions (Shipman and Marshall 1999). For example, physical interaction through circulation of paper charts and paper prescriptions among team members allows impromptu interpersonal interactions (Luff and Heath 1998), while a shift to greater use of EHR is often coupled with time spent in isolation at the computer (Poissant et al. 2005), reducing mobility (Richardson and Ash 2008), and hindering interpersonal communication (Tang and Carpendale 2008).

Formal and Informal Work

The use of technology in healthcare settings has been criticized for a tendency toward "formalizing" work practices, such as increasing the structuralization of information representation, and making work processes standardized and rigid (Bowers et al. 1995; Dourish 2003; Shipman and Marshall 1999). Therefore, team members may have to rely on informal practices to leverage the flexible and spontaneous aspects of collaborative work (Isaacs et al. 1997; Kraut et al. 1990; Mejia et al. 2007; Nardi et al. 2000; Whittaker et al. 1994). Informal practices identified in the literature include impromptu human interactions and the use of tools outside of the central system (Kraut et al. 1990; Mejia et al. 2007; Nardi et al. 2000; Whittaker et al. 1994), such as face-to-face conversations, instant messaging, and text messaging which overcome the rigidity and formality of EHR systems (Brown et al. 2009; Ellingson 2003; Lee et al. 2012).

In practice, clinicians frequently adopt informal workarounds beyond the standard operations of health applications and HIT (Koppel et al. 2008) in order to circumvent problems that emerge when a newly deployed IT system disrupts workflows and interferes with task performance or goal attainment (Azad and King 2008; Zhou et al. 2011). These workarounds can be new or reconfigured tools, artifacts, or ways of interacting with an EHR system (Ash et al. 2004; Campbell et al. 2006; Handel and Poltrock 2011; Park and Chen 2012; Tang and Carpendale 2008). Well-documented examples of workarounds are the use of "*scraps*" or "*paper notes*" (Chen 2010; Fitzpatrick 2004; Hardey et al. 2000; Hardstone et al. 2004; Tang and Carpendale 2008) and clinicians' avoidance of documenting social-psycho-emotional information in EHRs (Ames 1993; Zhou et al. 2009).

In healthcare settings, organizational culture and policy determine the kind of information an artifact should contain and who may view or alter this information. Some information artifacts are meant to be maintained permanently as the official legal record of care. Other information artifacts are created for temporary and informal use, to mediate work processes (Gorman et al. 2000) or transmit sensitive information (Ames 1993), only to be disposed of afterwards. Clinicians often use a variety of informal, sometimes individualized information tools to represent information in ways that support specific tasks, in addition to the official, archival EHR record. Temporary storage on paper or personal computing devices may be used to gather fragments of information found in different information systems or in fragmented locations within a single EHR. Portable and temporary forms of information may support tasks and work activities or support certain activities that EHRs fail to support. These informal artifacts have been pervasively used by clinicians and play a vital role in coordinating healthcare work (Fitzpatrick 2004; Hardey et al. 2000; Hardstone et al. 2004; Sexton et al. 2004; Tang and Carpendale 2007, 2008).

Previous studies also found that clinicians often chose to refrain from entering social-psycho-emotional information regarding a patient's care in EHR systems, as this type of subjective information often conflicts with the objective and factual requirements of EHR-based formal documentation (Ames 1993; Mentis et al. 2010; Zhou et al. 2009). Thus, informal artifacts such as the "kardex" are frequently used for sharing work-related information including subjective patient care information during shift transitions (Fitzpatrick 2004; Gorman et al. 2000; Hardey et al. 2000; Hardstone et al. 2004; Tang and Carpendale 2008) and they carry flexible and work-in-progress notes that are not ready to be documented in archival format in the EHR (Chen 2010; Park and Chen 2012; Tang and Carpendale 2008).

Visible and Invisible Work

Current HIT is primarily designed for performing explicit, visible tasks and supporting visible roles, but healthcare work also involves important but less visible roles and tasks (Spence and Reddy 2007). The concept of visible and invisible shares some similarities to the front-stage-back-stage concept; an explication of the latter is presented in the second case study at the end of the chapter. Examples of invisible tasks include those performed by nurses to conduct comfort work (Strauss et al. 1985) and secretaries to coordinate patient transfer (Bossen et al. 2012; Holten Møller and Vikkelsø 2012). These tasks are not recorded, thus become invisible, in patient medical records, but these invisible tasks are important, and often indispensible, for work accomplishment. However, invisible work has been overlooked in the design of many IT systems (Star and Strauss 1999).

Thus, the design of complex collaborative systems should recognize and represent all invisible roles, tasks, and processes in the collaboration process (Nardi and Engestrom 2001; Suchman 1995). This goal of making work visible is difficult to achieve, however, with EHR designs that are focused primarily on explicit tasks and documentation. For example, non-clinical or unlicensed staff in hospitals and clinics such as clerical personnel, social workers and case managers, or medical assistants often remain invisible in systems, and the critical roles they play in providing and coordinating care may not be taken into account in the IT infrastructure (Bossen et al. 2012; Holten Møller and Vikkelsø 2012; Spence and Reddy 2007). Other important work processes are also neglected. In particular, EHRs often display aggregated tasks without showing and tracking the multiplicity of individual work tasks involved (Chen 2010). The lack of a systems-level representation of these invisible but critical steps can result in serious collaboration breakdowns.

Furthermore, system design has to balance visibility and invisibility among different team members so that individuals will not be overwhelmed by specific details that are not related to their work (Star and Strauss 1999), e.g., keeping backstage work invisible and providing different levels of granularity to different roles. Yet, current EHRs sometimes present the exact same view to team members with different information and communication needs, e.g., physicians and nurses likely require and use information differently but the information display in current EHRs are typically the same (Park and Chen 2012).

10.2.2   Supporting Team Collaboration with New Technologies

Research on collaborative work in healthcare investigates how current practices are conducted in specific settings or examines the impact of new technologies in

supporting collaborative work *in situ*. These studies have often led to new implications for supporting collaborative work practices or insights for improving
current HIT. In this section, we briefly review new technologies developed in
supporting collaborative work in healthcare. Of special note, there are only a
handful of studies that actually designed and deployed new technologies for real
use, which is largely due to the high threshold of safety control and regulations in
healthcare settings.

10.2.2.1   Technology for Supporting Distributed Communication

Collaborative healthcare practices often require that workers have timely access to
people, information, and resources (Bardram and Bossen 2005). However, competing tasks as well as spatial and temporal distribution of team members create
barriers or delays in communication. Mobile wearable communication devices
(e.g., Vocera) provide voice-operating connectivity for ad hoc communication
among team members that can improve communication and reduce their spatial
movements (Hanada et al. 2006; Tang and Carpendale 2009a). In particular, such
devices allow clinicians to continue with a current task while communicating with
team members about other patients or tasks, improving the efficiency and the
quality of patient care (Tang and Carpendale 2009a). Similarly, Richardson and
Ash (2008) found that the use of hands-free communication devices in clinical
settings provided clinicians with better communication access and also better
control over the information they could access.

10.2.2.2   Technologies for Supporting Coordination in Medical Work

Other than supporting point-to-point direct communication, technologies have also
been developed to support social awareness that underpins collaborative work. In
particular, Bardram and Hansen (2004) developed the AWARE architecture that
offered a platform for supporting context-mediated social awareness for mobile and
distributed teams. AwarePhone was a context-aware technology designed to support awareness among hospital clinicians and AwareMedia was developed on a
large interactive display that supports social, spatial, and temporal awareness with a
shared messaging system (Bardram et al. 2006). These technologies provided new
ways for promoting awareness in hospital work and their deployment showed
promising results in enhancing communication.

Moreover, supporting the coordination of actual work tasks among collaborators
is crucial for team-based practices, and a special challenge when task scheduling
must be dynamically changed in response to changing needs. For example, surgical
operations require careful planning of resources and personnel including the operating room, equipment, specialized surgeons, anesthesiologists, and nurses, taking
account of their availability, schedule, and constraints. In fact, coordination and

scheduling are often tightly coupled and are necessary for achieving collaborative healthcare work. However, in practice, these tasks are non-trivial and often challenging as resource optimization, a key goal for hospital efficiency, must be balanced against changing patient care needs and competing demands on personnel (Bardram and Hansen 2010). Thus, a variety of new technologies such as electronic whiteboards and scheduling systems have been developed and deployed to facilitate the coordination of team-based activities. For example, a study conducted in an emergency department found that the use of an electronic whiteboard improved work efficiency and communication quality among clinicians (France et al. 2005). Wong et al. (2009) conducted a survey and found that 71 % of the respondents considered that the whiteboard helped improve their team-based communication and 62 % agreed that they were able to retrieve patients' medical information faster with the whiteboard. Moreover, a prototypical Patient Scheduler deployed in a surgical unit was also found to help facilitate patient scheduling, and temporal coordination of the collaborative work and allocation of resources in the hospital (Bardram 2000).

10.2.2.3 Technology for Supporting Information Access

Most modern healthcare settings are equipped with an EHR system to facilitate the retrieval and use of medical information for improving the quality of patient care. Mobile devices have been introduced to support flexible bedside access to the EHR and other information, including tablets (Silva et al. 2006; Zamarripa et al. 2007) and computers-on-wheels (Tang and Carpendale 2008). Though potentially helpful, challenges have been documented including mechanical flaws and perceived intrusiveness into the nurse-patient relationship as the nurse shifted focus to the computer screen (Fig. 10.1) (Tang and Carpendale 2008). The nurses were also found to continue to use paper notes that they had always created and used for their shift work despite the availability of the mobile computers-on-wheels intended for information access at bedside.

Based on their longitudinal field studies in a hospital, including the computers-on-wheels study previously described, Tang and Carpendale (2009b) developed a prototype technology that made use of digital pen and paper that allowed nurses to continue to use their familiar pen and paper to create their paper notes. The handwritten notes could be easily transformed into digital texts for documentation without navigating the hierarchical EHR system. The integrated paper-and-digital design was based on the findings that clinicians strongly preferred handwritten notes to the digital information in the EHR system. The feedback for this prototype gathered from six focus groups with nurses was generally encouraging and design guidelines were proposed for further development of the prototype to support both clinicians' preferred practices and the use of EHRs intended by the hospital. In a related study, a mobile digital pen meant to allow more flexible and mobile record keeping was viewed positively by nurses, but used little because of mechanical or physical limitations of the device (Yen and Gorman 2005). If these issues are

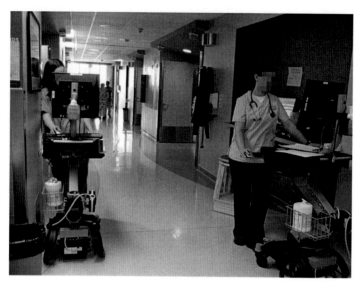

Fig. 10.1 The use of computer-on-wheels weakened interpersonal interaction (Source: Tang 2009)

addressed, these novel designs can be useful in a variety of healthcare settings including hospitals, primary care clinics and community health centers.

10.2.3 Case Studies of Teamwork

As described above, communication and coordination of healthcare teams play a crucial role in achieving quality patient care. Therefore, two case studies on different healthcare teams in different contexts are presented below. The first case study presents communication challenges encountered by healthcare teams dynamically and ephemerally formed in an ED, primarily for stabilizing the patients such that they can be quickly transferred out of the ED. The second case study describes the use of information artifacts and the communication processes during medical rounds that took place in a Pediatric Intensive Care Unit (PICU).

10.2.3.1 Communication Challenges for Loosely Formed Collaboration Teams

The following vignette was abstracted from our field study in an ED to show how mobile phones adopted in the ED failed to support the distributed teamwork.

> While Paul, a nurse in the ED, was at bedside drawing a blood sample from a patient, his mobile phone vibrated. Not knowing what the call was about, Paul decided to ignore it. This

phone call turned out to be an emergency call to help with a critically ill patient in another room. Paul later commented why he didn't pick up the call "...when you are at the bedside with the patient, it [the mobile phone] rings; you pick it up to answer it. Sometimes they [the patients] may think it's rude. I don't think the patients know it's a work phone. I think they think it's a personal phone. Or it's ringing, ringing, ringing and you are in the middle of doing IV. The patients can go like 'okay it's ringing.' So that is a problem!"

Although mobile phones are highly appreciated in many other fields for the convenience it offers to distributed team members, clinicians in the ED actually often ignored mobile phone calls. Instead, they generally preferred to use overhead pagers to communicate work-related information inside the ED. This is because communication via mobile phones did not provide sufficient group awareness information for the patient care team members, which often led to unwanted interruptions at patients' bedside. More importantly, it failed to support role-based communication, which is important to the dynamic collaborative healthcare work that sometimes requires personnel of a specific role instead of a specific named person. The lack of role-based communication has caused considerable challenges in the ED teamwork communication since the team members are often formed dynamically and ephemerally in the ED (Fig. 10.2).

Our analysis of communication breakdowns in the ED revealed a unique characteristic of the collaborative teamwork that we regarded as *loosely formed* team collaboration. Specifically, patient care teams in the ED differ considerably from those in other medical wards, as ED care teams are often dynamically and quickly assembled upon patient arrival and the heterogeneous team members must

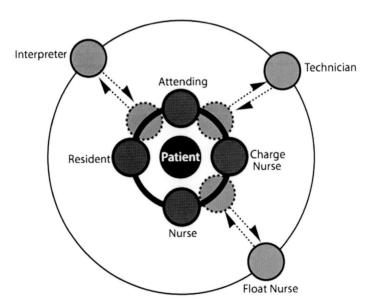

Fig. 10.2 The formation and disassembly of a loosely formed patient care team. *Dark and light grey* indicate core and peripheral members respectively. The *dotted circles* show that peripheral members join the care team temporarily (Source: Lee et al. 2012)

immediately engage in interdependent and complex care activities, since ED patients often require care from different providers including ED doctor, nurses, and various specialists. These team members come together dynamically and work with various collaborators for patients with different needs. Variations in shift cycles, temporal horizons, and collaborators' job nature further complicate the collaborative work. For example, ED nurses and residents have different shift cycles. ED nurses work on 12-h cycles and their bed assignment usually changes every 4 h, whereas ED residents work on 8–12 h shifts with different starting times. Thus, the residents may have to work with different nurses for a single patient during a shift, complicating the work collaboration. When individual care team members simultaneously work in multiple patient cases, the complexity in collaboration becomes highly intertwined and significantly more challenging. Finally, when an ED patient is stabilized, the responsible team dissolves right away. The coordination required for achieving this kind of fluid work practice is highly challenging, and thus susceptible to breakdowns. In particular, the frequently changing collaborative teams require substantial spatial movement for collaboration, temporal coordination of the collaborative tasks, effective handling of unpredictable interruptions, and coordination across multiple healthcare teams comprising of team members of different roles and each team member may be concurrently involved in multiple patient cases.

The team members' spatial distribution explains why mobile phones were not preferred in the ED since each team member has to be reached separately. Moreover, sometimes when personnel of a particular role, such as a technician, instead of a specific person are needed, the current communication system did not support locating team members by their role. In addition, calls may interrupt patient care activities at the bedside, as mobile phones used in the ED did not provide any caller information. In contrast, overhead pagers allowed ED-wide broadcasts alerting all team members at the same time. However, they might run the risk of disclosing private patient information over an open link. Hence, the findings from this study pointed to the need for designing future communication technologies to meet the needs of loosely formed collaborative environments by providing team-based communication with lightweight feedback and point-to-point information transparency while preserving patient privacy.

10.2.3.2 Information Arena to Support Team Rounding in a Pediatric Intensive Care Unit

Hospital rounds are multi-disciplinary meetings convened at regular times (often daily), partly for purposes of coordinating care among workers. The complexity of hospital care (Strauss et al. 1985) has made such rounds ever more essential for the safety and quality of care received by the patients. Hospital rounds are an example of teamwork for exchanging and updating critical information and responsibility under time constraints. Therefore, it is important for participants to select the most relevant details while providing an overall assessment. The following dialogue presents a typical segment from a "walking" round in a surgical Intensive Care Unit (ICU) during which the participants often ambulate. The information artifacts are underlined.

> Resident: Mr. VVV is a 52-year old male with… His white cell count is continuing to increase. He is on antibiotics. Plan for him … [Resident provides a summary of the patient's current condition using her summary sheet while the attending looks at the computer for getting an update on patient's status]
> Attending: Why don't we change his antibiotics to antibiotic x?
> Pharmacist: Because he is allergic to Penicillin.
> Attending: OK.
> Resident: He has also developed a high fever last night.
> [The charge nurse interrupts the conversation and asks]
> Charge nurse: Excuse me Dr. B (the attending), how many empty beds will we have for today's admissions?
> [Attending and the charge nurse walk together from the bedside to the whiteboard to check]

This case study highlights the findings of several studies on communication and coordination during rounds conducted in different settings (Fig. 10.3) including a pediatric intensive care unit (Cardarelli et al. 2009) and a trauma specialty hospital (Sen et al. 2009). A large number of physical artifacts (e.g. lists, bed boards, notes, charts) are used by round participants, both as memory aids for relevant patient information and as a record of goals and to-do lists (Fig. 10.3, left). Participants also spend considerable amount of time in preparing for information exchanges during rounds so that they can quickly transfer information about status and tasks to another in order to sustain effective performance across task boundaries (Gurses et al. 2006, 2009).

The information processes that took place during rounds were found to be multi-threaded and overlapping. Hence a "front-stage-back-stage" model was developed for capturing the choreographing of discourse and interaction with the information artifacts. Information processes were considered front-stage when they were part of verbal exchanges or shared visual exchanges occupying the conversation "floor"

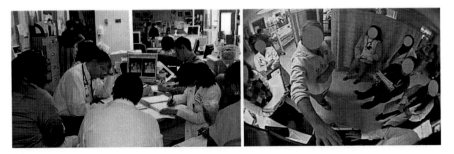

Fig. 10.3 (*Left*) Sit-down rounds in a pediatric intensive care unit: multi-disciplinary meetings convened for daily management of patient care. Note information objects scattered around the workplace and manipulated by participants (e.g., X-rays on computer terminals, notes, papers on the wall, charts in binders); (*right*) A surgeon pointing at a chest X-ray on the computer

whereas back-stage processes were those not occupying the floor, mostly non-verbal occasional side interactions or gestures, as well as private interactions between participants and their information sources and computer terminals. Below we illustrate the use of the front-stage-back-stage model in capturing the interactions between the multi-threaded information processes and discuss the model's implications on designing computing support for the information arena.

1. *Front-stage activities driving front-stage activities* can be exemplified by a resident physician presenting data that the attending physician regards as a good teaching point and interrupts the presentation to launch into a didactic discussion.
2. *Front-stage activities driving back-stage activities* are most commonly represented by attending physicians filling in their personal notes (back-stage) as the presenting resident physician reads the data values out loud to the group (front-stage).
3. *Back-stage activities for supporting front-stage activities* include a resident on the computer listening to the presentation and locating relevant patient data on the computer while the resident later interjects to provide the latest values (e.g., laboratory results).
4. *Back-stage activities driving other back-stage activities* happen when a note-taking resident has difficulty keeping up with the presented data, conferring with another participant nearby. They would quietly exchange information as the round proceeds without interrupting the front-stage activities.

Based on the information arena just described, our field studies offer several implications for designing support for the interactions between activities in the front and the back stages. As the back-stage activity interacts with the front-stage both as an information contributor (e.g., during case presentation) as well as an information receiver (e.g., transcribing into personal notes), there is a potential to increase the "information density" of discourse. Newman and Smith (2006) observed a similarly high requirement for ease of information access, beyond which people tended to disengage from the conversation. We thus speculate that the use of the front-stage may be improved with computing tools to support back-stage preparation and visual presentation in the front-stage so that communication of precise information (such as data value or medication dosages) may be more reliable. A major role of back-stage activities is to assist in developing a common information space by packaging and organizing relevant information (Bannon and Bodker 1997; Fields et al. 2005) and to provide an annotated environment for fixing inadequacy in the physical space, artifacts, and technology (Coiera 2013) for facilitating front-stage information exchange. We believe that the front-stage-back-stage model provides useful guidance for both studies of critical discourse as well as the design of supporting tools.

10.3   Conclusions

Healthcare is a team activity, which entails intense coordination and collaboration among heterogeneous personnel who are typically distributed, both spatially and temporally. Healthcare teams exist in different types depending on individual teams' structural context and its functioning. An organization with a strong organizational shell, well-formulated team structures, and well-designed technology support is associated with lower coordination needs (Ginnett 1993). Yet, teamwork constantly faces a variety of challenges in the dynamic, information-rich, time-critical, and complex healthcare settings.

Recent developments in the use of HIT including the EHR systems and various mobile devices for enhancing real-time information access were discussed as new opportunities to enhance collaborative activities in healthcare. Given the complexity and diversity of healthcare settings, it is crucial to consider relevant sociotechnical issues when designing and deploying HIT for practical use in specific healthcare settings. These issues include design considerations to facilitate dynamic communication behaviors in healthcare settings and the use of medical records for enhancing collaborative healthcare teamwork through supporting relational coordination and social interactions, formal and informal work, and visible and invisible work. Recent technological development for supporting distributed healthcare teamwork was also described. Finally, two case studies on different healthcare teams in different contexts were presented to offer practical challenges in team communication in an ED and the complex information arena and processing involved in team-based medical rounds in an ICU. Both case studies concluded with design implications for supporting technologies.

Discussion Questions
1. What are the communication challenges facing healthcare providers using EHR systems?
2. What are the advantages of dashboard displays showing patient status in an ED?
3. How can EHR engage family members to be part of the care team for a patient in an ICU?

Additional Readings

Gorman, P., Ash, J., Lavelle, M., Lyman, J., Delcambre, L., Maier, D., Weaver, M., & Bowers, S. (2000). Bundles in the wild: Managing information to solve problems and maintain situation awareness. *Library Trends, 49*(2), 266–289.

Lee, S., Tang, C., Park, S. Y., & Chen, Y. (2012). Loosely formed patient care teams: Communication challenges and technology design. In *Proceedings of the 2012 ACM conference on computer supported cooperative work* (pp. 867–876). New York: ACM.

Xiao, Y., Schenkel, S., Faraj, S., Mackenzie, C. F., & Moss, J. A. (2007). What whiteboards in a trauma center operating suite can teach us about emergency department communication. *Annals of Emergency Medicine, 50*(4), 387–395.

References

Abraham, J. (2013). Re-coordinating activities: An investigation of articulation work in patient transfers. In *Proceedings of the 2013 ACM conference on computer supported cooperative work* (pp. 67–78). New York: ACM.

Abraham, J., & Reddy, M. (2008). Moving patients around: A field study of coordination between clinical and non-clinical staff in hospitals. In *Proceedings of the 2008 ACM conference on computer supported cooperative work* (pp. 225–228). New York: ACM.

Ackerman, M. S., Halverson, C. A., Erickson, T., Kellogg, W. A., Reddy, M., & Dourish, P. (2008). Representation, coordination, and information artifacts in medical work. In *Resources, co-evolution and artifacts* (pp. 167–190). London: Springer.

Ames, S. A. (1993). *Multiple spoken and written channels of communication: An ethnography of a medical unit in a general hospital*. Ann Arbor: UMI Dissertation Services.

Aronsky, D., Jones, I., Lanaghan, K., & Slovis, C. M. (2007). Supporting patient care in the emergency department with a computerized whiteboard system. *Journal of the American Medical Informatics Association, 15*(2), 184–194.

Ash, J. S., Berg, M., & Coiera, E. (2004). Some unintended consequences of information technology in health care: The nature of patient care information system-related errors. *Journal of the American Medical Informatics Association, 11*(2), 104–112.

Azad, B., & King, N. (2008). Enacting computer workaround practices within a medication dispensing system. *European Journal of Information Systems, 17*(3), 264–278.

Baldwin, L., & McGinnis, C. (1994). A computer-generated shift report. In *Nursing Management, 25*(9), 61–64. Wolters Kluwer.

Bannon, L., & Bodker, S. (1997). Constructing common information spaces. In *Proceedings of the ECSCW* (pp. 81–96). Dordrecht: Kluwer Academic Publishers.

Bannon, L., & Schmidt, K. (1992). Taking CSCW seriously: Supporting articulation work. *Computer Supported Cooperative Work, 1*, 7–40.

Bardram, J. (2000). Temporal coordination: On time and coordination of collaborative activities at a surgical department. *Journal of Computer Supported Cooperative Work, 9*(2), 157–187.

Bardram, J. E., & Bossen, C. (2003). Moving to get ahead: Local mobility and collaborative work. In *Proceedings of the eighth conference on European conference on computer supported cooperative work 2003* (pp. 355–374). Dordrecht: Kluwer Academic Publishers.

Bardram, J. E., & Bossen, C. (2005). Mobility work: The spatial dimension of collaboration at a hospital. *Computer Supported Cooperative Work, 14*(2), 131–160.

Bardram, J., & Hansen, T. (2004). The AWARE architecture: Supporting context-mediated social awareness in mobile cooperation. In *CSCW'04: Proceedings of the 2004 ACM conference on computer supported cooperative work* (pp. 192–201). New York: ACM.

Bardram, J., & Hansen, T. (2010). Why the plan doesn't hold: A study of situated planning, articulation and coordination work in a surgical ward. In *Computer supported cooperative work* (pp. 331–340). New York: ACM.

Bardram, J., Hansen, T., & Søgaard, M. (2006). AwareMedia: A shared interactive display supporting social, temporal, and spatial awareness in surgery. In *Computer supported cooperative work* (pp. 109–118). New York: ACM.

Bates, W. D., Cohen, M., Leape, L. L., Marc Overhage, J., Michael Shabot, M., & Sheridan, T. (2001). Reducing the frequency of errors in medicine using information technology. *Journal of the American Medical Informatics Association, 8*(4), 299–308.

Bates, D. W., Ebell, M., Gotlieb, E., Zapp, J., & Mullins, H. C. (2003). A proposal for electronic medical records in U.S. Primary Care. *Journal of the American Medical Informatics Association, 10*(1), 1–10.

Benham-Hutchins, M. M., & Effken, J. A. (2010). Multi-professional patterns and methods of communication during patient handoffs. *International Journal of Medical Informatics, 79*(4), 252–267.

Berg, M. (1996). Practices of reading and writing: The constitutive role of the patient record in medical work. *Sociology of Health & Illness, 18*(4), 499–524.

Berg, M. (1999). Accumulating and coordinating: Occasions for information technologies in medical work. *Computer Supported Cooperative Work, 8*(4), 373–401.

Berg, M., & Bowker, G. (1997). The multiple bodies of the medical record. *Sociological Quarterly, 38*(3), 513–537.

Berg, M., Pirnejad, H., & Stoop, A. P. (2006). Bridging information gaps between primary and secondary healthcare. *Studies in Health Technology and Informatics, 124*, 1003–1008.

Bossen, C. (2002). The parameters of common information spaces: The heterogeneity of cooperative work at a hospital ward. In *Proceedings of the conference on computer-supported cooperative work* (pp. 176–185). New York: ACM.

Bossen, C., Jensen, L., & Witt, F. (2012). Medical secretaries' care of records: The cooperative work of a non-clinical group. In *Proceedings of the 2012 ACM conference on computer supported cooperative work* (pp. 921–930). New York: ACM.

Bowers, J., Button, G., & Sharrock, W. (1995). Workflow from within and without: Technology and cooperative work on the print industry shopfloor. In *Proceedings of the first conference of European conference on computer supported cooperative work* (pp. 51–66). Dordrecht: Kluwer Academic Publishers.

Brown, J. B., Lewis, L., Ellis, K., Stewart, M., Freeman, T. R., & Kasperski, M. J. (2009). Mechanisms for communicating within primary health care teams. *Canadian Family Physician, 55*(12), 1216–1222.

Cabitza, F., Sarini, M., Simone, C., & Telaro, M. (2005). When once is not enough: The role of redundancy in a hospital ward setting. In *Proceedings of GROUP* (pp. 158–167). New York: ACM.

Campbell, E. M., Sittig, D. F., Ash, J. S., Guappone, K. P., & Dykstra, R. H. (2006). Types of unintended consequences related to computerized provider order entry. *Journal of the American Medical Informatics Association, 13*(5), 547–556.

Cardarelli, M., Vaidya, V., Conway, D., Jarin, J., & Xiao, Y. (2009). Dissecting multidisciplinary cardiac surgery rounds: Data, wisdom, time and money. *Annals of Thoracic Surgery, 88*(3), 809–813.

Chen, Y. (2010). Documenting transitional information in EMR. In *Proceedings of the 2010 ACM conference on human factors in computing systems* (pp. 1787–1796). New York: ACM.

Coiera, E. (2013, September 4). Communication spaces. *Journal of American Medical Informatics Association, 21*(3), 414–422. doi:10.1136/amiajnl-2012- 001520.

Coiera, E., & Tombs, V. (1998). Communication behaviours in a hospital setting – An observational study. *British Medical Journal, 316*, 673–677. BMJ Publishing Group Ltd.

Collins, S., Stein, D. M., Vawdrey, D. K., Stetson, P. D., & Bakken, S. (2011). Content overlap in nurse and physician handoff artifacts and the potential role of electronic health records: A systematic review. *Journal of Biomedical Informatics, 44*, 704–712.

Currie, J. (2002, June). Improving the efficiency of patient handover. *Emergency Nurse, 10*(3), 24–27.

Dietz, A. S., Pronovost, P. J., Mendez-Tellez, P. A., Wyskiel, R., Marsteller, J. A., Thompson, D. A., & Rosen, M. A. (2014). A systematic review of teamwork in the ICU: What do we know about teamwork, team tasks, and improvement strategies? *Journal of Critical Care, 29*(6), 908–914. doi:10.1016/j.jcrc.2014.05.025.

Dourish, P. (2003). The appropriation of interactive technologies: Some lessons from placeless documents. *Computer Supported Cooperative Work, 12*(4), 465–490.

Ebright, P. R., Urden, L., Patterson, E., & Chalko, B. (2004). Themes surrounding novice nurse near-miss and adverse-event situations. *Journal of Nursing Administration, 34*(11), 531–538.

Edinger, T., Cohen, A. M., Bedrick, S., Ambert, K., & Hersh, W. (2012). Barriers to retrieving patient information from electronic health record data: Failure analysis from the TREC medical records track. In *AMIA annual symposium proceedings* (pp. 180–188). Chicago, IL: American Medical Informatics Association.

Ellingson, L. L. (2003). Interdisciplinary health care teamwork in the clinic backstage. *Journal of Applied Communication Research, 31*(2), 93–117.

Fields, B., Amaldi, P., & Tassi, A. (2005). Representing collaborative work: The airport as common information space. *Cognition, Technology & Work, 7*(2), 119–133.

Fitzpatrick, G. (2004). Integrated care and the working record. *Health Informatics Journal, 10*(4), 291–302.

France, D., Levin, S., Hemphill, R., Chen, K., Richard, D., Makowski, R., Jones, I., & Aronsky, D. (2005). Emergency physicians' behaviors and workload in the presence of an electronic whiteboard. *International Journal Medical Informatics, 74*(10), 827–837.

Gandhi, T. K. (2006). Fumbled handoffs: One dropped ball after another. *Annals of Internal Medicine, 142*(5), 352–358.

Ginnett, R. (1993). Crews as groups: Their formation and their leadership. In E. Weiner, B. Kanki, & R. L. Helmreich (Eds.), *Cockpit resource management* (pp. 71–97). London: Academic.

Gittel, J. (2002). Coordinating mechanisms in care provider groups: Relational coordination as a mediator and input uncertainty as a moderator of performance effects. *Management Science, 48*(11), 1408–1426.

Grudin, J. (1988). Why CSCW applications fail: Problems in the design and evaluation of organizational interfaces. In *Proceedings of the 1988 ACM conference on computer-supported cooperative work* (pp. 85–93). New York: ACM.

Gurses, A. P., Xiao, Y., Gorman, P., Hazelhurst, B., Bochicchio, G., Vaidya, V., & Hu, P. (2006). A distributed cognition approach to understanding information transfer in mission critical domains. In *Proceedings of the human factors and ergonomics society annual meeting* (pp. 924–928). San Francisco, CA: Sage

Gurses, A. P., Xiao, Y., & Hu, P. (2009). User-designed information tools to support communication and care coordination in a trauma hospital. *Journal of Biomedical Informatics, 42*(4), 667–677.

Hanada, E., Fujiki, T., Nakakuni, H., & Sullivan, C. (2006). The effectiveness of the installation of a mobile voice communication system in a university hospital. *Journal of Medical Systems, 30*, 101–106.

Handel, M. J., & Poltrock, S. (2011). Working around official applications: Experiences from a large engineering project. In *Proceedings of CSCW 2011* (pp. 309–312). New York: ACM.

Hardey, M., Payne, S., & Coleman, P. (2000). 'Scraps': Hidden nursing information and its influence on the delivery of care. *Journal of Advanced Nursing, 32*(1), 208–214.

Hardstone, G., Hartswood, M., Procter, R., Slack, R., Voss, A., & Rees, G. (2004). Supporting informality: Team working and integrated care records. In *Proceedings of the 2004 ACM conference on computer-supported cooperative work* (pp. 142–151). New York: ACM.

Hatten-Masterson, S. J., & Griffiths, M. L. (2009). SHARED maternity care: Enhancing clinical communication in a private maternity hospital setting. *Medical Journal of Australia, 190* (11 Suppl), S150–S151.

Havens, D. S., Vasey, J., Gittell, J. H., & Lin, W. T. (2010). Relational coordination among nurses and other providers: Impact on the quality of patient care. *Journal of Nursing Management, 18*, 926–937.

Henneman, P. L., Marquard, J. L., Fisher, D. L., Bleil, J., Walsh, B., Henneman, J. P., Blank, F. S., Higgins, A. M., Nathanson, B. H., & Henneman, E. A. (2012, December). Bar-code verification: Reducing but not eliminating medication errors. *Journal of Nursing Administration, 42* (12), 562–566.

Holten Møller, N. L., & Vikkelsø, S. (2012). The clinical work of secretaries: Exploring the intersection of administrative and clinical work in the diagnosing process. In J. Dugdale, C. Masclet, M. A. Grasso, J.-F. Boujut, & P. Hassanaly (Eds.), *From research to practice in the design of cooperative systems: Results and open challenges* (pp. 33–47). London: Springer.

Horwitz, L. I., Meredith, T., Schuur, J. D., Shah, N. R., Kulkarni, R. G., & Jenq, G. Y. (2009). Dropping the baton: A qualitative analysis of failures during the transition from emergency department to inpatient care. *Annals of Emergency Medicine, 53*, 701–710.

Isaacs, E. A., Whittaker, S., Frohlich, D., & O'Conaill, B. (1997). Informal communication re-examined: New functions for video in supporting opportunistic encounters. In K. Finn, A. Sellen, & S. Wilbur (Eds.), *Video-mediated communication*. Mahwah: Lawrence Erlbaum.

Kerr, M. (2002). A qualitative study of shift handover practice and function from a socio-technical perspective. *Journal of Advanced Nursing, 37*(2), 125–134. Wiley-Blackwell.

Koppel, R., Wetterneck, T., Telles, J., & Karsh, B. (2008). Workarounds to barcode medication administration systems: Their occurrences, causes, and threats to patient safety. *Journal of the American Medical Informatics Association, 15*(4), 408–423.

Kovalainen, M., Robinson, M., & Auramaki, E. (1998). Diaries at work. In *Proceedings of CSCW* (pp. 49–58). New York: ACM.

Kraut, R., Egido, C., & Galegher, J. (1988). Patterns of contact and communication in scientific research collaboration. In *Proceedings of computer supported cooperative work* (pp. 1–12). London: Routledge.

Kraut, R. E., Fish, R. S., Root, R. W., & Chalfonte, B. L. (1990). Informal communication in organizations: Form, function, and technology. In *People's reactions to technology in factories, offices, and aerospace* (pp. 145–199). Thousand Oaks: Sage.

Luff, P., & Heath, C. (1998). Mobility in collaboration. In *Proceedings of the 1998 ACM conference on computer supported cooperative work* (pp. 305–314). New York: ACM.

Luff, P., Heath, C., & Greatbatch, D. (1992). Tasks-in-interaction: Paper and screen based documentation in collaborative activity. In *Proceedings of computer supported cooperative work* (pp. 163–170). New York: ACM.

MacMillan, J., Paley, M. J., Levchuk, Y. N., Entin, E. E., Serfaty, D., & Freeman, J. T. (2002). Designing the best team for the task: Optimal organizational structures for military missions. In M. McNeese, E. Salas, & M. Endsley (Eds.), *New trends in cooperative activities: System dynamics in complex settings*. San Diego: Human Factors and Ergonomics Society Press.

Mejia, D. A., Morán, A. L., & Favela, J. (2007). Supporting informal co-located collaboration in hospital work. In *Proceedings of the 13th international conference on groupware: Design implementation, and use* (pp. 255–270). Berlin: Springer.

Mentis, H. M., Reddy, M., & Rosson, M. B. (2010). Invisible emotion: Information and interaction in an emergency room. In *Proceedings of the 2010 ACM conference on computer supported cooperative work* (pp. 311–320). New York: ACM.

Morán, E., Tentori, M., González, V., Favela, J., & Martinez-Garcia, A. (2007). Mobility in hospital work: Towards a pervasive computing hospital environment. *International Journal of Electronic Healthcare, 3*(1), 72–89.

Nardi, B. A., & Engestrom, Y. (2001). A web on the wind: The structure of invisible work. *Computer Supported Cooperative Work, 8*(1), 1–8.

Nardi, B. A., Whittaker, S., & Bradner, E. (2000). Interaction and outeraction: Instant messaging in action. In *Proceedings of the 2000 ACM conference on computer supported cooperative work* (pp. 79–88). New York: ACM.

Newman, W., & Smith, E. L. (2006). *Disruption of meetings by laptop use: Is there a 10-second solution?* (pp. 1145–1150). New York: ACM.

Orlikowski, W. J., & Hofman, J. D. (1997). An improvisational model for change management: The case of groupware technologies. *Sloan Management Review, 38*(2), 11–22.

Orlikowski, W. J., & Scott, S. V. (2008). Sociomateriality: Challenging the separation of technology, work and organization. *The Academy of Management Annals, 2*(1), 433–474.

Park, S. Y., & Chen, Y. (2012). Adaptation as design: Learning from an EMR deployment study. In *Proceedings of the 2012 ACM conference on human factors in computing systems* (pp. 2097–2106). New York: ACM.

Patterson, E. S., Watts-Perotti, J., & Woods, D. D. (1999). Voice loops as coordination aids in space shuttle mission control. *Computer Supported Cooperative Work: The Journal of Collaborative Computing, 8*(4), 353–371.

Patterson, E. S., Roth, E. M., Woods, D. D., Chow, R., & Gomes, J. O. (2004). Handoff strategies in settings with high consequences for failure: Lessons for health care operations. *International Journal for Quality in Health Care, 16*(2), 125–132.

Paul, S., Das, A., & Patel, V. (2003). Specifying design criteria for electronic medical record interface using cognitive framework. In *AMIA annual symposium proceedings* (pp. 594–598). Washington, DC: American Medical Informatics Association.

Poissant, L., Pereira, J., Tamblyn, R., & Kawasumi, Y. (2005). The impact of electronic health records on time efficiency of physicians and nurses: A systematic review. *Journal of the American Medical Informatics Association, 12*(5), 505–516.

Randell, R., Wilson, S., Woodward, P., & Galliers, J. (2010). Beyond handover: Supporting awareness for continuous coverage. *Cognition, Technology & Work, 12*(4), 271–283.

Reddy, M., & Dourish, P. (2002). A finger on the pulse: Temporal rhythms and information seeking in medical work. In *Proceedings of the 2002 ACM conference on computer supported cooperative work* (pp. 344–353). New York: ACM.

Reddy, M., Pratt, W., Dourish, P., & Shabot, M. (2002). *Asking questions: Information needs in a surgical intensive care unit.*

Reddy, M., Dourish, P., & Pratt, W. (2006). Temporality in medical work: Time also matters. *Computer Supported Cooperative Work, 15*(1), 29–53.

Richardson, J., & Ash, J. (2008). The effects of hands free communication devices on clinical communication: Balancing communication access needs with user control. In *AMIA annual symposium proceedings* (pp. 621–625). Washington, DC: American Medical Informatics Association

Riesenberg, L. A., Leisch, J., & Cunningham, J. M. (2010). Nursing handoffs: A systematic review of the literature. *American Journal of Nursing, 110*, 24–34.

Salas, E., Dickinson, T. L., Converse, S., & Tannenbaum, S. I. (1992). Toward an understanding of team performance and training. In R. W. Swezey & E. Salas (Eds.), *Teams: Their training and performance* (pp. 3–29). Norwood: Ablex.

Schmidt, K., & Bannon, L. (1992). Taking CSCW seriously: Supporting articulation work. *Computer Supported Cooperative Work (CSCW): An International Journal, 1*(1), 7–40.

Sen, A., Xiao, Y., Lee, S., Hu, P., Dutton, R. P., Haan, J., O'Connor, J., Pollak, A. P., & Scalea, T. (2009). Daily multi-disciplinary discharge rounds in a trauma center: A little time, well spent. *Journal of Trauma, 66*(3), 880–887.

Sexton, A., Chan, C., Elliott, M., Stuart, J., Jayasuriya, R., & Crookes, P. (2004). Nursing handovers: Do we really need them? *Journal of Nursing Management, 12*, 37–42. Wolters Kluwer.

Shipman, F. M., & Marshall, C. C. (1999). Formality considered harmful: Experiences, emerging themes, and directions on the use of formal representations in interactive systems. *Computer Supported Cooperative Work, 8*(4), 333–352.

Silva, J., Zamarripa, M., Strayer, P., Favela, J., & Gonzalez, V. (2006). Empirical evaluation of a mobile application for assisting physicians in creating medical notes. In *Proceedings of the 12th Americas conference on information systems*, Acapulco, Mexico.

Spence, P. R., & Reddy, M. C. (2007). The "active" gatekeeper in collaborative information seeking activities. In *Proceedings of the 2007 international ACM conference on supporting group work* (pp. 277–280). New York: ACM.

Staggers, N., & Jennings, B. M. (2009). The content and context of change of shift report on medical and surgical units. *Journal of Nursing Administration, 39*(9), 393–398.

Star, S. L., & Strauss, A. (1999). Layers of silence, arenas of voice: The ecology of visible and invisible work. *Computer Supported Cooperative Work, 8*(1–2), 9–30.

Strauss, A., Fagerhaugh, S., Suczek, B., & Wiener, C. (1985). *Social organization of medical work.* Chicago: University of Chicago.

Strople, B., & Ottani, P. (2006). Can technology improve intershift report? What the research reveals. *Journal of Professional Nursing, 22*(3), 197–204. Elsevier.

Suchman, L. (1995). Making work visible. *Communication of the ACM, 38*(9), 56–64.

Tang, C. (2009). *Studying nurses' information flow to inform technology design*. Ph.D. dissertation, Department of Computer Science, University of Calgary, AB, Canada.

Tang, C., & Carpendale, S. (2007). An observational study on information flow during nurses' shift work. In *Proceedings of the ACM conference on human factors in computing systems* (pp. 219–228). New York: ACM.

Tang, C., & Carpendale, S. (2008). Evaluating the deployment of a mobile technology in a hospital ward. In *Proceedings of the 2011 ACM conference on computer supported cooperative work* (pp. 205–214). New York: ACM.

Tang, C., & Carpendale, S. (2009a). A mobile voice communication system in medical setting: Love it or hate it? In *Proceedings of the ACM conference on human factors in computing systems* (pp. 2041–2050). New York: ACM.

Tang, C., & Carpendale, S. (2009b). Supporting nurses' information flow by integrating paper and digital charting. In *Proceedings of the European conference on computer supported cooperative work* (pp. 43–62). Heidelberg: Springer.

Vuckovic, N., Lavelle, M., & Gorman, P. N. (2004). Eavesdropping as normative behavior in a cardiac intensive care unit. *JHQ Online, W5*, 1–6.

Whittaker, S., Frohlich, D., & Daly-Jones, O. (1994). Informal workplace communication: What is it like and how might we support it? In *Proceedings of the 1994 ACM conference on human factors in computing systems* (pp. 131–137). New York: ACM.

Wilson, S., Galliers, J., & Fone, J. (2006). Not all sharing is equal: The impact of a large display on small group collaborative work. In *Proceedings of computer supported cooperative work* (pp. 25–28). New York: ACM.

Wong, H., Caesar, M., Bandali, S., Agnew, J., & Abrams, H. (2009). Electronic inpatient whiteboards: Improving multidisciplinary communication and coordination of care. *International Journal of Medical Informatics, 78*(4), 239–247.

Xiao, Y., Lasome, C., Moss, J., & Mackenzie, C. (2001). Cognitive properties of a whiteboard: A case study in a trauma centre. In *Proceedings of European computer supported cooperative work* (pp. 259–278). Bonn: Kluwer Academic Publishers.

Xiao, Y., Parker, S. H., & Manser, T. (2013). Teamwork and collaboration. *Reviews of Human Factors and Ergonomics, 8*(1), 55–102.

Yen, P. Y., & Gorman, P. N. (2005). Usability testing of a digital pen and paper system in nursing documentation. In *Proceedings of AMIA annual symposium* (pp. 844–848). Austin, Texas: American Medical Informatics Association.

Zamarripa, M., Gonzalez, V., & Favela, J. (2007). The augmented patient charts: Seamless integration of physical and digital artifacts for hospital work. In C. Stephanidis (Ed.), *Universal access in HCI, Part III, HCII 2007, LNCS 4556* (pp. 1006–1015). Berlin/New York: Springer.

Zerubavel, E. (1979). *Patterns of time in hospital life: A sociological perspective*. Chicago: University of Chicago Press.

Zhou, X., Ackerman, M. S., & Zheng, K. (2009). I just don't know why it's gone: Maintaining informal information use in inpatient care. In *Proceedings of the 2009 ACM conference on human factors in computing systems* (pp. 2061–2070). New York: ACM.

Zhou, X., Ackerman, M. S., & Zheng, K. (2011). CPOE workarounds, boundary objects, and assemblages. In *Proceedings of ACM on Human Factors in Computing Systems (SIGCHI '11)* (pp. 3353–3362). ACM Press.

Chapter 11
The Unintended Consequences
of the Technology in Clinical Settings

Amy Franklin

11.1 Introduction

Unintended consequences (UCs) are direct and indirect outcomes that are outside of
expectation. In the context of healthcare, this includes the unanticipated impact of
health information technology (HIT) on clinical practice. For example, although
electronic health record (EHR) systems may improve access to information through
the use of standardized fields, the increased documentation demands may cause
busy doctors to enter data into free text fields rather than attempt to search for the
"right" location in a structured field. Downstream effects of this extra burden of
documentation include additional effort required for subsequent users of that data
by other stakeholders. This is because other users must either assume that the
information is unavailable or search for the information outside its expected
location.

The recent surge in HIT, particularly EHR systems, has spurred discussion and
research into the potential consequences of its use including unanticipated outcomes. From physician complaints and praise of EHRs to patients' reports regarding the impact on visits, interaction with HIT has altered healthcare processes.
Headlines in the popular media have pointed out the changes to how medicine is
practiced in the digital age (Campbell 2014a, b; Meisel 2011). One often cited
example of unintended consequences in HIT is the changing dynamics of the
doctor-patient interaction when using an EHR system. It is no longer just the doctor
and the patient in the room: EHRs add a "third party", the computer, to the patient
visit. This results in changes to workflow, including alteration of the patient's
narrative (Lown and Rodriguez 2012) as well as changes in communication behaviors such as eye contact (Al-Jafar 2013). All of these may adversely impact the

A. Franklin, Ph.D. (✉)
School of Biomedical Informatics, University of Texas Health Science Center at Houston,
7000 Fannin St, Suite 165, Houston, TX 77030, USA
e-mail: Amy.Franklin@uth.tmc.edu

© Springer International Publishing Switzerland 2015
V.L. Patel et al. (eds.), *Cognitive Informatics for Biomedicine*, Health Informatics,
DOI 10.1007/978-3-319-17272-9_11

quality of patient care and patient satisfaction. These are **unintended consequences** of technology that are not intended in its design.

Although HIT systems, including EHRs, have great potential for improving healthcare quality and safety, it is necessary to elucidate and manage the outcomes that were not foreseen or intended in the design and implementation of the system. Unintended consequences, though commonly thought of as being unexpected *problems* created by a system, are not always negative. Technology may provide benefits beyond their intended design. Serendipitous benefits may include repurposing of tools beyond their original purpose. For example, Kuziemsky et al. (2012) provide examples in which physicians found a new use for their data entry and process monitoring system developed for palliative care. By leveraging the features that helped physicians visualize data for developing care plans, doctors found that sharing the visual depictions of patient's disease progression (e.g., medication needs, pain reports) aided difficult conversations with family members regarding end of life decision-making.

In this chapter, we discuss the unintended consequences (UC) of HIT in clinical practice. We begin with examples of how computerized physician order entry (CPOE) created unforeseen outcomes in clinical care. Following a review of literature, we use these instances to drive a discussion of the nuances of different frameworks for classifying UCs. Next, we consider potential mechanisms underlying UCs and touch on issues regarding the constraints of human cognition, usability of devices, and work processes described in other chapters of this volume. Finally, we look at reported issues on common UCs in EHR systems and outline proposed solutions. Through a better understanding of UCs, particularly those generated through human computer interaction (HCI), we can build systems that mitigate negative UCs and reap the benefits of serendipity in unanticipated positive outcomes.

11.2 Defining Unintended Consequences

The idea of unexpected outcomes is not unique to healthcare nor is it always mediated by technology. The disciplines of philosophy, sociology, and even economics have discussed unintended consequences over the course of recent centuries (see for example Adam Smith's The Theory of Moral Sentiments (Smith 1759)). An analogous phenomenon is commonly observed in biological systems. For example, introducing new sources of food such as rabbits or new crops can solve a short-term food supply problem, while leading to long-term issues including the disruption of the ecosystem (e.g., lack of predation leads to overpopulation of rabbits that decimate other food sources such as crops). The first modern definition of UCs as direct and indirect outcomes not intended by purposeful action was popularized in the 1930s by the sociologist Robert Merton (1936). Through his research, Merton attempted to explain why human actors were unable to anticipate outcomes in complex systems. Although Merton's argument was a philosophical discussion regarding the limitations of human reasoning, his ideas have been applied in other domains for understanding outcomes that are outside of expectation.

Merton's treatise centered on understanding UCs via potential sources of causation. UCs could be understood as leading from errors in assumptions, (un)-informed tradeoffs in short versus long term gain, and the impact of culture/policy. This theme of classifying UCs by causation re-emerges in later frameworks. However, Merton's ideas on UCs continued to evolve over time to include other components. For example, rather than focusing solely on causation, other frameworks have separated UCs along dimensions of outcome (e.g., negative or positive results, expected or unanticipated from design).

Research by Ash and colleagues (2007) provides the seminal framework for unintended consequences in HIT. In their hierarchy, the singular notion of unintended consequences has been broadened. First, consequences are split into those that were **anticipated** or **unanticipated**, i.e., *not predicted*, outcomes. Next, the dimension of the **desirability** of the outcome is included. This allows for the traditional negative/undesirable, unanticipated and thus unintended consequence as well as unexpected and yet desirable outcomes of serendipity. The inclusion of desirability shifts the focus from prediction (i.e., anticipation) of the outcome to a new examination of the actual outcomes themselves (i.e., positive or negative results). In this framework, expected negative outcomes can be thought of as **risks or tradeoffs** (*undesired but anticipated results*), which differ substantively from the negative surprises of UCs.

Figure 11.1 depicts the hierarchy created by Ash et al. (2007) expressing both benefits and negative consequences through direct processes measures as well as indirect outcomes. In this framework only consequences that are both unanticipated and undesired are deem unintended. Although this hierarchy focused on CPOE use, the attributes of anticipation, desirability and direct/indirect outcomes can be generalized to classifying consequences in other domains (including those outside HIT). The above hierarchy highlights both the positive and negative consequences; however, much of the literature (and the popular press) has focused on *unintended adverse consequences*.

Campbell et al. (2006) provide a typology for looking just at these negative outcomes, again with a CPOE focus.[1] Campbell and her team interviewed and observed clinicians (including physicians, nurses, pharmacists, and allied health care providers) at five hospital sites. Using a grounded theory approach and card sorting techniques, they first distilled shared themes from across observations and interviews. Next, in the card sort, with clinician assistance, they grouped the ideas presented into nine classes of negative unanticipated outcomes. These categories, organized as a typology, add a finer grade of classification to the discussion of UCs.

---

[1] CPOE is often the HIT component under study given its rich and tangible connection between design and potential safety events such as medication errors.

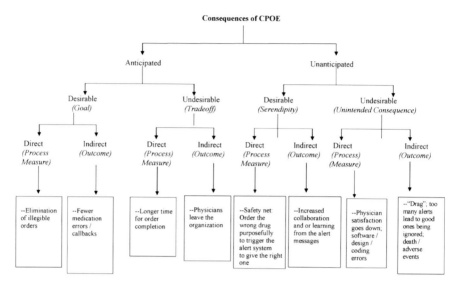

Fig. 11.1 Ash et al.'s (2007) hierarchy [Reprinted with permission]

Campbell's typology included categories for generalizing across problems, and mapped UCs to their underlying outcomes. For example, the additional work generated by technologies can vary from transformed work practices and workflow to additional required effort (e.g., documentation, the handling of new decision support alerts). When compared to the paper-based clinical practice at sites within their study, respondents noted, there is simply more work to be done. Other classes of UCs include a poor fit between the human-computer interface and the context of use, unintended overload of individual cognitive and collective work processes, and changes to coordination and communication practices. Of course, at this point in time, some of those consequences can be construed as anticipated. As with Ash et al.'s hierarchy, several instances within this typology are extensible to other forms of healthcare products beyond CPOE, including medical devices, communication tools and other technology.

While the above typologies focus on an expectation of outcomes, socio-technical models reevaluate UCs through a systems' lens. Rather than focusing only on the technology, these models were developed with foundations in systems research, and were based on the idea that the impact of HIT can only be understood while considering its social, organizational and technical context of use (Fox 1995; Cummins and Srivastva 1977). They depict complex and interdependent components of the health care system including users' characteristics, workflow, organizations, and policy along with the health information technology itself.

In Harrison et al.'s Interactive Socio-technical Analysis (ISTA) (Harrison et al. 2007), UCs were not seen as created by the HIT system (e.g., failure to fully understand the impact of design); instead the consequences were understood as resulting from different types of interactions. ISTA depicts the emergent relationships between HIT, clinicians and workflows. Technology is viewed as part of the complex system that is shaped by the technical and physical infrastructure within which it resides. The system as a whole is understood as the interaction and interdependence among its components. UCs in this framework are not solely classified by *anticipation* of their design (e.g., anticipated use/unanticipated outcomes), rather ISTA considers how HIT is actually *used* within a given context. Thus, interaction type is used to define UCs rather than the intent or outcome. The five interaction types include: (1) new HIT changes existing social system, (2) technical and physical infrastructure mediates HIT use, (3) social system mediates HIT use, (4) HIT-in-use changes social systems, and (5) HIT-social system interactions engender HIT redesign. Instances of new HIT changing the existing social system include UCs such as new/more work on tasks such as documentation, changes to informal interactions yielding communication changes, or alterations in workflow such as shifts in roles and responsibilities. As illustrated in Table 11.1, Harrison et al. incorporate both Campbell's typology (Campbell et al. 2006) as well as the work on communication and information transfer by Ash et al. (2007, 2009) into their interaction types. Importantly, ISTA shifts the focus from causation or outcome of UCs to pointing out the impact and differences of *systems in use* from the ways in which the *systems were designed*. Harrison's framework offers a richer and more nuanced analysis, and provides significant potential for remediation through redesign.

The 2009 American Medical Informatics Association (AMIA) Annual Health Policy meeting focused on outlining "outcomes of actions that are not originally intended in a particular situation (e.g., HIT implementation)." The resulting publication (Bloomrosen et al. 2011) from a panel of experts considered another perspective on sociotechnical systems and consequences. In their article, Bloomrosen et al. put forth a model with inputs and outputs that span domains including:

- *Technology*: hardware and software systems that are implemented and the constraints they impose.
- *Human factors and cognition*: thought processes, habits of behavior, and mental capabilities that humans bring to the use of HIT tools and processes.
- *Organization*: embedding of technology in the complex environment of healthcare organizations.
- *Fiscal/policy and regulation*: the legislative and regulatory environment governing the design, implementation, and use of HIT such as HIPPA requirements, indicators of meaningful use and standards for health information exchange.

In this input-output model, interactions define the model as they did in ISTA. The domains of technology, organization and human factors along with the addition of policy and regulations converge into a sociotechnical system with an even broader scope and in which HIT resides. Complicated interactions yield outcomes that can be understood in terms of types of consequences and the affected stakeholders. Like the ISTA framework, Bloomrosen's efforts frame UCs as a study of interactions. The input-output model specifies stakeholders (i.e., inputs) as well as

Table 11.1 Unintended consequences by ISTA type

ISTA type	Unintended consequences[a]
1. New HIT changes social system	***More/new work for clinicians***[b]
	Physicians spend more time on documentation and justification
	Changes in communication patterns and practices
	Introduction of IT leads to decline of vital interactions among care providers, ancillary services and units[c]
	IT system eliminates informal interactions and redundant checks that help catch errors[c]
	Workflow
	CPOE undermines informal gatekeeping by clerk who decided whether patients really needed daily x-rays
2. Technical and physical infrastructure mediate HIT use	***Paper persistance***[b]
	Paper used to solve problems of lack of integration of CPOE and other clinical information systems
3. Social system mediates HIT use	***New types of errors***[b]
	Busy physicians enter CPOE data in miscellaneous section rather than scrolling for optimal location. Improper placement can impede use by other physicians and by CPOE systems
	Causing Cognitive Overload by Overemphasizing Structured and "Complete" Information Entry or Retrieval[d]
	Fragmentation
	Distribution of information over several screens sometimes leads busy physicians to miss key parts of record, such as interpretations or reports by other types of physicians
	Structure, overcompleteness
	Extensive reporting requirements lead physicians to cut and paste whole reports, rather than extracting pertinent facts
	Paper persistence[b]
	Counter to hospital directives and recommended IT practice, MDs who prefer paper records annotate CPOE printouts and place these in patient charts as formal documentation
	Misrepresenting collective, interactive work as linear, clear cut, predictable workflow[d]
	Inflexibility: Transfers: Inflexible EHR reporting requirements generate failures to record clinically appropriate drug administration and cause difficulties in managing patient transfers
	Urgency: Nurses and Physicians refuse to follow data-entry rules requiring physician pre-authorization for urgent care

(continued)

Table 11.1   (continued)

ISTA type	Unintended consequences[a]
	Workarounds: Physicians and nurses provide urgent care by working around cumbersome procedures
	Misrepresenting communication as information transfer[d]
	Decision support overload: Alert fatigue: physicians ignore warnings and reminders
	Loss of communication: Urgent requests and some test results from accident and emergency, admissions are never viewed on ward terminal
	Loss of feedback: Nurses initial orders on receipt, rather than administration, so physicians cannot tell if orders have been carried out
	Human-computer interface unsuitable for highly interruptive context[d]
	Juxtaposition errors
	Entry of orders for or on behalf of the wrong person
4. HIT-in-use changes social system	***Changes in the power structure[b]***
	Narrow, role-based authorizations redistribute work – requiring physicians to enter orders directly
	Remote monitoring by the organizations undermines physicians' autonomy
	IT, quality assurance departments, administration gain power by requiring physician to comply with CPOE-based directives
	In decentralized systems, internal variations in CPOE uses and configurations increase interdepartmental conflicts and competition
5. HIT-social system interactions engender HIT redesign	***Never-ending system demands[b]***
	As implemented CPOE systems evolve, users rely more on the software, demand more sophisticated functionality, & customize software (e.g., physicians create their own order sets). New features must be added to original software. Interactions among multiple variations of the software in use make CPOE system unmanageable & require replacement with newer versions

Reprinted with permission from Harrison et al. (2007)
[a]Types of consequences cited by Campbell et al. (2006)
b Campbell et al. (2006)
[c] Instances also treated in Ash et al. (2003)
[d] Ash et al. (2003)

results or outcomes as components within the sociotechnical system. The complexity of the system underscores the need to understand points of input to the unintended consequences. For example, poor usability of an interface can increase the cognitive burden on the clinicians by requiring searching for a returned laboratory value in a sea of electronic, scanned, and paper data. Cognitive factors such as limited memory and attention coupled with a poorly designed or cluttered

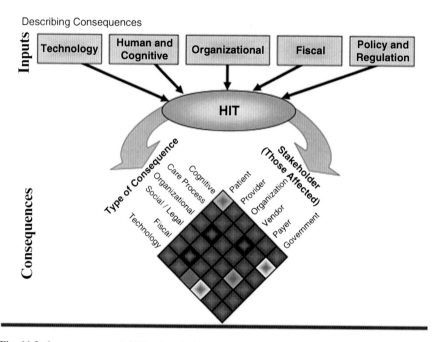

Fig. 11.2 Input-output model [Reprinted with permission from Bloomrosen et al. (2011)]

interface may engender potential UCs. These inputs can lead to output (i.e., consequences) that may impact both cognitive (e.g., diagnostic reasoning) and care processes for patients and providers. At another level of analysis, organization policy may serve to mitigate or exacerbate these consequences. In this example, documentation requirements could lead to workflow changes generating further unanticipated outcomes.

This multi-faceted model depicted in Fig. 11.2 underscores the shifting view of UCs as an individual problem to a perspective in which UCs is considered as complex and situated in system-wide issues. Embedding HIT into sociotechnical frameworks highlights the need to consider all the interactions of inputs and products of work in design.

11.3 Exploring Unanticipated Consequences

The potential unintended impacts of HIT in clinical settings are wide ranging, including risk of harm to patients and inefficiencies in work practices. Just as UCs can occur with technology (Tenner 1997), introducing new devices, or new processes, have the potential for both gainful and harmful effects beyond the expectation of the product developers. CPOE-based problems are some of the best documented, and are some of the most documented issues related to unintended consequences of the use of healthcare technology (Ash et al. 2003, 2007, 2009; Campbell et al. 2006, 2007; Koppel et al. 2005; Weiner 2007).

Some of the technology-induced errors are derived from the user interface. Reckmann and colleagues' (2009) review identified problems created by poor usability including incorrect drug selection induced by lengthy drop down menus (Shulman et al. 2005), and duplicate orders or failures to discontinue medications (Koppel et al. 2008). Subsequent problems also arose when unexpected consequences led to downstream issues. For example, Computers on Wheels (CoW) were used to seamlessly move computers to the patient's bedside. Having a computer at the point of care can potentially prevent errors in identification, reduce interruptions, and improve the completeness of procedures such as documentation. Combined with bar code technology, CoW can improve medication administration by reducing medication errors (i.e., scan the patient, scan the medication to prevent errors). However, Koppel et al. identified 15 kinds of modified workflows in use while using the barcode medication administration technology (19). For example, the authors identified an instance where the potential benefits of bar code/CoW systems were thwarted when these units were too large to fit into the patients' rooms. Rather than scanning patient wrist identification at the *bedside*, nurses would print out extra bar codes *outside* the room. Such alterations to clinical practice can have downstream effects and, in fact, can lead to identification errors this technology was originally intended to prevent.

Similarly, HIT may not function as expected in the realm of Clinical Decision Support (CDS) alerts. Alerts for drug-drug or drug-allergy problems can be triggered during the prescribing process. If too many alerts are delivered, clinicians may fail to acknowledge the appropriate and relevant alerts. Additionally, the high rate of potential notifications can lead to *alert fatigue* (Steele and DeBrow 2008), and subsequently to technology-induced errors. For example, many studies found that drug-drug and drug-allergy alerts were often overridden. Payne et al. (2002) found an 88 % override rate for drug interaction alerts, and a 69 % override rate for drug-allergy alerts. Similarly, Weingart et al. (2003) found ambulatory physicians overrode 91 % of drug-allergy alerts, and 89 % of high-severity drug-drug interaction alerts. A percentage of these alerts may have provided limited detail (e.g., notifying the physician that no drug information was available in system) and perceived to be uninformative, presented information with unknown clinical significance (e.g., lacking indicators of the severity of an interaction), or may have repeated the content of previous messages.

In a 2013 case study, Carspecken et al. (2013) described an instance where a 2-year-old child was admitted to a pediatric intensive care unit (PICU) with a documented antibiotic allergy. Over a 1-month period, more than 100 alerts related to a drug-allergy cross reactivity were overridden, as the treatment was deemed as a requirement for the patient's condition (i.e., ignoring what was considered an inappropriate alert). Over time it was determined the child did in fact have an allergic hypersensitivity, and his medical record was eventually amended. However, even after this change, the now appropriate alert (i.e., acknowledging that the child does have an allergy) was *still* overridden. Due to the routine rejection of the alert, clinical staff had become de-sensitized to drug-allergy alerts in this child's case.[2]

There are multiple issues at the heart of this example. First, the unintended consequence of new/additional work led to an increased burden on the physicians. Subsequently, the repeated alerts decreased clinicians' sensitivity to the message resulting in inappropriate persistence of behavior (i.e., continued override of the alert.) Additionally, the EHR did not make the addition/change to the allergy list salient to the users of the system. Finally, the unintended changes to the workflow, particularly around communication practices regarding medications, may have led to less feedback and decreased opportunities to prevent this error.

We can break the case down into its component parts to situate it within the previously described UC frameworks. Within Campbell's CPOE typology and Ash's work on communication, this case study includes communication failures (e.g., misrepresenting communication as information transfer (Ash et al. 2003)), demonstrates new types of errors not found in paper-based systems, and shows how changes to communication practices can lead to unanticipated outcomes. Sociotechnical system models could also include discussion regarding how the social system mediated HIT use including changes in assignment of roles (i.e., who maintains the allergy list and notifies others) as well as workflows. To prevent these types of errors in the future, changes to the work system would be necessary to provide a more nuanced and context-sensitive decision support. This would include having appropriate content, including severity of interactions, visible changes for new alerts and appropriate timing of alerts in the decision process.

Ongoing research shows potential improvement in adherence to alerts (rather than overriding them) through improving the relevance of alert messages (Weingart et al. 2011). Shah et al. (2006) found that with appropriate design it is possible to generate high rates of alert acceptance by clinicians. In their study of 18,115 drug alerts generated during a 6-month study period, 67 % of *interruptive* but informative alerts were accepted in spite of its impact on workflow.

Modifying a system to prevent or fix an existing problem can introduce other unintended consequences as well. For example, Strom et al. (2010) identified the complexities surrounding the unintended consequences of trying to prevent errors in a CPOE system that in turn created new problems. In this study, a hard stop, or a required step in the ordering process by which no further action can occur until a response is produced, was added to the ordering process. It was intended to promote adherence to decision support by preventing concomitant orders for a known hazardous sulfa drug interaction (i.e., warfarin and trimethoprim-sulfamethoxazol). Their clinical trial exploring the effectiveness of this hard stop was in fact halted when it was determined that four patients received delayed treatment as a consequence of changes to the medication-ordering process. In those cases, concurrent prescribing was in fact appropriate and the hard stop should have been overridden.

---

[2] This case has additional complications regarding the appropriateness of sulfonamide allergies. Please see the original publication for details.

Like the pediatric study, this case provides an example of the complicated process for determining system rules, workflows, and challenges to anticipating all potential outcomes for decision support choices. Other ways in which unintended consequences emerge are through workarounds or additional unplanned innovations (Strauss et al. 1997). When systems fail to support workflow in an acceptable fashion, users may innovate and introduce new paths for completing their tasks and goals.

Just as with consequences, workarounds can have positive or negative impacts (See Chap. 10, this volume for a detailed discussion on workarounds). For example, Vogelsmeier et al. (2008) studied five nursing homes to uncover workaround practices related to electronic medication administration records. They found two types of workarounds: those associated with the system interface, and those related to organizational processes. For example, when the CDS alerted that a medication was "excessive" in dose, nurses entered multiple within-range doses in order to measure up to the requested dose (rather than directly speaking with a physician or pharmacist). Other system requirements were managed by a "flouting" policy. For example, in these nursing homes, there was a requirement for separate documentation, one for preparation of medication and one subsequent to the administration of the medication. Nurses would often only note the process prior to administration of medication, and ignore the post-administration records. If delays occurred, or if the medication was not actually administered, it would not be accurately reflected on the patient record. Similarly, when voluminous printouts of medication orders were required to complete the policy-driven fax for prescription, nurses often elected to follow a speedier (but not supported) process of calling-in medication orders.

The above cases are complex events for which it may be difficult to define a singular unintended outcome, potential cause, or solution. As Bloomrosen's input-output model suggests, to understand the triggers of these events, and to work towards managing such outcomes, the inputs (clinicians, technology, organizational policy and the social structure), interactions, and outputs must all be considered in the system in which the work occurs. In these circumstances, triggers to the event include the changes to the interactions of the nurses and physicians, adaption of clinicians to technology, workers negotiating organizational policy and the social structure that guides their actions. All of these contribute to the "excessive" dose workaround. The way in which a nurse enters drug information is only one of the many problems. Solutions to these kinds of cases are not as straightforward as changing specific algorithms in decision support systems. Rather, consideration should be given to the communication practices and policies that lead to these events, as well as the HIT demands.

At a more basic level, outside the nuances of specific drug interactions or dosing rates, there are basic computer functions that lead to significant confusion. For example, the onerous demands of documentation are an often-touted (perhaps, even shouted) unintended consequence of EHR implementation. All of that new work could be supported by judicious copy and paste within clinical notes. Seventy four to ninety percent of physicians use the copy-paste function in their EHRs, and between 20 and 78 % of physician notes are copied text (Bowman 2013). However, many are concerned that this function is not being used appropriately (Hripcsak et al. 2011; Hirschtick 2006). Issues with copied text include the potential for lost information as reviewing notes becomes a hunt for new or different information. In addition, other clinicians caring for the same patient may elect not to read the patient notes which contain copious amounts of redundant or uninformative text. There is also a concern that copying and pasting could lead to inappropriate billing (McCann 2013). The American Health Information Management Association (AHIMA) provides a stakeholder perspective on the issues of copy and paste. As the association for health information management (as compared to clinicians using the health record system), this organization has a broad interest in the use of these basic computer functions. In their position paper (40), AHIMA proposes that copy and paste (i.e. cloning, identical documentation) should be used only under technical and administrative control and with well trained users, potentially limiting the adverse outcomes of this function. This example also demonstrates how multiple sources (i.e. stakeholders) have to be considered as input to both the event and the solution. While copy and paste may be an activity of the individual, organizational policy, technological constraints and socio-cultural practice can define (or even regulate) how this activity is completed. Copy and paste could well be an issue within the EHR systems that may someday be constrained by Federal regulation.

Paper persistence, similar to copy and paste, offer short-term solutions to HIT problems that may have an impact on long-term consequences. The inability to satisfy the demand of having access to an EHR system, as well as simple preference for physical documents can lead to the persistence of paper in the presence of electronic solutions. Some people like that napkin as a note tucked in their pocket, while others are forced to create paper based workarounds due to the constraints of their HIT systems. In a study on consultation practices at a Veterans Affairs Medical Center, Saleem et al. (2011) explored the ways in which paper persisted as a means of communicating and coordinating between physicians even in the presence of electronic consultation tools. They found that the use of paper documents and informal notes persisted for a 5-year period where electronic processes were already in place. Coordination workarounds were a common response to limitations in the EHR system, for example, delays in notifying primary care physicians that a consult report was available. Preferences for homegrown solutions such as compact spreadsheets listing multiple patients and individual checklists were also common workarounds.

Concerns for these behaviors include maintenance of dual paper and electronic records: paper persistence engenders the potential consequence that handwritten information may not become part of the electronic record and gaps in information retrieval may occur as individuals may not be exhaustive in their search for information. When evaluating the differences across paper and electronic sources, Kannampallil et al. (2013) found that a process of local optimization drove the information-seeking process across paper and electronic documents. Physicians gathered information from sources that maximized their information gain even though it required significantly more cognitive effort. Given the argument that unintended consequences are derived from poorly supported cognitive processes, it is necessary that we seek solutions that better support work processes including information search.

11.4   Human Factors Models

The sociotechnical frameworks for understanding UCs focus on the systems in which technology is used. Macroergonomic models that emerged from a human factors engineering approach to patient safety (including UCs) similarly embrace a systems-centered perspective (Carayon et al. 2014). Karsh et al.'s Human Factors (HF) Paradigm (Karsh et al. 2006) is exemplified by a principle that the goal should be to *"design work systems that support and enhance work process performance"* and that safety, risk, and all other outcomes then flow from the accommodation of the system to this work. Well-designed systems would then not only support typical efforts but also should be robust and resilient enough to reinforce work under *challenging conditions*, such as high patient load. Although the HF paradigm focuses on error and harm (the worrisome potential outcomes of UCs), Holden (2011) suggests that the way that HIT improves or worsens outcomes is dependent on how that system impacts cognitive performance. In his extension of this paradigm to EHRs, Holden proposes that cognitive performance processes are the mediating mechanism between a work system and outcomes. Rather than saying failures in design lead to error, harm or unintended consequences, Holden outlines how the work system either positively or negatively affects cognitive performance.[3] The resulting themes from Holden's interviews of clinicians surface many of the same unintended consequences previously outlined in the UC literature such as the burden of extra cognitive effort generated from poor displays, impacts on workflow including extra steps, and communication changes including simply less face-to-face time. Likewise, the SEIPS (Systems Engineering Initiative for Patient Safety) (Carayon et al. 2006; Carayon and Smith 2000) model echoes many of the components of Bloomrosen's Input-Output model in that they both share the idea of interacting components encompassing clinicians, technology, human interaction, and external factors such as policy. Importantly, the SEIPS model includes feedback loops between the work system and care processes, and between the work system and outcomes that provide support for redesign. These human factors engineering models provide a means for discussing potential interventions to systems to safeguard patient safety. More direct and immediate methods for assessing the risk of UCs have been recently provided through federal programs (see next section for a brief overview).

---

[3] In line with Hollnagel and Woods, all performance, or work, in healthcare is considered cognitive, from procedures to decision-making, including the cognitive processes of mental, physical, social, and behavioral activities.

11.5   Solutions

Finding productive means to manage unintended consequences can take many forms. As Holden (2011) suggests, redesign of work systems to support cognitive processes is necessary. We view that this redesign would include not only features of the technology but also the social and organizational structures. As Bloomrosen et al. (2011) suggest, regulation and policy may also play a role. Funding through the Office of the National Coordinator (ONC) and the Agency for Healthcare Research and Quality (AHRQ) has spawned research programs along the development of guidelines to understand and mitigate UCs. Examples of the output from these efforts are the 2011 AHRQ *Guide to Reducing Unintended Consequences of Electronic Health Records* (Jones et al. 2011) and the *Safety Assurance Factors for EHR Resilience (SAFER) Guides*. The AHRQ Guide provides detailed support in understanding and identifying unintended consequences in EHR systems as well as suggestions for remediation. Through a series of case studies, this guide highlights 15 areas of concern and provides references regarding research in each area. For example, the guide describes a case in which the implementation of a nursing documentation system unintentionally duplicated efforts (both paper and electronic forms were completed) as part of a policy requirement for a specific type of documentation (here, patient social function). Process assessment and redesign are provided as suggested solutions.

As Jones et al. suggest in this guide (Jones et al. 2011), corrective actions may fall into one or more broad categories: (a) software change, (b) training for local IT staff, (c) configuration change, (d) custom programming, (d) care process change and (e) policy change. As these corrective actions may be costly both in terms of time and effort, remediation plans detailing the problem, its impact, the scope of the request, stakeholder involvement as well as benefits from change may all be necessary to justify the price of change. Such plans may therefore vary in their ranking of importance for patient safety, user satisfaction and desirability for corrective action.

The *SAFER* guidelines, also put out by ONC and AHRQ, are designed to help care delivery organizations conduct self-assessments of recommended practices in those areas important to the safe use of health information technology. These efforts are part of the HIT Patient Safety Action and Surveillance Plan. Some of the guides such as those targeting CPOE and Lab results detail unintended consequences in these systems and provide assessments of system function.

Other federal efforts include ONC initiatives for EHR certification requirements for usability testing with public reporting. These requirements have increased the dialogue regarding user and system performance. Summative testing is one way of uncovering unintended consequences in ready-to-deploy or implemented products. The potential inclusion of formative testing requirements as part of the 2015 rule may prevent some UCs from reaching end users through discovery and recovery during development. Regional Extension Centers (RECs) and Health Information Technology Research Centers (HITRC) are other programs funded by ONC which may help in supporting UC capture and remediation by providing support directly to providers.

Professional organizations such as the American Medical Informatics Association (AMIA), Healthcare Information and Management Systems Society (HIMSS) and American Health Information Management Association (AHIMA) have also sponsored efforts supporting HIT implementation and the identification of unintended consequences.

11.6 Conclusions

To understand and support HIT in clinical practice, we must recognize the impact of the complex sociotechnical system of healthcare in both contributing to unintended consequences as well as discovering solutions to managing these emerging issues. Through better understanding of UCs, particularly those generated through human computer interaction, we can build systems that mitigate negative UCs and reap the benefits of serendipity in unanticipated outcomes.

Discussion Questions
1. How do we design systems such that we mitigate negative unintended consequences while engendering positive unexpected outcomes? Are the solutions for remediating unintended consequences similar to the processes necessary to create serendipitous outcomes? Explain.
2. Sociotechnical models highlight the interwoven factors of individual, organizational, and technical components surrounding unintended consequences (UCs). Do solutions for UCs necessarily have to bridge domains? That is, can solutions occur at only one level such as the technical component, or does the management of UCs require responses from multiple inputs?

Additional Readings

Bloomrosen, M., Starren, J., Lorenzi, N., Ash, J. S., Patel, V. L., & Shortliffe, E. (2011). Anticipating and addressing the unintended consequences of health IT and policy: A report from the AMIA 2009 Health Policy Meeting. *Journal of the American Medical Informatics Association, 18*(1), 9.

Carayon, P., Wetterneck, T. B., Rivera-Rodriguez, A. J., Hundt, A. S., Hoonakker, P., Holden, R. J., et al. (2014). Human factors systems approach to healthcare quality and patient safety. *Applied Ergonomics, 45*(1), 14–25.

Harrison, M. I., Koppel, R., & Bar-Lev, S. (2007). Unintended consequences of information technologies in health care an interactive sociotechnical analysis. *Journal of the American Medical Informatics Association, 14*, 542e9.

Patel, V. L., & Kannampallil, T. G. (2014). Human factors and health information technology: Current challenges and future directions. *International Medical Informatics Association (IMIA) Yearbook of Medical Informatics*, 58–66.

References

Al-Jafar, E. (2013). Exploring patient satisfaction before and after electronic health record implementation: The Kuwait experience. *Perspectives in Health Information Management, 10*(Spring), 1c.

Ash, J. S., Berg, M., & Coiera, E. (2003). Some unintended consequences of information technology in health care: The nature of patient care information system-related errors. *Journal of the American Medical Informatics Association, 11*(2), 104–112.

Ash, J. S., et al. (2007). Categorizing the unintended sociotechnical consequences of computerized provider order entry. *International Journal of Medical Informatics, 76*(Suppl 1), S21–S27.

Ash, J. S., et al. (2009). The unintended consequences of computerized provider order entry: Findings from a mixed methods exploration. *International Journal of Medical Informatics, 78* (Suppl 1), S69–S76.

Bloomrosen, M., et al. (2011). Anticipating and addressing the unintended consequences of health IT and policy: A report from the AMIA 2009 Health Policy Meeting. *Journal of the American Medical Informatics Association, 18*(1), 9.

Bowman, S. (2013). Impact of electronic health record systems on information integrity: Quality and safety implications. *Perspectives in Health Information Management, 10*, 1c.

Campbell, K. R. (2014a). Embrace the age of digital medicine. In K. R. Campbell (Ed.), *KevinMD. com* [cited 2014 8/29/2014] Available from: http://www.kevinmd.com/blog/2014/06/embrace-age-digitalmedicine.html

Campbell, K. R. (2014b). *Practicing medicine in the digital age: Challenges & opportunities of the virtual encounter* [cited 2014 8/29/2014]. Available from: http://www.eplabdigest.com/blog/Practicing-Medicine-Digital-Age-Challenges-Opportunities-Virtual-Encounter

Campbell, E. M., et al. (2006). Types of unintended consequences related to computerized provider order entry. *Journal of the American Medical Informatics Association, 13*(5), 547–556.

Campbell, E. M., et al. (2007). Overdependence on technology: An unintended adverse consequence of computerized provider order entry. In *AMIA Annual symposium proceedings* (pp. 94–98).

Carayon, P., & Smith, M. (2000). Work organization and ergonomics. *Applied Ergonomics, 31*(6), 649–662.

Carayon, P., et al. (2006). WORK system design for patient safety: The SEIPS model. *Quality & Safety in Health Care, 15*(Suppl 1), i50–i58.

Carayon, P., Xie, A., & Kianfar, S. (2014). Human factors and ergonomics as a patient safety practice. *BMJ Quality Safety, 23*(3), 196–205.

Carspecken, C. W., et al. (2013). A clinical case of electronic health record drug alert fatigue: Consequences for patient outcome. *Pediatrics, 131*(6), e1970–e1973.

Cummins, T. S., & Srivastva, S. (1977). *Management of work: A sociotechnical systems approach.* San Diego: University Associates.

Fox, W. (1995). Sociotechnical system principles and guidelines: Past and present. *The Journal of Applied Behavioral Science, 31*(1), 91–105.

Harrison, M. I., Koppel, R., & Bar-Lev, S. (2007). Unintended consequences of information technologies in health care – An interactive sociotechnical analysis. *Journal of the American Medical Informatics Association, 14*(5), 542–549.

Hirschtick, R. E. (2006). A piece of my mind. Copy-and-paste. *JAMA, 295*(20), 2335–2336.

Holden, R. J. (2011). Cognitive performance-altering effects of electronic medical records: An application of the human factors paradigm for patient safety. *Cognition, Technology & Work, 13*(1), 11–29.

Hripcsak, G., et al. (2011). Use of electronic clinical documentation: Time spent and team interactions. *Journal of the American Medical Informatics Association, 18*(2), 112–117.

Jones, S. S., et al. (2011). *Guide to reducing unintended consequences of electronic health records.* Rockville: Agency for Healthcare Research and Quality (AHRQ).

Kannampallil, T. G., Franklin, A., Mishra, R., Almoosa, K. F., Cohen, T., & Patel, V. L. (2013, January). Understanding the nature of information seeking behavior in critical care: Implications for the design of health information technology. *Artificial Intelligence in Medicine, 57,* 21–29. doi:10.1016/j.artmed.2012.10.002. http://dx.doi.org/10.1016/j.artmed.2012.10.002

Karsh, B. T., et al. (2006). A human factors engineering paradigm for patient safety: Designing to support the performance of the healthcare professional. *Quality & Safety in Health Care, 15* (Suppl 1), i59–i65.

Koppel, R., et al. (2005). Role of computerized physician order entry systems in facilitating medication errors. *JAMA, 293*(10), 1197–1203.

Koppel, R., et al. (2008). Identifying and quantifying medication errors: Evaluation of rapidly discontinued medication orders submitted to a computerized physician order entry system. *Journal of the American Medical Informatics Association, 15*(4), 461–465.

Kuziemsky, C. E., et al. (2012). The nature of unintended benefits in health information systems. *Studies in Health Technology and Informatics, 180,* 896–900.

Lown, B., & Rodriguez, D. (2012). Lost in translation? How electronic health records structure communication, relationships and meaning. *Academic Medicine, 87*(4), 3.

McCann, E. (2013). *EHR copy and paste? Better think twice.* Healthcare IT NEws.

Meisel, Z. F. (2011, January 12). *The health IT paradox: Why more data doesn't always mean better care* [cited 2014 8/29/2014]. Available from: http://content.time.com/time/health/article/0,8599,2041900,00.html

Merton, R. K. (1936). The unanticipated consequences of purposive social action. *American Sociological Review, 1*(6), 894–904.

Reckmann, M. H., et al. (2009). Does computerized provider order entry reduce prescribing errors for hospital inpatients? A systematic review. *Journal of the American Medical Informatics Association, 16*(5), 613–623.

Saleem, J. J., et al. (2011). Paper persistence, workarounds, and communication breakdowns in computerized consultation management. *International Journal of Medical Informatics, 80*(7), 466–479.

Shah, N. R., et al. (2006). Improving acceptance of computerized prescribing alerts in ambulatory care. *Journal of the American Medical Informatics Association, 13*(1), 5–11.

Shulman, R., et al. (2005). Medication errors: A prospective cohort study of hand-written and computerised physician order entry in the intensive care unit. *Critical Care, 9*(5), R516–R521.

Smith, A. (1759). *The theory of moral sentiments* (S. M. Soares, Ed.). MetaLibri, 2005.

Steele, A. M., & DeBrow, M. (2008). Efficiency gains with computerized provider order entry. In K. Henriksen (Ed.), *Advances in patient safety: New directions and alternative approaches (Vol. 4: Technology and medication safety).* Rockville: Agency for Healthcare Research and Quality (AHRQ) US. Available from: http: //www.ncbi.nlm.nih.gov/books/NBK43766/

Strauss, A., et al. (1997). *Social organization of medical work.* London: Transaction Publishers.

Strom, B., et al. (2010). Unintended effects of a computerized physician order entry nearly hard-stop alert to prevent a drug interaction: A randomized controlled trial. *Archives of Internal Medicine, 170*(17), 1578–1583.

Tenner, R. (1997). *Why things bite back: Technology and the revenge of unintended consequences.* New York: Random House.

Payne, T. H., et al. (2002). Characteristics and override rates of order checks in a practitioner order entry system. In *Proceedings of the AMIA symposium* (pp. 602–606).

Vogelsmeier, A. A., Halbesleben, J. R., & Scott-Cawiezell, J. R. (2008). Technology implementation and workarounds in the nursing home. *Journal of the American Medical Informatics Association, 15*(1), 114–119.

Weiner, J. P. (2007). "e-Iatrogenesis": The most critical unintended consequence of CPOE and other HIT. *Journal of the American Medical Informatics Association, 14*(3), 387–388. discussion 389.

Weingart, S., et al. (2003). Physicians' decisions to override computerized drug alerts in primary care. *Archives of Internal Medicine, 163*(21), 2625–2631.

Weingart, S., et al. (2011). Electronic drug interaction alerts in ambulatory care: The value and acceptance of high-value alerts in US medical practices as assessed by an expert clinical panel. *Drug Safety, 34*(7), 587–593.

Chapter 12
The Role of Human Computer Interaction in Consumer Health Applications: Current State, Challenges and the Future

Holly B. Jimison, Misha Pavel, Andrea Parker, and Kristin Mainello

12.1 Introduction

Health technologies for use by consumers and patients run the gamut from Web pages for browsing health information, to disease management systems involving real-time measurement and tailored feedback on a mobile phone. In this chapter, we will consider consumer health applications to be the set of technologies used by consumers to promote their health and wellbeing. One of the distinctions of this chapter, from the rest of the medical informatics applications described in this book, is that the primary user of the technology is the consumer or patient. Interactive consumer health technologies offer a scalable and potentially cost-effective mechanism for engaging individuals in their own care, certainly an important component of healthcare reform, as healthcare becomes more proactive and takes place outside the hospital and clinic.

In contrast to medical technologies designed for specific clinicians with common training and level of education, with consumer health applications we find additional challenges in designing for a broad base of consumers with varying educational, cultural, language and literacy levels. Then the need to communicate medical and health information in lay language and meaningful graphics adds another level of complexity. The following sections will provide an overview of the field, as well as background and guidance on addressing the needs of specific populations of consumers of healthcare.

H.B. Jimison (✉) • M. Pavel • A. Parker • K. Mainello
College of Computer and Information Science and College of Health Sciences, Northeastern University, Boston, MA, USA
e-mail: h.jimison@neu.edu; m.pavel@neu.edu; a.parker@neu.edu; k.mainello@neu.edu

© Springer International Publishing Switzerland 2015
V.L. Patel et al. (eds.), *Cognitive Informatics for Biomedicine*, Health Informatics,
DOI 10.1007/978-3-319-17272-9_12

12.1.1   Overview of Consumer Health Informatics

Interactive consumer health technology applications are increasingly recognized as an important component of healthcare services. The Institute of Medicine's (IOM) report on Crossing the Quality Chasm (Committee on Quality Health Care in America 2001) discusses fostering self-management support by encouraging providers to use education and other supportive interventions in order to systematically increase patients' skills and confidence in managing their health problems. Two of their recommended initiatives refer to patient-centered care and informatics. Patient-centered care is aligned with consumer health informatics in that it aims to inform and involve patients and their families in their decision-making and self-management, apply principles of disease prevention and behavioral change appropriate for diverse populations, and understand patients' concepts regarding their illness and their cultural beliefs. They additionally recommended informatics approaches to communicate, manage knowledge, and support decision-making using information technology (Committee on Quality Health Care in America 2001). Examples of consumer-facing technologies for health include searchable Web portals for health information (e.g., WebMD.com or MayoClinic.com) and Web access to newspaper and magazine health articles. These are currently perhaps the most commonly used consumer health applications. However, systems that adapt to individual users' inputs and provide tailored responses or advice can be much more powerful (Jimison et al. 2008). For example, such interactive health technologies may include home monitoring sensors with interactive disease-management or self-management technology, educational or decision-aid software that is interactively tailored to a patient's needs, online patient support groups, tailored interactive health reminder systems where interactions are linked with electronic medical records, and patient-physician electronic messaging (Jimison et al. 2008).

Johnson et al. used a framework of modes of engagement to categorize basic types of consumer health informatics applications, with categories of communication, data storage, behavior management, and decision support. Table 12.1, adapted from their chapter in Shortliffe and Cimino's book on Biomedical Informatics Computer Applications in Health Care and Biomedicine (Johnson et al. 2013), provides definitions and examples of such systems. This framework and classification scheme shows that consumer health applications range from simple browsing for health information to interactive systems that provide tailored advice and interventions. In the category of Communication, we include online support groups and social networking sites that deal with health issues.

For example, a person interested in learning about multiple sclerosis (MS) could find structured background information at a Web site like Healthline.com (Healthline Multiple Sclerosis). The first steps would be viewing the section on Learning the Basics, which would cover symptoms, vocabulary, causes, risk factors, tests and diagnoses, and complications of the disease. The use of video, graphics, simple language and a clear organization can help users successfully

Table 12.1 Categorization of types of consumer health informatics applications

Mode of engagement	Definition	Examples
Communication	Support for patient-to-patient, computer-to-patient and patient-to-provider communication or information dissemination	Patient portals
		Patient-physician secure email
		Online support groups
		Social networking sites
Data storage	A patient-centered and managed repository for patient-entered data	Personal health records
		Data portals for home monitoring devices
Behavior management	Tools to support personal health goals, often by combining data storage, care protocols, information dissemination, and communication	Weight management tools
		Physical activity tools
		Medication reminder systems
Decision support	Tools to prepare patients to participate in 'close call' decisions that involve weighing benefits, harms, and uncertainty	Interactive tools for treatment decisions for Breast Ca, Prostate Ca, Back Pain, End of Life, Heart Disease

Adapted from Johnson et al. (2013)

navigate these sites and help them obtain the information they need. Further sections on treatment options, finding a doctor, advice on managing the condition, and links to ongoing clinical trials become important for those diagnosed with MS. Many health Web sites with disease specific information also offer online support groups. Continuing with the Healthline.com example for MS, there are several ways in which patients can reach out to one another online. The site offers a location where patients can rate their therapies and share results, a place to load and share video testimonials, a place to share tips for living with MS, a set of MS patients' blogs, and also an online support group that links to Facebook. Some organizations offer online support groups with expert moderators, such as WebMD's MS Community. Both types of services serve important functions. Much of the care for chronic conditions, such as MS, occurs at home and has to do with managing symptoms and adhering to treatment goals. Oftentimes, other patients who have long-term experience with a condition can be most helpful. Additionally, the health benefits of social support from patients in the same situation can be very powerful (Umberson and Montez 2010). Researchers have found improved quality-of-life outcomes not only for patients enrolled in face-to-face support groups for diagnoses like breast cancer (Würtzen et al. 2013), but also for online patient support groups (Klemm et al. 2003). The social support provided by patients with similar issues can serve to provide empathy and encouragement in a way that is difficult for clinicians or even family members. Additionally, patients who have already learned to cope with self-management challenges can offer just-in-time information to patients struggling to cope. An online venue makes these connections more accessible and convenient. Additionally, the anonymity encourages a more honest and open dialogue (Hsuing 2000). It is important that the computer interface design of the online systems facilitate these important features for patients. Representative interface design issues include clearly communicating the level of privacy and security of the data being shared, and helping the consumer in distinguishing advertising from legitimate health information.

Other examples of consumer health applications include personal health records, decision support tools and health behavior change systems. Personal health records offer users a mechanism to store and retrieve their health information. Those that are linked to specific health systems often additionally offer secure patient-physician email, appointment setting, and medication renewals. Decision support tools for patients have run the gamut from early interactive video systems designed to integrate patient preferences on potential health outcomes into medical treatment decisions such as prostate or breast cancer treatments to Web-based systems that led patients through background material and assessments for tailored feedback on their health care decisions (O'Connor et al. 1999). Finally, systems that offer monitoring and performance feedback (i.e., Fitbit.com for activity monitoring or Beddit.com for sleep monitoring) can be clustered in Table 12.1 under Health Behavior Change systems. User feedback from the monitoring itself has been shown to influence behavior change (Bravata et al. 2007), but for many chronic conditions such as diabetes, asthma and heart failure, it is important to have sophisticated behavior change protocols in consumer systems that can be facilitated by a coach or nurse care manager (Demiris et al. 2008). Changing health behaviors is challenging, and user interface design for the necessary prompts and reminders becomes critical to the success of these systems.

Consumer health applications may be implemented on a variety of platforms using Web/Internet technology, desktop computer applications, touch screen kiosks, cell phones, smart watches, or combinations of the above. The human computer interaction implications of deploying these types of health interventions on varying display devices with varying types of consumers generates many challenges for designers. The subsequent sections further elucidate these challenges and offer potential design guidance.

12.1.2 *Needs Assessment as Part of Interface Design for Consumers*

Interface design for a new health information technology must originate with a careful needs assessment and understanding of goals and tasks to be performed. In the case of designing a system for consumers, it is important to anticipate whether the intended users will be from varying age ranges, different cultures, and different education levels. It is important to determine whether there will be separate systems for use by specific groups or whether the interface and content need to be adapted to the type of user (See Chap. 7, this volume, for a more detailed description). Needs assessment techniques such as focus groups and interviews with stakeholders can provide feedback to inform these design choices. An example of an iterative needs assessment is described in Jimison's study on multimedia tools for informed consent (Jimison et al. 1998). The initial challenge was to address the needs of patients with decisional capacity but varying forms of cognitive impairment. Standard consent materials were often written at above the college level when considering trials with complex protocols. The researchers selected consent procedures associated with trials for patients with schizophrenia, depression, and newly diagnosed patients with breast cancer. Design specifications for a tool to help patients decide whether or not to volunteer for a trial were developed with input from a series of focus groups with representative patients with experience in these types of trials. The resulting prototype was then tested again as stimulus material with similar focus groups, followed by usability testing of a following iteration and then a trial comparing paper consents to the multimedia decision aid. Breast cancer patients were found to be the most decisionally impaired, wanting almost uniformly to defer to their doctor. Patients with schizophrenia were better able to focus with a tool that kept the amount of material on any one screen minimal and let patients browse for further information, then bring them back to the main points. A needs assessment with users, encouraging participatory design, is helpful, especially for rapidly changing technologies.

12.2   How Culture Influences Design Choices

Culture is an umbrella term used to refer to a multi-layered construct influenced by language, education, societal rules and religion (The Providers Guide to Quality and Culture; McCrickard et al. 2012). Designing user interfaces for people with different cultural and health beliefs requires adapting and incorporating a variety of factors. People from different countries/cultures use interfaces in different ways, prefer different graphical layouts and have different expectations in how the health technology interacts (McCrickard et al. 2012). Therefore, user interfaces should be designed to accommodate the cultural differences of the target end users to provide an optimum user experience (McCrickard et al. 2012). If you have ever tried to assemble furniture produced in another country using instructions roughly translated to your language, you probably have a sense of the frustration or confusion non-native consumers have when using health information systems that have been crudely adapted to their language using word-by-word translations instead of looking for the cultural meaning to convey. The success of a consumer health intervention in a new culture critically depends on careful and meaningful message adaptation. Additionally, visuals containing graphics with colors may seem to have an agreed upon interpretation for many people in the United States with common experiences, but quite different when shown to immigrant populations or subgroups with a nonstandard exposure to the media.

As an example of the benefits of user testing of health content, the Los Angeles Cancer Education Project conducted a learner verification of a number of national and local publications with potential users from the Hispanic community (Briceno and Killam). The materials were found to be unsuitable "because they dealt with facts rather than with people and their concerns," meaning that the patients' emotional responses were felt to be more salient and of concern than finding out medical facts about cancer. The feedback from this resulted in a new publication based on one extended family's experiences with cancer: Hablaremos Sobre Cancer de la Familia (Let's Talk About Cancer Among the Family) (Briceno and Killam). This became the centerpiece for a comprehensive community effort to detect early cancer. Family participation for cancer detection was more culturally appropriate than individual participation. Culture involves common beliefs, values, traditions, lifestyle, communication, region, and the way you look at the world. Another interesting location requiring multiple styles of communication and influencing interface design occurs in the Hawaiian Islands. There are several ethnic subcultures there, including Hawaiian, Portuguese, Chinese, Japanese, Korean, Caucasian, Filipino, Vietnamese, Samoan, and other Pacific Island ethnic groups, often identified as native Hawaiian. Each group, on average, has different cultural expectations for communication styles and this influences how best to use (or not use) technology to communicate health messages (e.g., screening for cancer or appointments) (Evercare; Goebert et al. 2007). Chinese and Caucasian cultures tend to prefer a more direct style, Japanese a more formal style, and native Hawaiians a more indirect approach that first addresses social needs. It is important for designers of health technology tools to consider communication styles as part of the human computer interaction design process.

12.2.1 Designing for Populations with Health Disparities

There are several subpopulations in the United States who are predisposed to worse health outcomes than other groups. For example, African Americans when compared to non-Hispanic white Americans, have higher rates of obesity, hypertension, cardiovascular disease and are disproportionately affected by increased rates of HIV, especially among African American women (Braveman et al. 2005). Similarly, Hispanic populations also have worse health outcomes when compared to whites. Latino and Hispanic populations have higher incidences of diabetes, hypertension and obesity in addition to double the amount of cervical cancer among Latino/Hispanic women (Braveman et al. 2005).

When designing user interfaces for these groups, there are several key considerations to address (Reinecke and Gajos 2011). Disparities in education and income levels are intertwined with health disparities. Approximately 16 % of African Americans and Hispanics live below the federal poverty line. 37.7 % of Hispanics and 16.1 % of African Americans aged 25 and older did not complete high school (Braveman et al. 2005). Additionally, studies have shown that design technologies for African American youth should also be "cool" (Reinecke and Gajos 2011). This includes interfaces that are "rebellious, authentic, rich and innovative" (Reinecke and Gajos 2011). For many populations, studies show interfaces that contain culturally appropriate content are more effective than solely language translations (Chang and Yu 2012; Kreuter and McClure 2004). It is important that design be able to bridge digital divides and embrace disenfranchised populations or those who are medically underserved.

12.2.2 Access Issues and the Digital Divide

The access to technology for consumer health information and patient-facing interventions has presented a challenge to researchers, policy makers and clinicians with an interest in the equitable delivery of care. Populations who most need health information often lack the means, knowledge, and skills necessary to benefit from Internet health resources (Smith and Zickhur 2012). In a recent Pew Internet and American Life Project, they found that more than one quarter of U.S. adults had no online presence, and many Americans used a slow-speed Internet connection (Smith and Zickhur 2012). Non-users were more likely to be poor, less educated, over the age of 65, disabled, members of ethnic minorities, and nonnative English speakers (Smith and Zickhur 2012). This lack of access to health information and management tools has direct implications on general access to health care services, as more and more care will be provided with the use of Internet technologies.

The design choices that developers of consumer health informatics systems make with regard to media and format have a direct impact on the degree of use by populations of interest. Access by definition affects degree of use. Even though conventional access to health information through more traditional Web interfaces on desktop computers may have less use in minority populations, a design choice to use mobile phones to communicate may actually increase use above the norm in targeted populations. Many developers are surprised to learn that according to a recent Nielsen study of smartphone sales, it was found that White consumers were less likely than Blacks, Asians or Hispanics to have a smartphone (Nielsen Report). In fact, only 42 % of White consumers purchasing a mobile phone chose a smartphone over a feature phone, whereas the percentage choosing a smartphone was higher for minority populations (44 % for African Americans, 56 % for Hispanics, and 60 % for Asian and Pacific Islanders).

12.3 Design Considerations According to Age

The population of older adults in the U.S. is increasing dramatically. In 2010, there were 40 million people age 65 and older, accounting for 13 % of the total U.S. population. The Older Americans report of 2012 projects an increase of 32 million people in this segment by the year 2030 (20 % of total U.S. population) (Older Americans 2012). In parallel to this trend is the projected increase in healthcare expenditures for older adults. According to the Centers for

Disease Control, Medicare spending has grown in the past 25 years, increasing from $37 billion to $336 billion, a trend that is expected to continue due to the increases in aging populations (Healthy Aging Improving and Extending Quality of Life Among Older Americans).

Empowering patients will apply to all ages, but age must be taken into account in addition to all other user characteristics in order to optimize the user experience with consumer health technologies. There are age-related declines in several cognitive and sensory-motor skills. For example, psychomotor skills such as dexterity and hand–eye coordination decline with age and these limitations can make it more challenging for older users to learn to use a keyboard or control a mouse device (Hedden and Gabrieli 2004). Age-related declines in working memory and divided attention have very direct implications for interface design (Fisk et al. 2009). Interface content must be much simpler and less cluttered to allow older users to attend to pertinent material. Rogers and Fisk have found that older adults are limited in their ability to develop automated responses (Rogers and Fisk 1991), which also has implications for needing to keep interface designs simple and easy to learn. Further, it is important to minimize tasks that might maintain a high cognitive load over time without the development of an automated response. Although there are several types of age-related declines, and many are quite severe with the onset of various pathologies, such as dementia, healthy older adults are quite adaptive in compensating and can continue to perform interactive tasks with technology quite successfully (Rogers and Fisk 1991).

An equally important aspect of the design is matching the communication style of the interface to that of the users, as vocabulary changes over time. The communication styles vary significantly across generations and ages, but are very important in creating trust and acceptance on the part of the users. The rapid evolution of communication styles is greatly influenced by the advances in communication technology including email, short message service (SMS) and various social media. Even adults in their 30s and 40s have a hard time keeping up with the new tech lingo of the next generation. Language is dynamic and technology content must match the vocabulary of the targeted audience.

The matching of communication styles is not limited to the textual information, but rather generalizes to all modalities. In particular, audio and pictorial representation as well as icon-based systems must be adjusted in accordance with the expected age and style of the users. Figure 12.1 shows a simple example of various choices of icons to represent a phone call. The icon on the left is recognizable to older adults, however, most young people will never have seen a dial phone, or perhaps even a land line. Additionally, with the advent of smartphones, physical keypads on a cell phone may not look familiar to some.

Given the effectiveness of video-based communication as demonstrated by YouTube and similar sites, it is expected that this style of information communication will find increasing applicability in the domain of consumer health informatics. Much like the text-based communication, these video-based approaches are likely to comprise a wide range of styles, ranging from cartoon animation, to interactive avatars and human actors.

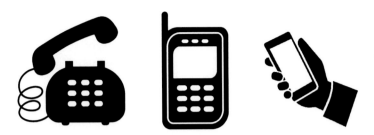

Fig. 12.1 Examples of phone icons, showing how the choice of a visual icon may be different for different age groups (Courtesy dreamstime.com)

In summary, the dynamics of the cognitive and sensory-motor skills combined with the heterogeneity in users' knowledge present significant challenges to the developers of interactive systems. Although consumer health information technology has the potential to empower patients to become more active in the care process, the elderly may be disadvantaged unless the designers of both software and hardware technology consider their needs explicitly (Fisk et al. 2009). The mitigation of these challenges in designing for consumer health technologies across ages and skill levels will be addressed in the section on the Future of Human Computer Interaction for Consumer Health. Despite the concerns addressed in this section, there is evidence suggesting older adults are connecting with technology more than ever before. According to a GE market research report, of the more than 53 % of older adults who use the Internet or email, 70 % report using the Internet regularly. However, a majority of older adults preferred simpler technology with fewer features (Care Innovations).

12.3.1 Additional Design Considerations Based on Chronic Conditions

If designed appropriately, health technology interventions for older adults could contain the costs burden on the healthcare system while simultaneously improving health outcomes for this population. Older populations also experience higher incidences of chronic conditions, and many of these conditions affect a user's ability to interact successfully with health information technology unless specific adaptations are in place. For example, approximately a third of adults between ages 65 and 74 have hearing loss, and most people notice visual problems around the age of 40 (Care Innovations). Having adaptable visual and auditory interfaces as options for technology addresses much of the problem. For example, varying font size and contrast options can often address the needs of individuals with mild to medium vision impairment. Common tools with many computers include auditory feedback and screen magnifying software. There are also several software packages for screen reading, converting text to speech. The American Foundation for the

Blind provides a review of 18 such systems (American Foundation for the Blind). An additional visual factor related to designing consumer health systems is that about 8 % of the population (mostly males) has a form of color blindness, and confuse either red and green and/or blue and green. The implication here is that interfaces should not rely on just color to convey information.

Arthritis is another common condition that affects users' ability to interact with keyboards, mouse devices and small phone interfaces. Arthritis is a leading cause of work disability, and those with the disease may have difficulty performing physically demanding jobs, and may select jobs that appear less strenuous but require intensive computer use. In 2010–2012, arthritis was the most frequently occurring chronic condition among older persons. 50 % of people over 65 were diagnosed with arthritis (U.S. Department of Health & Human Services 2013). A recent study of 315 arthritis patients found that 84 % percent of respondents reported a problem with computer use attributed to their underlying disorder and 77 % reported some discomfort related to computer use, mainly reporting problems with finding a comfortable position while using the computer and in manipulating the keyboard and mouse. Newer speech interfaces may serve to alleviate these issues. For example, voice browsers for the Web usually adhere to the World Wide Web Consortium guidelines (World Wide Web Consortium) and use Voice Dialog Extensible Markup Language (VoiceXML) to interpret and encode the Hypertext Markup Language (HTML) of a Web page. Voice browsers serve to both interpret human speech with speech recognition software and generate text-to-speech while interacting with a given Web page.

12.4 Health Literacy

Health literacy of the target population is a key concern for the design of both the content and interface of consumer health informatics systems. The lack of understanding of the material will hinder both the use and usefulness of a system. Health Literacy, defined by an IOM report as "the degree to which individuals have the capacity to obtain, process, and understand basic health information and services needed to make appropriate health decisions," is measured across the following domains: (1) cultural and conceptual knowledge, (2) oral literacy, including speaking and listening skills, (3) print literacy, including writing and reading skills, and (4) numeracy (Baker 2006; Schillinger et al. 2002). Individual health literacy is most commonly assessed by using the Rapid Estimate of Adult Literacy in Medicine (REALM) and Test of Functional Health Literacy in Adults (TOFHLA) tests. Both these instruments measure reading skills, word recognition, vocabulary, reading fluency and to some extent numeracy (Baker 2006). The impact of low health literacy, while a general concern, is particularly important to address when designing for groups with known literacy problems. For example, low health literacy is common among racial and ethnic minorities, older adults, and patients with chronic conditions (Jimison et al. 2008; Eysenbach 2001). Nearly 9 of 10 adults have trouble using the everyday health information that is routinely available in our healthcare facilities, retail outlets, media, and communities (Smith and Zickhur 2012). Among adult age groups, those aged 65 and older have the smallest percentage of people with proficient health literacy skills and the largest percentage with "below basic" health literacy skills (Jimison et al. 2008).

There are several tools for helping designers of consumer health applications to provide appropriate text content. For example, Web sites like The Readability Test Tool and ReadabilityScore.Com provide measures of the reading grade level of any English language text submitted. These tools typically include several standard measures, such as

- Flesch Kincaid Reading Ease (Kincaid et al. 1988)
- Flesch Kincaid Grade Level (Kincaid et al. 1988)
- Gunning Fog Score (The Gunning's Fog Index)
- Coleman Liau Index (Coleman and Liau 1975)
- SMOG Index (Hedman 2008)
- Automated Readability Index (Senter and Smith 1967)

The guidelines for developing patient education materials call for maintaining a reading level of grade 5 or below (Ochsner Health System). This can sometimes be quite challenging for designers not trained in writing at this level. FirstClinical.com has a Web tool that assists in this process by providing a glossary of simple health terms (First Clinical Research Glossary) and a document analysis tool (First Clinical Research Document Analysis) to ensure readability by a majority of the population.

When considering human computer interaction design in consumer health applications, it is also important to consider what has been termed "eHealth" literacy. The term eHealth refers to health interventions or information using Internet, wireless services, and related technologies (Demeris and Eysenbach 2002). These types of consumer-oriented applications are used to engage consumers in managing their own health care, communicating with clinicians, making health decisions, and adhering to their health behavior change goals (Jimison et al. 2008). Several researchers have proposed methods for measuring eHealth literacy. For example, vander Vaart et al. use eHEALs, an 8-item scale that measures perceived skills in finding, evaluating and applying electronic health information to health problems (van der Vaart et al. 2011). Chan and Kaufman created a theoretical framework for evaluating eHealth literacy (Kaufman et al. 2003a). They first considered the dimensions proposed by Norman and Skinner (2006) consisting of computer literacy, information literacy, media literacy, traditional literacy and numeracy, science literacy and health literacy. They then integrated a second model to include variation in task performance along a continuum of cognitive demands (e.g., remembering, understanding, applying, analyzing, evaluating, and creating). The goal of this new framework was to elucidate the barriers to effective user performance on intended health management tasks. Given that self-management and consumer engagement are critical to the success of our new models of care, it is now well recognized that we must address the barriers of health literacy and eHealth literacy more specifically as part of healthcare services. This is increasingly recognized as a problem that impacts healthcare quality and costs.

12.5 The Future of Human Computer Interaction for Consumer Health

One important, but often ignored, aspect of interface design involves the consequences of rapid advances in technologies that affect the design approaches. We see several important trends in the development of systems used to communicate health information to consumers. First, the interfaces and user designs will be tailored to target populations and potentially to individuals as well. More importantly, these interfaces will continuously adapt to changing user needs, for example, as a consequence of the aging process. Secondly, we will be conducting real-time remote usability testing using video-conferencing techniques for protocol analysis and ecological momentary assessment using just-in-time feedback from mobile phones. Lastly, we see that the move toward pervasive and ubiquitous computing will impact the design of consumer health systems, especially our notion of user interface design and usability testing (Chap. 13 provides an overview of the design considerations for mobile technology in healthcare).

12.5.1 Approaches to Developing Adaptive User Interfaces

Throughout this chapter, we noted that interfaces for consumer health informatics systems need to be user specific. In particular, the effectiveness of interactions depends on how closely the interface style is matched to that of the users. In addition, the state, ability and functionality of the user are not constant over time. Some of these changes are predictable; others are highly variable. For example, it is well documented that an individual's perceptual, cognitive and physical functionality declines with aging (Jimison et al. 2008; Hedden and Gabrieli 2004; Fisk et al. 2009; Rogers and Fisk 1991). In contrast, users' health literacy is likely to improve with exposure to information. Less well documented is the short-term variability, for example, as function of the daily variability in the quality of sleep (Hedden and Gabrieli 2004). Given the dynamics of users' characteristics, an important question faced by the designer is how to optimize interfaces with respect to these characteristics. There are many options, but two approaches stand out. The first is based on a prior, population-based characterization of the users, perhaps by clustering them with respect to their age, functionality, communication styles, demographics, socio-economic status, etc. The interface design would then be tailored to the cluster and its characteristics. Individual users would be categorized and assigned to the most appropriate interface. Recent advances in commercial systems (e.g., Amazon.com) have demonstrated the potential of adaptation strategies. For example, a number of Internet-based marketing strategies use history of users' visits to various sites and the targets of their prior clicks. Much like these commercial approaches, using algorithms for collaborative filtering, one could develop interfaces that adapt their style, knowledge level and information content to the specific user. Collaborative filtering methods (Su and Khoshgoftaar 2009) are based on using large amounts of information on users' quantifiable characteristics, behaviors, activities or preferences and determining similarity among users that is then used to infer their preferences and aspects of interactions. Some early work in this area is described by Yue et al. 2014, where researchers used collaborative clustering to anticipate users' intended tasks. We note that this type of implementation would require more basic research concerning the types of data and their implication on the interactions before it can be used as a standard interface design practice.

In an alternate approach, interfaces would be designed to adapt to the communication styles and task-specific information processing capabilities, e.g., domain-specific health literacy of the individual users. A user may be relatively naïve about health issues in general, but in short time acquires significant information about a specific health issue. For example, following a diagnosis of diabetes, an individual may acquire a sophisticated diabetes-related vocabulary. The recent advances in sensor technology, networking and inference algorithms open the opportunity to monitor users' interactions and make inferences about the individuals' states. These inferences can then be used to adapt aspects of the interfaces. Examples of such adaptive actions can be found in the commercial settings where advertisements are geared to the search activities of the users. Emotional responses, as assessed by physiological measurements, can be used to modify consumer information delivery and presentation. In the field of education, interfaces have been adapted in real time through signals of pressure-sensitive mouse devices and wrist sensors for heart rate variability and galvanic skin response. Research versions have been used to categorize level of understanding for users of interactive educational materials (tentative movements and pressure correspond to low levels of understanding, and firm clicks and movements to higher levels of understanding) (Viadero 2010). There is also indication that in the more distant horizon it is likely that brain-computer interfaces will enable even finer adaptation and thus track the changing functionality of elderly users. This fits within the field of Neuroergonomics – the study of the human brain in relation to performance in everyday settings, including interactions with devices and systems (Parasuraman and Rizzo 2008; Parasuraman 2011). One of the objectives of this nascent discipline is to enhance our understanding of how humans interact with technology and thereby improve the scientific underpinning of user interface design.

12.5.2 Remote Usability Testing of Consumer Health Systems

Given that most consumer health systems are used in the home or workplace, it is important that future usability testing occur in these naturalistic settings and occur in real-time. Traditional usability testing takes place in a controlled laboratory setting where a sample of users are asked to perform representative tasks with the technology being tested, typically while talking aloud as in protocol analysis or task analysis. The advantages to this approach have been that video recordings of the user's face, speech, and interactions with the technology can be carefully recorded and later analyzed. However, the set of interactions tested can be quite limited and typically do not have normal background distractions or a normal context. Early attempts at remote usability testing of naturally occurring interactions with Web sites used sequences and timings of user clicks to infer intent and to look for potential misunderstandings. The advantages were that the data collection was inexpensive and it was possible to test all users of a site. The downside was not truly knowing what users were thinking or whether they were successful. For mobile phone health interventions it is possible to use the newer techniques of Ecological Momentary Assessment (EMA) (Dunton et al. 2012; Heron and Smyth 2010) for testing some aspects of usability. EMA is used more generally for health assessments, where questions are sent to a user's phone based on time, location, and/or context. These questions can be adapted to verify a system's inference on context, intended task, and other aspects that influence the content and interface. This was an important aspect to the participatory design of Goodman et al.'s work on technology for older adults in the home (Goodman et al. 2002).

Kaufman et al. used a more thorough approach to field testing their diabetes technology in the homes of older adults (Kaufman et al. 2003b). The researcher participated in the usability testing in the home environment with cameras recording the user, the researcher and the screen interactions. The usability testing was coupled with cognitive walkthrough analysis of the telemedicine system. Researchers at the Oregon Center developed a novel approach to usability testing for Aging & Technology. They developed and evaluated remote usability testing on an ongoing basis (without researchers in the home) for participatory design. An initial implementation of the approach involved a cohort of older adult participants in their "Living Lab" (a group of approximately 50 cognitively healthy adults over 70 years of age living independently in their homes) (Jimison and Pavel 2008). As part of a study of health coaching technology, as well as sensors for monitoring of movement, sleep, socialization, medication management, physical exercise and cognitive exercise, these seniors were used to using Web cameras and Skype as part of their coaching and socialization interventions with family members. Usability researchers in a central academic setting used the seniors' Web cameras with video conferencing software and screen capture software to conduct low-cost iterative usability tests of new software while users remained in their homes using their own computers, as shown in the diagram in Fig. 12.2.

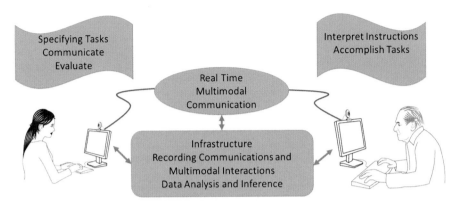

Fig. 12.2 Schematic of the video conferencing set-up for remote usability testing from the research lab to the home (Figure rendered by Jesse Pavel of Electrika, Inc)

Testers were able to remotely control the computer in the home and obtain video (face and computer screen) and audio recordings of talk-aloud task analyses as subjects used the technology in their familiar setting (Yu 2010). Recordings of the computer screen during the test were synced with the Web camera recording of the participant's facial expressions and audio for later analysis. This form of user testing could be performed quickly and conveniently, allowing for frequent iterations of software design with user participation and immediate feedback. It also allows the user to feel more comfortable in their own environment with a familiar computer. The convenience on the part of the developers and usability testers, being able to conduct the tests from their office or home, is also important in encouraging frequent iterations to optimize the interface. These remote usability approaches allow researchers and developers to perform frequent low-cost remote usability tests of new screen designs and content as part of a participatory iterative design process.

12.5.3   New Horizons: Human Computer Interaction with Distributed Computing

The advances in technology, computation and engineering alluded to in the section on adaptive interfaces have much farther-reaching implications than those discussed thus far. Perhaps for the first time in history, we have access to technology that is capable of monitoring, inference and interpretation of behaviors, ranging from physical activity to emotional responses. We are in the midst of a rapid expansion in the availability of sensors to measure motion, acceleration, location, sleep quality and many physiological quantities. These sensors are now smaller and cheaper than ever before. There have been advances in energy harvesting, and enhancing battery life will continue to make these more convenient to use in wearable versions.

These sensors add to our ability to collect routine physiological measures in the home, such as blood glucose for diabetes, peak flows for asthma, and blood pressure for cardiovascular disease. The new wearable sensors now allow us continuous and unobtrusive monitoring, and thereby provide more effective tailored interventions in a variety of areas ranging from cardiovascular monitoring to physical exercise and weight management. Among the consequences of this technological revolution is the rise of movements such as "Quantified Self" (Adventures in Self-Surveillance) on the monitoring side and "PatientsLikeMe" (Wicks et al. 2010) on the networking side. Both of these directions are suggestive of future trends in consumer health informatics that incorporate behavioral inferences, social connectivity and big data analytics, but will require appropriate human computer interfaces and data visualization. The raw data from monitoring converted to information will be increasingly useful in matching consumer needs with available sources of information and knowledge.

The concurrent rising ubiquity of smartphones will also play a large role in the future of interface design. In fact, for many, smartphones are the main method of interfacing with the Internet. The user interface issues in attempting to convey complex information on a small screen will remain a challenge. However, more importantly, users will likely be interacting with displays of varying sizes throughout their environment, much as the newer displays on cars now can show applications from the driver's mobile phone. Linking to displays in varying locations and of varying dimensions will offer a potentially much improved user experience and certainly convenience. The sophistication of user interface algorithms will necessarily grow, making this a fertile area for discovery and innovation.

Overall, user interfaces and user-centered design more generally will play a large role in the success of health interventions in the future, as more healthcare is provided in the home and environments outside a hospital or clinic. The challenges in designing systems for a highly variable set of consumers are great, but the opportunities provided by new monitoring and communications technologies are also great. This will certainly be a dynamic field for both research and development of successful systems for consumers of healthcare.

Discussion Questions

1. Imagine that you are working for a clinic that provides consumer technology for diabetes care in the home, consisting of blood glucose meters, a Web site with educational material, and automated reminders by cell phone. You have been asked to develop design specifications to adapt it for a low-income Spanish-speaking immigrant population living in an urban setting. Describe your process in adapting this set of technology for this new population.
2. For a new era of pervasive computing, where sensors and communication displays are distributed throughout the home, workplace, and general environment, describe the challenges and potential solutions to usability testing of a new device or tailored health communications tool.

Additional Readings

Agency for Healthcare Quality and Research. *Designing consumer health IT: A guide for developers and systems designers.* http://healthit.ahrq.gov/sites/default/files/docs/page/designing-consumer-health-it-a-guide-for-developers-and-systems-designers.pdf

Johnson, K., Jimison, H., & Mandl, K. (2013). Chapter 17: Consumer health informatics. In E. H. Shortliffe & J. J. Cimino (Eds.), *Biomedical informatics computer applications in health care and biomedicine* (4th ed.). New York: Springer.

Reinecke, K., & Gajos, K. Z. One size fits many Westerners – How cultural abilities challenge UI design. http://reinecke.people.si.umich.edu/Publications_files/CulturalAbilities.pdf

References

Adventures in Self-Surveillance, aka The Quantified Self, aka Extreme Navel-Gazing. Forbes. April 7, 2011.

American Foundation for the Blind. *Review of screen readers.* http://www.afb.org/prodBrowseCatResults.asp?CatID=49

Baker, D. (2006, August). The meaning and the measure of health literacy. *Journal of General Internal Medicine, 21*(8), 878–883.

Bravata, D. M., Smith-Spangler, C., Sundaram, V., et al. (2007). Using pedometers to increase physical activity and improve health: A systematic review. *The Journal of the American Medical Association, 298*(19), 2296–2304.

Braveman, P. A., Cubbin, C., Egerter, S., Chideya, S., Posner, S., Marchi, K. S., Metzler, M. (2005, December 14). Socioeconomic status in health research: One size does not fit all. *The Journal of the American Medical Association, 294*(22), 2879(10).

Briceno, C., & Killam, B. *Designing an effective web presence for the hispanic audience.* http://www.upa-dc-metro.org/Resources/Documents/conference/2011/Presentations/UsabilityofHispanicWebsites_09_16_2011(2)-1.pdf

Care Innovations. *Older populations have adopted technology for health: People over 65 will use remote care technology to take better care of themselves.* http://www.careinnovations.com/resources/Guide_WhitePaper_OlderPopulationsHaveAdoptedTechForHealth.pdf.   Last viewed September 13, 2014.

Chang, C. L., & Yu, Y. (2012, July). Cross-cultural interface design and the classroom-learning environment in Taiwan. *TOJET: The Turkish Online Journal of Educational Technology, 11*(3).

Coleman, M., & Liau, T. L. (1975). A computer readability formula designed for machine scoring. *Journal of Applied Psychology, 60*, 283–284.

Committee on Quality Health Care in America. (2001). *Crossing the quality chasm: A new health system for the 21st century.* Washington, DC: Institute of Medicine.

Demeris, G., & Eysenbach, G. (2002). Internet use in disease management for home care patients: A call for papers. *Journal of Medical Internet Research, 4*(2), E6.

Demiris, G., Afrin, L. B., Speedie, S., Courtney, K. L., Sondhi, M., Vimarlund, V., Lovis, C., Goossen, W., & Lynch, C. (2008 January–February). Patient-centered applications: Use of information technology to promote disease management and wellness. *Journal of the American Medical Informatics Association, 15*(1), 8–13.

Dunton, G. F., Liao, Y., Kawabata, K., & Intille, S. (2012). Momentary assessment of adults' physical activity and sedentary behavior: Feasibility and validity. *Frontiers in Psychology, 3*, 260.

Evercare, Developing Cultural Proficiency: Understanding and serving the people of Hawai'i. https://www.uhccommunityplan.com/content/dam/communityplan/plandocuments/culturalcompetency/en/HI-Evercare-QExA-Cultural-Competency.pdf

Eysenbach, G. (2001). What is e-health? *Journal of Medical Internet Research, 3*(2), E20. http://www.jmir.org/2001/2/e20/

First Clinical Research Document Analysis. http://www.firstclinical.com/words/. Retrieved September 25, 2014.

First Clinical Research Glossary. http://firstclinical.com/icfglossary/. Retrieved September 25, 2014.

Fisk, A. D., Rogers, W. A., Charness, N., Czaja, S. J., & Sharit, J. (2009). *Designing for older adults: Principles and creative human factors approaches* (2nd ed.). Boca Raton: CRC Press.

Goebert, D., Morland, L., Frattarelli, L., Onoye, J., & Matsu C. (2007). Mental health during pregnancy: A study comparing Asian, Caucasian and Native Hawaiian women. *Maternal and Child Health Journal, 11*, 244–255. http://www.cinahl.com/cgibin/refsvc?jid=1602&accno=2009589404

Goodman, C. A., Jimison, H. B., & Pavel, M. (2002). Participatory design for home care technology. In *Proceedings of the 24th annual engineering in medicine and biology conference* (Vol. 3).

Healthline Multiple Sclerosis. http://www.healthline.com/health/multiple-sclerosis

Healthy Aging Improving and Extending Quality of Life Among Older Americans. At a Glance 2009. National Center for Chronic Disease Prevention and Health Promotion. Centers for Disease Control and Prevention.

Hedden, T., & Gabrieli, J. D. E. (2004). Insights into the ageing mind: A view from cognitive neuroscience. *Nature Reviews Neuroscience, 5*(2), 87–96.

Hedman, A. S. (2008, January). Using the SMOG formula to revise a health-related document. *American Journal of Health Education, 39*(1), 61–64.

Heron, K. E., & Smyth, J. M. (2010). Ecological momentary interventions: Incorporating mobile technology into psychosocial and health behaviour treatments. *British Journal of Health Psychology, 15*(Pt 1), 1–39.

Hsuing, R. C. (2000). The best of both worlds: An online self-help group hosted by a mental health professional. *CyberPsychology and Behavior, 3*(6), 935–950.

Jimison, H. B., & Pavel, M. (2008). Integrating computer-based health coaching into elder home care. In A. Mihailidis, J. Boger, H. Kautz, & L. Normie (Eds.), *Technology and aging*. Amsterdam: IOS Press.

Jimison, H. B., Sher, P. P., & LeVernois, Y. M. (1998). The use of multimedia in the informed consent process. *Journal of the American Medical Informatics Association, 5*(2). San Francisco: Jossey-Bass Publishers.

Jimison, H., Gorman, P., Woods, S., Nygren, P., Walker, M., Norris, S., & Hersh, W. (2008 November). Barriers and drivers of health information technology use for the elderly, chronically ill, and underserved. *Evidence Report/Technology Assessment (Full Rep), 175*, 1–1422.

Johnson, K., Jimison, H., & Mandl, K. (2013). Chapter 17: Consumer health informatics. In E. H. Shortliffe & J. J. Cimino (Eds.), *Biomedical informatics computer applications in health care and biomedicine* (4th ed.). New York: Springer.

Kaufman, D. R., Starren, J., Patel, V. L., Morin, P. C., Hilliman, C., Pevzner, J., Weinstock, R. S., Goland, R., & Shea, S. (2003a). A cognitive framework for understanding barriers to the productive use of a diabetes home telemedicine system. In *AMIA annual symposium proceedings* (pp. 356–360).

Kaufman, D. R., Patel, V. L., Hilliman, C., Morin, P. C., Pevzner, J., Weinstock, R. S., Goland, R., Shea, S., & Starren, J. (2003b). Usability in the real world: Assessing medical information technologies in patients' homes. *Journal of Biomedical Informatics, 36*(1–2), 45–60.

Kincaid, J. P., Braby, R., & Mears, J. (1988). Electronic authoring and delivery of technical information. *Journal of Instructional Development, 11*, 8–13.

Klemm, P., Bunnell, D., Cullen, M., Soneji, R., Gibbons, P., & Holecek, A. (2003, May–June). Online cancer support groups: A review of the research literature. *Computers, Informatics, Nursing, 21*(3), 136–142.

Kreuter, M., & McClure, S. (2004). The role of culture in health communication. *Annual Review of Public Health, 25*, 439–455.

McCrickard, S., Doswell, F., Barksdale, J., & Piggot, D. (2012, May 5–10). *Understanding cool and computing for African-American youth. CHI 2012*, Austin, TX, USA.

Nielsen Report. *State of hispanic consumer report.* http://es.nielsen.com/site/documents/Stateof_Hispanic_Consumer_Report_4-16-FINAL.pdf

Norman, C. D., & Skinner, H. A. (2006). eHealth literacy: Essential skills for consumer health in a networked world. *Journal of Medical Internet Research, 8*(2), e9.

O'Connor, A. M., Rostom, A., Fiset, V., Tetroe, J., Entwistle, V., Llewellyn-Thomas, H., et al. (1999). Decision aids for patients facing health treatment or screening decisions: Systematic review. *British Medical Journal, 319*, 731.

Ochsner Health System – Development Guidelines for Patient Education Materials. http://academics.ochsner.org/editingdyn.aspx?id=51327

Older Americans. (2012, June). *Key indicators of well-being.* Federal Interagency Forum on Aging-Related Statistics.

Parasuraman, R. (2011). Neuroergonomics: Brain, cognition, and performance at work. *Current Directions in Psychological Science, 20*(3), 181–186.

Parasuraman, R., & Rizzo, M. (2008). *Neuroergonomics: The brain at work.* Oxford/New York: Oxford University Press, Inc.

ReadabilityScore.Com. https://readability-score.com/. Retrieved September 25, 2014.

Reinecke, K., & Gajos, K. Z. (2011, May 7–12). *One size fits many Westerners: How cultural abilities challenge UI design, CHI 2011.* Vancouver.

Rogers, W. A., & Fisk, A. D. (1991). Age-related differences in the maintenance and modification of automatic processes: Arithmetic stroop interference. *Human Factors, 33*, 45–56.

Schillinger, D., et al. (2002). Association of health literacy with diabetes outcomes. *The Journal of the American Medical Association, 288*(4), 475–482.

Senter, R. J., Smith, E. A. (1967, November). *Automated readability index.* http://en.wikipedia.org/wiki/Automated_Readability_Index. Wright-Patterson Air Force Base (p. iii). AMRL-TR-6620. Retrieved September 25, 2014.

Smith, A., & Zickhur, K. (2012, April 13). *Digital differences.* Pew Research Center. http://pewinternet.org/Reports/2012/Digital-differences/Main-Report.aspx?view=all

Su, X., & Khoshgoftaar, T. M. (2009). A survey of collaborative filtering techniques. In *Advances in Artificial Intelligence* (p. 19).

The Gunning's Fog Index (or FOG) Readability Formula. *Readabilty formulas.* Retrieved September 10, 2014.

The Provider's Guide to Quality and Culture. http://erc.msh.org/mainpage.cfm?file=5.2.0h.htm&module=provider&language=English

The Readability Test Tool. http://read-able.com/. Retrieved September 25, 2014.

Umberson, D., & Montez, J. K. (2010). Social relationships and health: A flashpoint for health policy. *Journal of Health and Social Behavior, 51*, S54.

U.S. Department of Health & Human Services. (2013). *Administration on aging & administration for community services, A profile of older Americans.* http://www.aoa.gov/Aging_Statistics/Profile/2013/docs/2013_Profile.pdf

van der Vaart, R., van Deursen, A., Drossaert, C., Taal, E., van Dijk, J., & van de Laar, M. (2011 October–December). Does the eHealth literacy scale (eHEALS) measure what it intends to measure? Validation of a Dutch version of the eHEALS in two adult populations. *Journal of Medical Internet Research, 13*(4), e86.

Viadero, D. (2010). Scholars test emotion-sensitive tutoring software. *Education Week, 29*(16), 6.

WebMD's Multiple Sclerosis Community. http://exchanges.webmd.com/multiple-sclerosis-exchange

Wicks, P., Massagli, M., Frost, J., Brownstein, C., Okun, S., Vaughan, T., Bradley, R., & Heywood, J. (2010). Sharing health data for better outcomes on PatientsLikeMe. *Journal of Medical Internet Research, 12*(2), e19.

World Wide Web Consortium. www.w3.org. Last viewed October 30, 2014.

Würtzen, H., Dalton, S. O., Elsass, P., et al. (2013). Mindfulness significantly reduces self-reported levels of anxiety and depression: results of a randomised controlled trial among 336 Danish women treated for stage I-III breast cancer. *European Journal of Cancer, 49*(6), 1365–1373.

Yu, C. H. (2010). *Evaluation of remote usability techniques in an elderly cohort.* http://digitalcommons.ohsu.edu/

Yue, Y., Wang, C., El-Arini, K., & Guestrin, C. (2014). Personalized Collaborative Clustering. In *WWW '14 Proceedings of the 23rd international conference on world wide web* (pp. 75–84).

Chapter 13
Designing and Deploying Mobile Health Interventions

Albert M. Lai and Katie A. Siek

13.1 Introduction

Early uses of mobile devices in healthcare were provider focused that enabled physicians communicate and access electronic health records whenever and wherever they were. Most healthcare providers are highly mobile and constantly moving throughout the healthcare environment – moving from patient to patient, making diagnoses, making treatment decisions, administering medications, and performing procedures – all of which need documentation.

As healthcare has moved from being acute care and physician-focused to a more patient- and wellness-centric model, applications of mobile devices in healthcare have shifted in focus as well. Much of the exciting new innovations in the use of mobile devices have focused on targeting the healthcare consumer and enabling them to be better engaged in their own care and efforts to maintain their wellness. In this chapter, we introduce mobile technology, its use in healthcare, user interface aspects to consider when using mobile devices, and study design considerations.

We discuss a broad range of mobile devices – covering personal digital assistants, basic cellular phones, feature phones, smartphones, tablets, and wearable devices. Strongly relevant to this chapter is the exciting and emerging field of *mHealth*. mHealth is defined broadly as the use of mobile telecommunication devices for the delivery of healthcare services. The majority of the sections of this chapter are encompassed by the term mHealth, but we also cover mobile

A.M. Lai, Ph.D. (✉)
Department of Biomedical Informatics, The Ohio State University,
250 Lincoln Tower, 1800 Canon Drive, Columbus, OH 43210, USA
e-mail: albert.lai@osumc.edu

K.A. Siek, Ph.D.
School of Informatics and Computing, Indiana University, 919 E. 10th Street,
Bloomington, IN 47408, USA
e-mail: ksiek@indiana.edu

© Springer International Publishing Switzerland 2015
V.L. Patel et al. (eds.), *Cognitive Informatics for Biomedicine*, Health Informatics,
DOI 10.1007/978-3-319-17272-9_13

devices that are not telecommunication devices such as PDAs and wearable devices, and are not traditionally included under mHealth.

This chapter is largely targeted at researchers, but we also discuss ideas that designers, software developers, and informaticians need to consider when designing and implementing mobile health care solutions. We place these mobile devices into their historical context and while this chapter does not provide a comprehensive systematic literature review, we cover important representative research that has been conducted using the variety of mobile devices covered in this chapter.

13.2 An Evolution of Mobile Devices

Mobile technology has undergone rapid advances in the last 20 years and healthcare adoption of mobile technology, although somewhat slower, has been rapidly increasing since the early 1990s (See Fig. 13.1). In the early 1990s, the first truly portable, full-featured laptops were just beginning to come to market. In the mid 1990s, mobile devices that acted as a personal information manager, personal digital assistants (PDAs), and cellular phones were beginning to have commercial success. In the early 2000s, smartphones were gaining traction and by the late 2000s had become widespread. It is around this time that the mobile revolution really took off and by 2010, tablet computers became very popular and in demand by consumers. Each of these form factors will be discussed in detail in the following sections of this chapter.

13.2.1 Mobile Stand-Alone

Internet-connected mobile applications are becoming easier to develop thanks to readily available software libraries (e.g., touchdevelop.com) and the increasingly pervasiveness of wireless Internet access. Initial mobile prototypes however were typically stand-alone and not connected to the Internet. Internet connected applications required the following set of resources that (the designer, evaluator, and developer need to consider): (1) a mobile Internet accessible area (which is still challenging in some rural communities); (2) a server or trusted cloud service that hosts data; a mobile device that can easily access the Internet; (3) a data plan for each user to access the Internet; and – especially relevant in health applications, (4) a secure connection to share health information. If resources are restricted, then researchers may consider a mobile stand-alone application that hosts all of the data on the device. Researchers can download the data when they meet with the users, however they also need to inform users of contingency plans and design software that alerts participants if they are not receiving accurate information because they are not transferring data in real time.

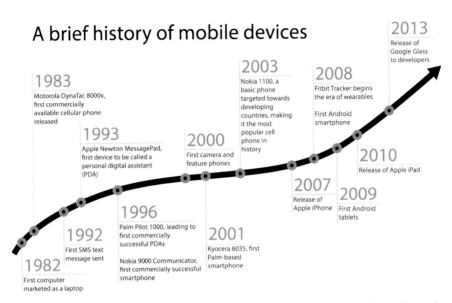

Fig. 13.1 As each of these form factors of devices became available, they were adopted for use in healthcare

An example of a stand-alone mobile application by Apple Research is a record keeping application to assist nurse midwives in rural India track the thousands of people that they must care for on a regular basis. The nurse midwives' responsibilities went beyond the typical ante and postnatal care to include treating injuries, vaccinating people, administering health tests, and providing health education. The researchers set out to design a mobile application to help the nurse midwives accurately and easily record health information so that it could readily be shared with government policy decision makers. The researchers spent significant time understanding the needs, expectations, and cultural issues surrounding the care and documentation of rural populations and ultimately designed an application that was informed by information resources the nurse midwives made for low literacy birth attendants. The researchers learned about the resources that the nurse midwives created after interviewing and shadowing participants (Grisedale et al. 1997). Researchers at Indiana University experienced a similar design issue when designing a dietary intake monitoring application (DIMA) for a low literacy, chronically ill population – participants preferred dietary feedback icons that looked similar to a cup that was used during their initial disease education meetings. Despite interviewing dietitians and nurses before designing the interfaces, it was not until the researchers presented the results to the health professionals that the similarity to the cup was mentioned (Siek et al. 2006). Based on these experiences, we encourage researchers to consider contextual inquiry methods (Holtzblatt et al. 2004) to learn about current processes and information resources so that the researcher can integrate these processes and artifacts earlier into their design and analysis cycle. Contextual inquiry methods typically include researchers interviewing (*the inquiry*) target users where they conduct the targeted activity (*the context*) and asking users to walk through typical activities to gain a better understanding of what is done when and how the process works. Researchers can gain rich data on users processes – specifically an understanding *if* technology is appropriate and *how* technology could enhance these processes.

Similar to the Apple Research example, DIMA researchers spent 2 years meeting with health professionals and patients in an iterative user-centered design process to design the application. The mobile application used icons, barcode scanning, and voice recording to provide users with an easy way to input what they ate and receive real-time feedback. In a pilot study, participants were able to successfully use DIMA and some noted that it helped them change their diet by becoming more compliant with their dietary restrictions (Connelly et al. 2012). Since the application needed to provide real time feedback, the researchers had to ensure that the database was primed with everything users could possibly input into the system. In addition, the authors had to iteratively design the interface because they were working with a low literacy population – a population often overlooked in the human computer interaction community. The research team had to consider everything from how to present dietary limits, organize food items (Siek et al. 2006), and the application's navigation structure (Chaudry et al. 2012).

13.2.2   Text Messaging

Text messaging – also known as Short Message Service (SMS) – uses standardized communication protocols to send short text messages via Web or mobile communication systems. In everyday conversation, we typically say we texted a picture, video, or other multimedia, however technically messages with multimedia are called Multimedia Messaging Service (MMS). In this chapter, we broadly define text messaging interventions that provide information – textual or multimedia – to individuals. Text messaging interventions provide health informatics researchers with a low cost, quick way to send and receive data to consumers and health professionals. Currently, there are two main text messaging programs – *push programs* that deliver information to people and *two-way programs* that can deliver and receive information from people users.

13.2.2.1   Push Text Messaging Programs

Current mass consumption text messaging programs are *push* systems in that they *push* information to the public to inform them about specific health related issues, but do not expect user responses. Push systems are fairly straightforward to implement – researchers could choose to manually send text messages from a phone or text message app (e.g., iMessage). Alternatively, researchers could create a more robust and automatic system by maintaining an SMS gateway or using an

SMS gateway service (e.g., Twilio) to automatically send text message at specific times.

In the United States, the Department of Health and Human Services compiles a list of text messaging programs that aim to improve health (http://www.hhs.gov/open/initiatives/mhealth/projects.html). For example, text4baby (text4baby.org) provides thousands of moms with three free text messages per week about their baby's development from pregnancy through their first year. Smokefreetxt (smokefree.gov) is a freely available text messaging program for young adults and adults to aid them in quitting smoking by sending 1–5 text messages per day for the 2 weeks leading up to their quit date and 6 weeks after their planned quit date. Smokefreetxt provides users with the ability to gain more information about specific points in the message by texting back specific words to get more information on how to deal with that point (e.g., texting "Cravings" to learn how to deal with cravings after quitting smoking). Push text message programs are beneficial because they provide an easy mechanism to send health messages to people and alert them about specific health considerations, however they are limited because they may not be customized enough to be relevant to some of the users or the message may not be delivered at the appropriate time to encourage a change in decision. For example, imagine designing relevant information about infant development that is understandable to someone with an elementary school reading level and yet still beneficial to the woman with an advanced degree in business.

13.2.2.2 Two-Way Communication Programs

Some health text messaging programs provide *two-way* communication so that users can communicate with other users or healthcare professionals. Two-way communication is slightly more complex to implement than *push* programs because the researcher needs to use a SMS gateway service and program some logic into the system to accommodate the various inputs a user may send to the system.

An example of a two-way communication program would be SMARTDIAB that provides type 1 diabetes patients with the ability to send and receive information to their doctor to receive personalized feedback. SMARTDIAB is also integrated with a web portal and mobile application for the users to transmit secure messages and reflect on aggregate data (Bin-Sabbar and Al-Rodhaan 2013). Since SMARTDIAB has multiple ways for people to access information – text message, mobile app, web portal – it provides users with a lot of flexibility. Researchers should also understand that the more flexibility users have to input and view data, the more time they must spend in designing, evaluating, and ensuring the users can efficiently interact with the system to promote ongoing use. For example, researchers have to consider the interactions users will have with each interface – text messaging, mobile app, and web portal – and between the interfaces. Do users interact with the application similarly independent of the platform or are they expected to remember different interactions for each platform? Can users easily transfer information between the interfaces and receive immediate feedback on their progress? We understand that each platform has different input and output mechanisms, however the overall user experience has to be similar enough so that users are not overburdened.

Sometimes researchers choose to use text messaging as an easy way to simulate real-time feedback without a database or Internet connection. For example, Chick Clique was a mobile phone application for teens to log their daily step counts, reflect on their progress, and check in on how their clique of friends were doing in their walking progress. The mobile phone application used text messages from a specific phone number to update the step counts that were shown on the phone application (Toscos et al. 2006). Although the application seemed to provide real-time data, the developer spent significant time ensuring that the most current data was updating the interface to avoid critical section issues that happen when multiple pieces of data (e.g., the sent text messages) want to access a shared resource (e.g., the individual step counts of each teen on the mobile phone). In addition, the users had to be warned not to edit any of the text messages received from a specific phone number otherwise the phone app would not be able to interpret the data properly.

An example that is closely related to a two-way text messaging solution is @BabySteps, a low-overhead system that uses twitter for parents to manage their child's development. For example, BabySteps would tweet to a user, "Can your baby do a push-up when he's on his tummy? #baby2325." The user would respond with "#yes #Adam can do a push-up when he's on his tummy! #baby2325." In this example, the hashtag #baby2325 helps to identify which milestone is being tracked. The user's response could add other free text or additional hashtags in addition to the necessary response of #yes, #sometimes, #no. In a feasibility study, the researchers found that parents could learn to use the hashtags, however they plan to iterate on how many messages parents should receive to keep them engage without overburdening them. The study shows that although the use of hashtags in text or twitter messages provides an easy mechanism for researchers to parse data and provide customized feedback, researchers have to carefully consider how often the intervention should require input from users and how users want to provide that input (e.g., using a service they already use in their everyday lives like twitter instead of a new off-the-app-store app) (Suh et al. 2014).

13.2.3 Feature Phones

Feature phones are mobile phones that contain features in addition to voice calling and text messaging included in basic mobile phones. Many of these phones included features such as cameras, mobile broadband access, WiFi, PDA functionality (e.g., address book, calendar, and email), and music and video playback. While there is no standardized way to distinguish feature phones from smartphones, a major distinguishing factor has been the ability of the phone to run third party applications. Feature phones typically do not have the ability to run third party applications or applications not officially certified by the mobile carrier. Many of the feature phones use a more traditional touchtone telephone-style keypad, though in recent times, this has begun shifting to include touchscreen displays as well.

The major benefits that feature phones provide over smartphones are that they are less expensive, have a longer battery life, and are usually more durable. Another benefit is that since they tend to utilize a keypad that is close to that of traditional touchtone phones and basic phones that most individuals are used to, people less familiar with technology may be able to easily use the basic functions on feature phones, while adding a few additional features.

However, this same advantage also creates some challenges for using the more advanced features in feature phones. For example, it can be extremely challenging to type URLs and browse the web using the basic keypad available on the majority of feature phones. In addition, building on the two-way text messaging example we discussed earlier, feature phones are difficult to text on because users have to touch the same button multiple times to get a specific character. For example, if someone tried to text "no" using the phone shown in Fig. 13.2, they would have to push the number 6 twice to get the letter "n" and then wait for the screen cursor to move over before pushing the number 6 three times to get the letter "o".

Because feature phones tend to cost less and have longer battery life than smartphones, feature phones are still relatively popular in developing countries, such as China, India, and Africa, where cost and availability of power is a major consideration in comparison to more developed countries.

Attempts to use feature phones for clinical interpretation of ECGs has been tried. An emergency physician photographed ECGs using a mobile phone and sent to an interpreting cardiologist (Bilgi et al. 2012). The images were photographed using a

Fig. 13.2 Chick clique
interface

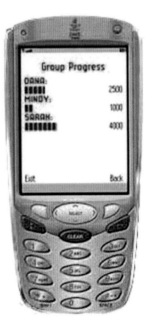

Nokia N93 mobile phone and sent via multimedia messaging system (MMS) to an identical phone used by an interpreting cardiologist. A separate cardiologist and an emergency physician interpreted the paper print out versions of the ECGs. While the cardiologist reading the paper printouts were deemed to have made the significantly fewer mistakes in interpretation than the cardiologist who read via the mobile phone and the emergency physician, the results of the cardiologist interpreting the ECG on the mobile phone screen were slightly better than those of the emergency physician who interpreted the ECG paper printouts. This suggests that sending the ECG images via MMS may be a cost effective telecardiology procedure, particularly when a cardiologist is not available in the emergency department.

13.2.4 Smartphones

A smartphone is a mobile phone with advanced computing capabilities and Internet connectivity. Modern smartphones enable web-browsing, installation of 3rd-party applications (apps), and since the introduction of the iPhone in 2007, frequently include a relatively large (approx. 3.5″–5″ or 90–130 mm when measured diagonally) color touchscreen display. With their ever-increasing computational capabilities, memory capacity, and ability to install applications, they are increasingly being viewed more and more like a handheld computer rather than just a mobile phone. The relatively compact form factor of smartphones makes them easily portable and are frequently carried almost everywhere the user goes. In addition smartphones typically come with the latest networking technology – from short-range wireless connections, such as Bluetooth, to wireless Internet. It is for these reasons that there has been a significant push to try to leverage them to enhance participatory healthcare (Boulos et al. 2011).

While smartphones are incredibly powerful portable devices, there are some major challenges due to the small form factor. Although the screens on smartphones tend to be larger than those on basic and feature phones, there is limited screen real estate compared to that of a desktop computer. This can create significant challenges for user interface designers, who then have to enable navigation through nested menus to fit all of the functionality onto a screen. Also, buttons in these user interfaces cannot be too small or they can be difficult to use for those with limited vision or dexterity as may occur with older adults or with other patients with health concerns. While enabling users to zoom into the user interface can compensate for some of these issues, the gestures required to zoom in can be challenging for users who are inexperienced with smartphones. In addition, some companies have strict design guidelines that limit designers' abilities to customize interface widgets and interactions.

Research regarding the performance of older adults when using touchscreen interfaces can provide some general guidance on the recommended button sizes for most effectively enabling older adults to use touchscreen enabled smartphones

(Motti et al. 2013). In a number of studies, researchers observed and measured the actions of study subjects on a variety of touch screen devices and user interfaces. In these studies, task completion times with various size buttons and gestures such as taps, drags, and pinching motions were studied.

Kobayashi et al. (2011) suggested that buttons should be at least 8 mm in size on smaller screens and targets that are located close to each other need to be larger. However, research has also shown that bigger is not always better. Jin et al. (2007) suggested that targets with 16.5 mm width and spacing between targets of 3.17 and 6.35 mm are appropriate for older users with good dexterity. For users with poor dexterity, larger target sizes of 19 mm in width and 6.35–12.7 mm spaces between targets are preferred. However, while increasing the button sizes and the space between buttons can increase performance, they can lead to higher response times, perhaps due to Fitts's Law. (Fitts's Law is a model of human movement that predicts the time required to rapidly move from one target area to another. This amount of time is proportional to the distance to the target and the size of the target.) Nischelwitzer et al. (2007) found that older adults preferred to tap on buttons rather than to use sliders or cursors buttons to select values. Accommodating these size requirements in an app can be difficult on the screen sizes typically found in smartphones.

Many early uses of smartphones in health care were focused on bringing clinicians mobile access to patient and reference information. One such example was the development of a web-based portal to a clinical information system called PalmCIS (Chen et al. 2004). PalmCIS was designed to be a wireless handheld extension to NewYork-Presbyterian Hospital's web-based clinical information system, WebCIS. PalmCIS was designed to be HIPAA compliant and to display as much clinical information as possible while still being easy to navigate and read. At the time, Palm OS devices were very popular and one of the earliest smartphones, the Kyocera QCP 6035 was chosen as hardware platform. One of the limitations of PalmCIS was due to the limited capabilities of mobile web browsers in the early 2000s. The web browser, EudoraWeb was limited to a subset of HTML and did not support images. Clinicians were able to view patient reports that summarized laboratory, cardiology, and radiology results for the current and previous days. Another interesting feature was that it also enabled clinician to query PubMed directly from the PalmCIS interface, allowing clinicians to quickly access relevant article abstracts and citations. A somewhat unique feature of the PalmCIS interface was how they chose to balance ensuring a high level of security while enabling ease of use (see Fig. 13.3). PalmCIS required two-factor authentication through the use of a user name, password, and SecurID token. The SecurID token was implemented using a series of checkboxes to help the user input the correct token. This authentication was only required once a week, enabling the provider to use PalmCIS throughout the week and not constantly interrupting the workflow of the clinician and making him or her log in at every use. This balance of ready access for the clinician while ensuring an appropriate level of security is an important factor to consider when designing clinical applications on mobile devices, as barriers to efficient clinical workflows will severely hamper adoption rates.

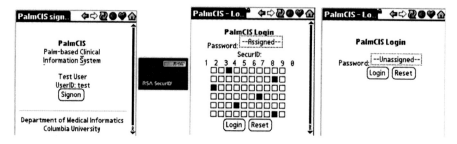

Fig. 13.3 Screenshots of PalmCIS Login Screens. Adapted by permission from BMJ Publishing Group Limited. PalmCIS: a wireless handheld application for satisfying clinician information needs, Chen, E. S., Mendonça, E. A., McKnight, L. K., Stetson, P. D., Lei, J., & Cimino, J. J. (2004). *Journal of the American Medical Informatics Association, 11*(1), 19–28

Another area of significant interest has been the use of smartphones for Personal Health Records (PHRs). There have been two main approaches to PHRs on smartphones—integrated and standalone. Within the category of integrated PHRs, they fall into two subcategories–those that integrate with EHRs and those that integrate with online PHR systems that contain data maintained by the patient. Integrated PHRs have been met with great interest and enable patients to access a subset of information that is stored in their health record that is maintained in their health care provider's EHR. They also frequently enable the patient to securely communicate with their provider. One such app is that of the MyChart for the iPhone from Epic Systems Corporation (see Fig. 13.4). There are a few PHR apps for smartphones that access information that are maintained by the patient themselves, but they have largely been unsuccessful due to the lack of adoption of these platforms, even on desktop computers (Kharrazi et al. 2012).

Despite the fact that smartphones have amazing capabilities, effort needs to be spent on making sure that interventions are designed appropriately and that the new capabilities of smartphones adds any substantive improvement in health care interventions over what is available in phones of lesser capabilities. Buller et al. (2014) performed a randomized trial of comparing the effectiveness of a smartphone mobile application to text messaging to support smoking cessation (Buller et al. 2014). Their smartphone application, REQ-Mobile had the ability to receive and send short messages, enabled smokers to create lists on the reasons for and benefits of quitting, had interactive tools, had support documents for strategies and benefits of quitting, and had audio testimonials from former smokers. They compared REQ-Mobile with the onQ text messaging system, which sent tailored automated messages to the text inbox of the participants. Their comparison of these two approaches showed that users of REQ-Mobile took longer to quit and fewer study subjects were abstinent at 6 weeks than those who were enrolled in the onQ text messaging approach. They also found that the audio testimonials were rarely used. One of the resulting hypotheses for why onQ may have been more effective than REQ-Mobile was that it delivered messages to the normal text messaging inbox rather than an inbox in the REQ-Mobile app. These results suggest that using

Fig. 13.4 Screenshot of Epic's MyChart on iOS. © 2014 Epic Systems Corporation. Used with permission

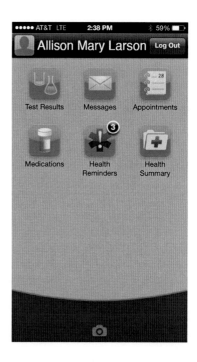

lesser technologies that are available in basic and feature phones, such as such text messaging, can be as effective if not more effective interventions than those that require smartphones, while enabling a wider audience to participate and lowering costs of the intervention.

Another major challenge can be deciding which platform or platforms to support. This used to be a much larger issue but as of early 2014, the leading two platforms are Google's Android and Apple's iOS, with a total of over 90 % of the worldwide market share. Researchers are also adopting platform independent solutions, such as PhoneGap (http://phonegap.com), that allow developers to create the app using web technologies and deploy the apps on multiple platforms. Most of the app functionality can be used offline, however researchers can benefit by being able to collect real time data when the smartphone can access the Internet.

13.2.5   Tablets

Modern tablet computers are typically similar to smartphones and are based on the same mobile operating systems as smartphones, but are larger with displays measured at 7″ (18 cm) or larger, diagonally. Another differentiation from smartphones is that while tablets may also have cellular connectivity, they usually do not have cellular calling as a feature and it can only be used as a data connection. The most typical form factors for tablets fall into two rough size categories: 7″ and 10″

(25 cm) displays. The 7″ size is obviously more portable and less costly, but the 10″ size offers more screen real estate, which can be highly desirable, particularly for individuals with lower levels of dexterity and vision. The larger form factor enables different user interface paradigms than are typically used on smartphones.

As discussed in the smartphone section, touch targets measuring between 16.5 and 19 mm in width and spacing between targets of 3.17 and 12.7 mm spaces between targets have been shown to be most appropriate in older adult populations. On screen buttons of these sizes in users interfaces are more easily accommodated on 7″ and 10″ tablets than on devices of smaller form factors. While the larger 10″ tablets can be very attractive from a user interface design and screen real estate perspective, a major downside is that because of their larger display size, they are less portable and are more costly. This has major implications for their use in healthcare interventions.

One application of tablets in the inpatient clinical environment is Epic Systems Corporation's MyChart Bedside (see Fig. 13.5). MyChart Bedside enables an admitted patient the ability to gain access to more information about his or her stay in the hospital, including knowing about the schedule of events for the day, who is on the care team, a dashboard of vital signs and lab results, and sending and receiving messages to/from the care team. As of this writing, MyChart Bedside is supported only on 10″ tablets because the interface requires a larger screen size. Because of the reduced hardware costs, support for 7″ tablets is planned for future releases. Some key issues to consider when deploying tablets to patients in the inpatient domain are who will deploy the devices to the patients, how to keep them

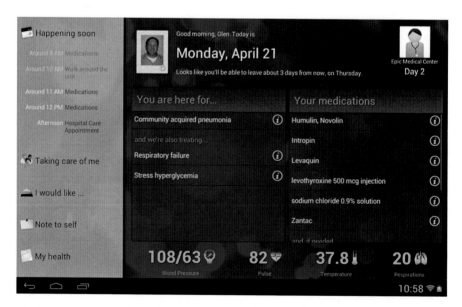

Fig. 13.5 Screenshot of Epic's MyChart Bedside. © 2014 Epic Systems Corporation. Used with permission

charged, how to secure the devices, who will reset the devices between patients, and who will disinfect the devices before redeployment to the next patient.

Another application of inpatient clinical use of tablets is for clinicians to access the medical record. There have been two primary approaches to this: native apps and thin client access. With native tablet apps, EHR vendors build apps that provide a subset of functionality that is available in the desktop applications. These apps frequently enable reviewing of patient's medications, lab results, and other data. In addition, some apps enable e-prescribing and charting functionality. The native apps however do not have the full functionality of the regular desktop application that providers are used to.

The other approach that has been used to enable clinicians to access the medical record is through thin client access software (such as Citrix). These thin client apps enable client devices such as tablets to access a remote virtual desktop hosted on a server. This allows tablets to access the full desktop application even though the application cannot run natively on the device. The main drawback of this approach is that the full desktop EHR applications are generally not designed for a touch screen interface or the screen resolution of the tablet, thus actions – such as right clicking – are difficult and can require a lot of scrolling to see the full interface. Display sizes less than 10″ will require extensive scrolling and zooming. Another significant challenge that is common with all thin client remote desktop systems is that one needs a relatively high bandwidth network with low latency for the user experience to be satisfactory. With poor quality networks, the screen refreshes can have a significant lag. When deciding between the two directions in tablet-based mobile EHR access, one needs to strongly consider whether full access to the EHR is necessary and whether or not the network environment can support thin-clients.

Botella et al. (2013) designed a virtual pillbox to help elderly patients with medication adherence. In their design process, they conducted a focus group with health professionals. In addition, they selected a patient and a caregiver to help with the design process. They started with the goal of developing for a mobile phone with a screen size of 3″ or more. After designing some initial prototypes, they decided to implement the virtual pillbox application for tablets of at least 7″. In their patient satisfaction studies with the tablet, 91.7 % found the tablet easy to use, and 87.5 % found the 7″ screen to be of adequate size (Botella et al. 2013).

Tablets and other mobile devices have been heavily used in time-motion studies studying clinical workflow (Lopetegui et al. 2014). Their portable form factor enables researchers to be mobile and more effectively collect data. One such time-motion tool is TimeCaT (Lopetegui et al. 2012). There were a series of crucial design decisions were made during the development of TimeCaT. One of the major architectural decisions was to make TimeCaT a web-based tool, rather than a native tablet or smartphone app. On one hand, making TimeCaT to be a web-based app instead of a native app, requires it to have a network connection to function. On the other hand, this choice enabled TimeCaT to be able to be used on a variety of mobile devices and platforms, including laptop computers, smartphones, and tablets. The decision to make TimeCaT a web-based tool resulted in a series of other design decisions that needed to be made. Traditional web-based applications have been designed around the idea of that a full page refreshes when data is submitted to a form. However, with the advent of Web 2.0-type technologies such as Ajax, full page reloads are no longer necessary, enabling web apps to have responsive behaviors similar to native applications. TimeCaT took advantage of these technologies, which improved the usability of the software and enabled users to collect data on short workflow activities that take less time than the time that it could take for a full page refresh in a web browser.

It was also determined that rather than to allow the client devices to manage the timestamps of the observed tasks, the time on the web server should be used. The main drawback of this design decision is that the latency of the network connection to the web server and the number of users increasing the load on the web server could perturb the accuracy of the timestamp. This decision enabled multiple users to simultaneously observe different aspects of the same environment and to more easily conduct inter-observer reliability studies.

Despite the ability to be used on a variety of devices, it was decided that the primary target platform for the web app was the tablet form factor. Since time motion studies tend to have observation times ranging on the order of an hour to a full workday, battery life and observer comfort is a major factor. The tablet form factor is nearly ideal for time-motion studies because the battery lives on tablets are approximately a full workday. In addition to the issue of battery life, tablets and smartphones have the advantage that they can be easily used while walking, unlike laptop computers. During the implementation of TimeCaT, it was discovered that the observers tended to use tablet-sized devices in landscape orientation. In addition, during longer observation sessions, the observers tended to cradle the tablet from behind with one hand and arm similar to how one would cradle a baby, minimizing the strain of carrying and using the device over long periods of time, while maximizing use of the other hand for capturing data. Researchers are strongly encouraged to look at how people not only interact with the software, but how they interact with the hardware to ensure the overall system can sufficiently meet the needs of the users.

13.2.6   Wearable Systems

There are many wearable systems that are designed, built, and evaluated in the health and wellness domains to assist users assess specific metrics. Wearable devices are broadly defined to include any computational device that an individual wears – from a pedometer that one clips onto their pants to a computationally enhanced contact lens. Popular off-the-shelf wearable systems provide users with instant feedback on various metrics – the most popular metrics are step counts and sleep – and usually with the ability to connect their data to their social networks. On the horizon are industry research into more integrated systems that enhance everyday objects such as watches, glasses, and contact lenses. Finally, we will review research activities that will further enhance our clothing and empower users to create their own wearable systems.

Wearable systems are interesting to evaluate because unlike traditional mobile systems where input and output is for the primary person interacting with the system, wearable systems may provide outputs that are observable not only by the primary wearer, but also anyone around the person. For example, if someone is wearing a running shirt that notes a runner's pace and heart rate, the runner and people around them can see this information (Mauriello et al. 2014). Thus, designers and evaluators must consider how they will evaluate observers in their study designs. In short – when does an observer become a study participant? If a user's pedometer posts weekly stats to a social networking site – is the friend who comments on the stat another study participant? Where is the line drawn? Researchers have discussed these issues related to ambient environment user studies (Hazlewood et al. 2011), but we have not investigated them fully in mobile, wearable systems for health.

13.2.6.1 Off-the-Shelf Usability

Currently, there seems to be a new off-the-shelf wellness monitoring system each week – from the long standing Fitbit (fitbit.com), Jawbone UP (jawbone.com/up), BodyMedia Fit (bodymedia.com), and Nike + Fuelband (nike.com/fuelband) to newer systems such as Misfit Shine (misfitwearables.com), Basis (mybasis.com) and Lumo (http://www.lumobodytech.com). The systems typically sense physical activity at a bare minimum and most also track sleep. Some push the market further to sense perspiration, skin temperature, heart rate, and posture. Most systems provide users feedback on the wearable system through an LED display, OLED display, or – in a small subset – vibrations. All of the systems provide aggregate data via a mobile application or website. Wearable systems are typically on the wrist, hip, neck, or upper arm – each of these decisions bring with them their own set of wear-ability issues. How professional does it look to have a glowing/blinking bracelet? What if a user's uniform cannot accommodate a clipped on wearable system – either because of appearance rules or the garment is not strong enough to hold the sensor properly?

When researchers choose to use an off-the-shelf wearable sensing system, they must consider the accuracy of the system, if users can use the system, and how the system may interfere with users' lives. For example, Chen et al. (2013) compared sleep tracking systems – two smartphone systems (an app that requires people to sleep with the phone to detect movements and an app that detects phone usage and ambient light to estimate sleep patterns) and two wearable systems (Jawbone and Zeo) – to better understand what users wanted from a sleep tracking system. They found that the wearable systems burdened users because the user had to set a sleep mode input or wear an additional sensor to help monitor sleep, whereas the smartphone applications required minimal user input. The authors acknowledge, however that the wearable sensors detected more information about the users' sleep. Overall, off-the-shelf wearable systems provide the health informatics community with a variable cost solution to get baseline data on users' specific health metrics. The study design does not necessarily need any development time, thus non-technical researchers could plan and facilitate the study design easily.

13.2.6.2 Enhanced Everyday Objects

Industry research labs and startups are introducing enhanced everyday objects that people readily wear to empower them to manage their health. Watches are the most pervasive example – from the community sourced (via kickstarter.com) Pebble (https://getpebble.com) to the watches proposed by Google, Motorola, and LG – the watch form factor ensures that updates are only a quick glance away. Currently, Pebble can track physical activity and cycling through apps on the users' smartphones. Users must currently have a smartphone or tablet device to send updates to the watches – thus the entire system cost must be considered in the study design.

Another enhanced everyday object is Google Glass (http://www.google.com/glass/start/), a pair of glasses that has an attached heads-up display to record what the user is seeing and provide feedback. Google Glass is currently being used in a small trial at Indiana University Health (IU Health) in some clinical environments to investigate how health professionals interact with patients to improve the quality of care and identify patients' emotional needs. Surgeons at The Ohio State University Wexner Medical Center are using Google Glass to consult with colleagues and teach students in real-time during surgery as shown in Fig. 13.6. The Australian Breastfeeding Association and Small World Social are currently conducting a small trial study where five mothers use Google Glass to help them with issues they encounter while learning to breastfeed their children – as shown in Fig. 13.7. Specifically, Google Glass provides the moms with the ability to get hands-free, step-by-step visual instructions and secure video conferencing with breastfeeding counselors to receive real-time, personalized feedback from professionals about issues they are encountering. Similar to the smart watches, Google Glass currently requires a smartphone to provide the user with full functionality, thus the cost and data plan for the entire system must be taken into account.

Google developed a contact lens that can measure one's glucose levels by sampling the user's tears via a wireless chip and glucose monitor sandwiched between two contact lenses (http://googleblog.blogspot.com/2014/01/introducing-our-smart-contact-lens.html). The researchers are investigating the accuracy of glucose readings in tears and how to communicate these levels to the user via LEDs. The current contact lens is in the early stages of clinical trials, however the technology is promising for future non-invasive ways to measure glucose levels.

Microsoft Research enhanced a bra to empower users to reflect on their own eating habits in relation to their mood. The bra form factor was selected because it provided an easy way to collect heart rate and respiration with an electrocardiogram (ECG) sensor; skin conductance with an electrodermal activity (EDA) sensor; and

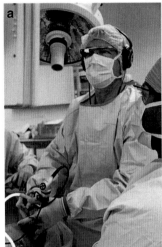
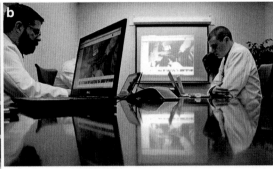

Fig. 13.6 (**a**) A surgeon at the Ohio State University Wexner Medical Center wearing Google Glass during surgery; (**b**) Ohio State University surgeons and students watch the surgery in real-time remotely

Fig. 13.7 A mother breastfeeds with the help of Google Glass, as part of the Breastfeeding Support Project trial run by Australian technology company, Small World Social

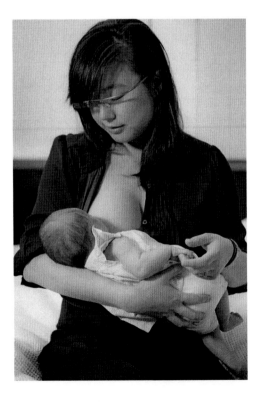

movement with an on-board 3-axis accelerometer without requiring participants to wear an extra piece of clothing. Researchers recruited a small, convenient sample for a feasibility study to investigate how accurately the system could infer that a user may be eating because of emotions. The researchers acknowledged that there were issues with battery length (the system had to be recharged every 3–4 h), comfort, and the need for the system to be worn by both genders (Carroll et al. 2013). Microsoft Research also has investigated providing feedback to users about their stress levels through Mood Wings, a wearable butterfly that moves its wings in relation to stressful feelings (MacLean et al. 2013). In a small study where users wore MoodWings while driving in a simulated environment, users were more aware of their stress and reported feeling more stressed, however they still thought the system was promising and researchers found that users needed more information on how to mitigate the noted stress.

Industry research continues to integrate intelligence into everyday artifacts to improve our physical, social, and emotional health. Most of the technology discussed here requires a smartphone, tablet, or computer to push information to the enhanced artifact. Thus, researchers must be careful to consider the cost (material, developmental, and maintenance) and user burden (e.g., putting on sensors, charging them, debugging the overall system) before deciding on a wearable system. Finally, the current technologies are in a nascent stage, thus they have smaller pilot user studies to assess how people would use the technology (Klasnja et al. 2011). Researchers who would like to use wearable technologies in large deployments should carefully consider if a wearable system is robust enough for general consumption.

13.2.6.3 Future Wearable Systems

Researchers in academia and industry continue to push the bounds about what we consider enhanced everyday artifacts. For example, researchers at the University of Minnesota are working on smart fabrics that will one day detect a user's gait, posture (Dunne et al. 2011), and joint angles (Gioberto et al. 2013). Indeed, the researchers used their techniques to sew conductive thread into stockings that provide a user with vibrotactile feedback if they are bending their knee incorrectly.

Researchers at the University of Colorado and Indiana University are creating a framework for designing wearable health systems that will empower laypeople to design and personalize interchangeable components to manage a specific health metric. For example, they investigated how a small, convenient sample could create their own system that tracks their outdoor exposure and visualizes their weekly progress on an ambient tree painting. Overall, participants were interested in crafting their own health sensing technologies, however the researchers acknowledge that more research has to be done to better understand what specifically people want to track and how to provide real-time feedback to them (Ananthanarayan et al. 2014).

Currently, wearable technologies require the user to wear another device (e.g., a fitbit) or an enhanced device that may be bulkier to accommodate the electronics and communication technology necessary to interface with various smart devices. In the future, researchers are working towards less bulky, more comfortable technologies that users can easily customize for their own sensing and feedback preferences. We decided to cover wearable technologies, a burgeoning booming field, in this mobile HCI section because mobile, which is traditionally thought of in terms of mobile computers and phones, is quickly morphing into smaller, wearable systems.

13.2.7 Mobile Digital Pens

Another enhanced mobile artifact, although not a wearable system per se, are mobile digital pens. These mobile digital pens try to bridge the paper and digital workflows. They act as an input device that captures the location and marks on paper and translates them as input into a digital system. Many of these pens use special paper with locator marks embedded into the surface that helps the pen better track the location and markings on the paper.

Sarcevic et al. (2012) developed a prototype system called TraumaPen that utilized an Anoto DP-201 digital pen that captured the user's writing and checkmarks and transmitted the information via Bluetooth to a nearby computer. TraumaPen was designed to be a system to help support situation awareness during trauma resuscitation. Information that was recorded through the pen was processed, interfaced with a flowsheet, and translated onto a wall display. Handwriting was processed by handwriting recognition software and mapped into relevant entries in their data model. One of the challenges with this approach was that the person recording the information, frequently needed to look up from the paper to the digital wall display to check the correctness of the data being captured, particularly with respect to handwritten notes. This would distract the recording nurses from their primary task of maintaining the documentation. TraumaPen's research results showed that handwriting recognition was not always accurate and moved to just simply displaying an image of the handwriting, but that resulted in some difficulties in reading the recording nurse's handwriting. The digital pen worked best for displaying information that was captured through checkboxes.

Similar to tablets, digital pens are helpful to researchers for *in situ* data capture during shadowing studies. Digital pens, such as Livescribe (www.livescribe.com), can record what is being said around a user. Thus, a researcher could make a quick mark in her notebook about something that a participant said or an interesting observation and later reflect on recording by either "playing back" the audio by touching the pen to the mark in her notebook or downloading the data from the digital pen and accessing it through the web interface.

13.2.8 A Summary of Mobile Technology

When selecting a mobile technology, researchers should consider mobility, input, output, uses, connectivity, and cost. We summarize these key points, as shown in Fig. 13.8, in relation to the technologies covered in this chapter. By mobility, we mean how often the technology will be available for participants to use – either all of the time or when an event occurs. Tablets are the only mobile devices that we would argue are mostly event driven because of their larger size – thus participants would be less likely to carry them around all of the time. Digital pens are sometimes used all of the time, thus the dotted line around the 24/7 icon, however they have mostly been used in event driven studies (e.g., in an emergency room during a trauma incident). Although we note that most mobile technology is available 24/7 to participants, most users want breaks from continuously being monitored or burdened with inputting something into a device. Thus, researchers should consider how much a sociotechnical intervention will burden the user and what implications could occur from having continuous monitoring. For example, are there repercussions for a user not being compliant? In addition, if continuous monitoring/input is part of the study, the researchers must seriously consider the robustness of the technology. Mobile devices with glass screens easily crack when dropped – thus a case may be needed (and a budget for fixing the device). Wearable technology must be comfortable and not get in the way of users' everyday activities. In addition, battery power is always a significant challenge when doing continuous monitoring because monitoring requires computation and computation requires power – thus, researchers must conduct small, beta tests to ensure the device can handle the continuous monitoring without burdening users to change batteries or recharge in the middle of the day.

Input mechanisms include buttons, touchscreen interaction voice, photos or videos, handwriting recognition via a stylus, touchscreen, or pen, and sensor input. All of the technologies discussed here with the exception of the digital pen can accept some sort of button input – whether it is a physical device button, touch screen button, or touch sensitive button on a wearable item. Only standalone devices, smartphones, and tablets have specific touch screen inputs. For voice input, we specifically meant that the voice can be recorded and acted on, thus only smartphones, tablets, and digital pens can use voice input in this way. Most higher end phone and tablets can take photos and videos for input. Handwriting recognition requires either a touch sensitive screen or camera embedded in the writing instrument, as is the case with digital pens. Only smartphones, tablets, and wearable systems have sensors for input.

Since we are working with mobile devices, the major output concern is how much screen space there is a small, medium, or large screen. Mobile devices can also provide vibrotactile or audio, lights/LEDs, and multimedia outputs. Most mobile devices can accommodate designs for small displays where information must be abstracted or divided into small, readable chunks. Some newer mobile devices, such as smartphones and tablets, have medium to large size displays, thus

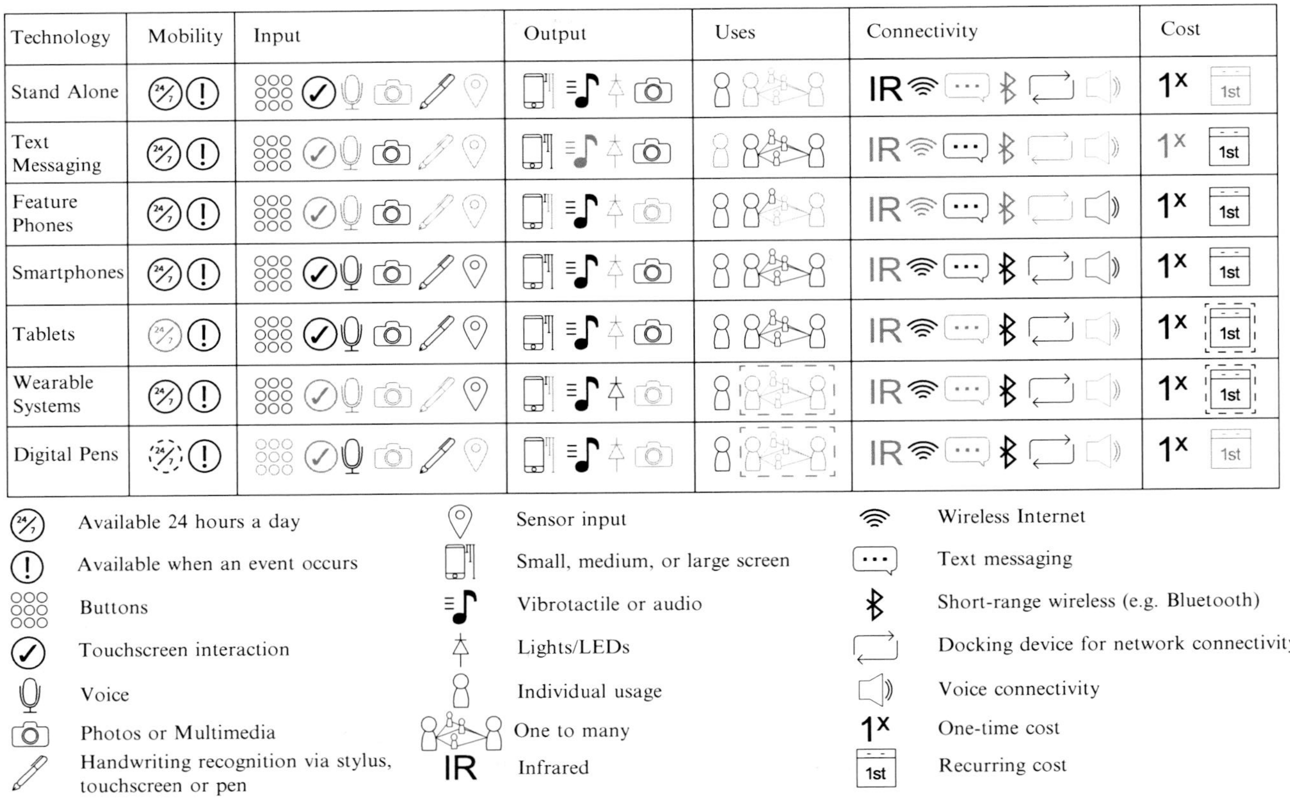

Technology	Mobility	Input	Output	Uses	Connectivity	Cost
Stand Alone					IR	1× / 1st
Text Messaging					IR	1× / 1st
Feature Phones					IR	1× / 1st
Smartphones					IR	1× / 1st
Tablets					IR	1× / 1st
Wearable Systems					IR	1× / 1st
Digital Pens					IR	1× / 1st

Legend:

- Available 24 hours a day
- Available when an event occurs
- Buttons
- Touchscreen interaction
- Voice
- Photos or Multimedia
- Handwriting recognition via stylus, touchscreen or pen
- Sensor input
- Small, medium, or large screen
- Vibrotactile or audio
- Lights/LEDs
- Individual usage
- One to many
- Infrared
- Wireless Internet
- Text messaging
- Short-range wireless (e.g. Bluetooth)
- Docking device for network connectivity
- Voice connectivity
- One-time cost
- Recurring cost

Fig. 13.8 An overview of mobile technology based on functionality. *Grey icons* mean that the functionality is typically not available. *Dashed icons* mean that the functionality is sometimes available

these technologies have more real estate to work with to design an interface with more information. All of the technologies except for text messaging and provide vibrotactile or audio feedback to the user. Stand alone, feature phones with screens, smartphones, and tablets can provide researchers with the ability to present multimedia information. Finally, wearable systems are currently the only systems that regularly use lights/LEDs to communicate information to users.

In terms of uses, we looked at what each technology performed best at – individual usage one-to-one, one-to-many, and many-to-one. The standalone, wearable, and digital pen technologies are best when used individually, however we do note that the latter two could connect one-to-many and many-to-one depending on connectivity (e.g., sharing over the Internet). Feature phones are good at individual or one-to-one communication since the device has limited inputs and connectivity. Finally, text messaging, smartphones, and tablets excel at one-to-many, one-to-one, and many-to-one communication because it is easy to communicate with multiple people using multiple connectivity mechanisms (e.g., text messages, emails, social networking). Researchers should consider the possible privacy issues that users may encounter when sharing information between various people – just because a technology provides users with the ability to easily *share* information does not necessarily mean that it is in the user's best interest to share information – especially information related to one's health.

We briefly note the type of connectivity each device has – infrared, wireless Internet, text messaging, short range wireless (e.g., Bluetooth), docking the technology to another device to connect the technology to a network, and voice, The connectivity is tightly tied to the cost of the technology – either a one-time cost or a reoccurring cost which can take the form of a monthly plan or a pay-as-you-go plan. All of the technologies with the exception of text messaging have a one time cost to purchase the device. Although it can be argued that text messaging requires a phone or computer to text message, we were looking at the costs of the specific technologies. If a researcher would like to automate text messaging, then in addition to the recurring text messaging costs, the researcher would have to pay for a text messaging gateway service – another reoccurring cost. Any technology that supports text messaging or voice connectivity has a reoccurring cost associated with it. We noted that tablets sometimes have a reoccurring cost because some tablets have data plans to receive Internet connectivity. We also identified that wearable systems sometimes have reoccurring costs because some systems are paired with a device, such as a smartphone, to connect to the Internet. Thus, in these wearable systems, researchers should be prepared for two one-time costs – the wearable costs and device cost – in addition to the reoccurring cost. Digital pens do not have a monthly or pay-as-you-go cost, but some may require special paper that has to be purchased or printed. Researchers should carefully consider the privacy and security of information when sharing information digitally – since mobile devices are small and computation drains batteries faster, information is typically not encrypted.

Based on the examples and overview provided in this section, researchers should be able to find a mobile technology that can meet their needs *if* their intervention truly needs to be relatively small, easy to carry, and available most of the time.

13.3 Methodological Considerations for Conducting Field Studies

There are a number of unique challenges with conducting studies with mobile devices. Many of the challenges are because (1) users are mobile and (2) capturing real world usage is challenging. Unlike capturing interactions on desktop computers, screen capture software generally cannot be used to conduct usability studies on phones and tablets. Problems with the screen capture approach include generally the lack of good software for the variety of mobile devices available in the ecosystem and that screen capture software cannot effectively capture the interactions of the user with the screen. When users interact with mobile devices, they frequently interact with touch screens. Without the ability to visually capture the user's finger taps on the screen, it can be difficult to determine whether or not some of the usability challenges are related to failure of the hardware device to pick up the user's taps or related to the design of the user interface.

To solve this issue, researchers have designed "sleds" to capture a user's interaction with the devices. These sleds usually have a camera focused on the mobile device and occasionally have an additional camera focused on the user (see Fig. 13.9). They attach to the mobile device to maintain a consistent view on the device, even when the user picks up the device to use it.

Fig. 13.9 Illustration of a low cost mobile usability sled. These sleds are frequently made from a sheet of acrylic and bent into shape

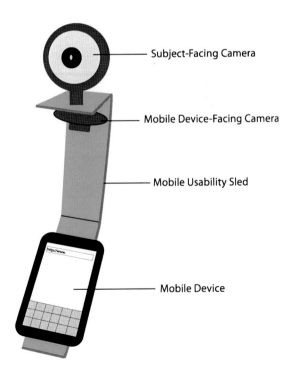

Subject-Facing Camera

Mobile Device-Facing Camera

Mobile Usability Sled

Mobile Device

When designing a user study to evaluate mobile systems in health informatics, researchers should carefully consider the goal of the mobile system and how it may impact the study. For example, if a dietary monitoring application was designed to help users be more compliant with specific dietary restrictions – such as the DIMA example we discussed earlier – then researchers must account for how the research team and users think about compliance. During the DIMA study, the research team found that some participants were not using the application frequently – initially they thought they had failed to design an application that met the *all* of the users' needs. It was not until after the study that the research team learned that a participant, who did not use DIMA often during the study, only used DIMA to find out what diet would keep him compliant and then he ate the same things each day until they got bored with the diet and then used DIMA to find a new diet that would help him stay compliant. He wanted to use DIMA after the study to help him decide what he could eat at upcoming holiday parties. This provided the research team with insights into their expectation of compliance – use the application at every meal – and the users' expectation of compliance – use the application when the user needs help being compliant.

This example also brings up another study design issue especially related to health and mobile systems – the time of year for the study. If a study is to investigate a groups' everyday diet, then the study should be planned around holidays where people may eat more than normal. If an intervention is aimed to increase physical activity, then the time of year and the weather during that year should be considered. If a study is being conducted in a clinical environment, then the unit and time of year should be considered. For example, conducting a study in pediatrics in August when children need physicals before school starts in comparison to the summer time when families are away or busy with summer activities.

We always encourage researchers to report on users' mobile system usage to provide the research community with an idea of how users appropriated the system into their daily lives. Usage statistics can take many forms – when the user opened the application; what screens they used most; how many items were input at one time; where did they navigate to (a normal navigation segment or are they getting "stuck" somewhere?). Returning to the example, the research team knew how often study participants were using DIMA and asked participants about any problems they were encountering with using the application and monitoring their diet. People who were not using DIMA as frequently as anticipated, in most cases, said that everything was fine. They enjoyed using the application – thus, the research team thought that the participants were possibly telling the researchers what they thought the researchers wanted to hear. Looking at the usage statistics during the study can help researchers ask personalized questions to participants to learn about their usage and acceptance of the system.

Another related issue to usage is to report on when participants used the system to help create a rich picture of the participants' interactions with the system. For example, if a participant was instructed to use a mobile system throughout the day, but only used the system once during a certain time period, then the research team has to acknowledge the possibility of recall bias. If participants only used the system when the research team contacted them – either to remind them of an upcoming meeting or right before a meeting – then the researchers have to acknowledge that usage spiked when the research team contacted the participants and the accuracy of the data may have been compromised. For example, Stone et al. coined the term "parking lot compliance" for when participants do their study participation in the parking lot of the building where they will meet the research team (Stone et al. 2003).

Since we use mobile systems to manage some health metric, we need to investigate ways to measure the metric through baseline data, validated instruments, physiological data, and self-report. For example, in the DIMA study, the research team conducted 24-h recalls and had permission to record patients' interdialytic weight gain in their medical files to compare with DIMA values. In the 24-h recall, participants reported what they had consumed in the last 24 h and the research team compared it with what was recorded in DIMA to note how accurate digital self report was to recalled, verbal self report. The research team used the interdialytic weight gain to calculate how much fluid participants' consumed and compare it with what DIMA recorded as participants' fluid consumption. These methods help us understand how accurate the system is and how accurate the self-reporting may be.

If a research team decides to use a fairly new mobile system, we would strongly recommend that they start the study with a small participant pool and a short duration– similar to the some of the studies discussed in this chapter. Although the results may not be generalizable and behavior will not change, researchers will have the opportunity to understand how and why people use the system and what changes are needed to provide easier interactions with the system. After the research team has assured that users want and can use the mobile system, they can decide to increase the study size and duration.

13.4 Conclusions

In this chapter, we provided a brief overview of how mobile technology has evolved over the last 20 years – from basic touch screens with infrared connectivity to wearable devices that can continuously sense information and share it with a larger community. For each technology, we presented examples from research, industry, and government to show best practices in design, implementation, and dissemination. We also closely examined the various functionality available in teach type of technology to assist researchers understand what types of mobile technologies they should consider for their own work. Finally, we concluded with some considerations one should make when designing and conducting studies related to healthcare with mobile technology. With the information in this chapter, researchers can make an informed decision about whether mobile technology is right for their system design, what technology they could use, and key considerations they must make when conducting their study.

Discussion Questions

1. Compare and contrast the similarities and differences in designing a system and study for a text messaging, smartphone, and wearable system intervention.
2. What are our responsibilities as researchers to consider:

   (a) How people want to use a mobile intervention in their everyday lives versus how the research team envisions the participants using the application?
   (b) What happens to the application after the study and funding is completed, but participants still want to use it?

Additional Readings

Klasjna, P., & Pratt, W. (2012). Healthcare in the pocket: Mapping the space of mobile-phone health interventions. *Journal of Biomedical Informatics, 45*(1), 184–198.

Motti, L. G., Vigouroux, N., & Gorce, P. (2013). *Interaction techniques for older adults using touchscreen devices: A literature review.* Paper presented at the 25ème conférence francophone sur l'Interaction Homme-Machine, IHM'13.

Siek, K. A., Hayes, G. R., Newman, M. W., & Tang, J. C. (2014). Field deployments: Knowing from using in context. In J. S. Olson & W. A. Kellogg (Eds.), *Ways of knowing in HCI* (pp. 119–142). New York: Springer.

References

Ananthanarayan, S., Lapinski, N., Siek, K. A., & Eisenberg, M. (2014). *Towards the crafting of personal health technologies.* Paper presented at the proceedings of the ACM conference on designing interactive systems, Vancouver, BC, Canada.

Bilgi, M., Gulalp, B., Erol, T., Gullu, H., Karagun, O., Altay, H., & Muderrisoglu, H. (2012). Interpretation of electrocardiogram images sent through the mobile phone multimedia messaging service. *Telemedicine Journal and e-Health, 18*(2), 126–131. doi:10.1089/tmj.2011.0108.

Bin-Sabbar, M. S., & Al-Rodhaan, M. A. (2013). Diabetes monitoring system using mobile computing technologies. *International Journal of Advanced Computer Science and Applications, 4*(2), 23–31.

Botella, F., Borras, F., & Mira, J. J. (2013). *Safer virtual pillbox: Assuring medication adherence to elderly patients.* Paper presented at the proceedings of the 3rd ACM MobiHoc workshop on Pervasive wireless healthcare, Bangalore, India.

Boulos, M. N., Wheeler, S., Tavares, C., & Jones, R. (2011). How smartphones are changing the face of mobile and participatory healthcare: An overview, with example from eCAALYX. *Biomedical Engineering Online, 10*, 24. doi:10.1186/1475-925x-10-24.

Buller, D. B., Borland, R., Bettinghaus, E. P., Shane, J. H., & Zimmerman, D. E. (2014). Randomized trial of a smartphone mobile application compared to text messaging to support smoking cessation. *Telemedicine Journal and e-Health, 20*(3), 206–214. doi:10.1089/tmj.2013.0169.

Carroll, E. A., Czerwinski, M., Roseway, A., Kapoor, A., Johns, P., Rowan, K., & schraefel, M. C. (2013). *Food and mood: Just-in-time support for emotional eating.* Paper presented at the IEEE affective computing and intelligent interaction, Geneva, Switzerland.

Chaudry, B. M., Connelly, K. H., Siek, K. A., & Welch, J. L. (2012). *Mobile interface design for low-literacy populations.* Paper presented at the proceedings of the 2nd ACM SIGHIT international health informatics symposium, Miami, FL, USA.

Chen, E. S., Mendonca, E. A., McKnight, L. K., Stetson, P. D., Lei, J., & Cimino, J. J. (2004). PalmCIS: A wireless handheld application for satisfying clinician information needs. *Journal of the American Medical Informatics Association, 11*(1), 19–28. doi:10.1197/jamia.M1387.

Chen, Z., Lin, M., Chen, F., Lane, N. D., Cardone, G., Wang, R., ... Campbell, A. T. (2013). *Unobtrusive sleep monitoring using smartphones.* Paper presented at the 2013 7th international conference on pervasive computing technologies for healthcare (PervasiveHealth), Venice, Italy.

Connelly, K., Siek, K. A., Chaudry, B., Jones, J., Astroth, K., & Welch, J. L. (2012). An offline mobile nutrition monitoring intervention for varying-literacy patients receiving hemodialysis: A pilot study examining usage and usability. *Journal of the American Medical Informatics Association, 19*(5), 705–712. doi:10.1136/amiajnl-2011-000732.

Dunne, L. E., Gioberto, G., & Koo, H. (2011). *A method of measuring garment movement for wearable sensing.* Paper presented at the 2011 15th annual international symposium on wearable computers (ISWC), San Francisco, CA.

Gioberto, G., Coughlin, J., Bibeau, K., & Dunne, L. E. (2013). *Detecting bends and fabric folds using stitched sensors.* Paper presented at the proceedings of the 2013 international symposium on wearable computers, Zurich, Switzerland.

Grisedale, S., Graves, M., & Grünsteidl, A. (1997). *Designing a graphical user interface for healthcare workers in rural India.* Paper presented at the proceedings of the ACM SIGCHI conference on human factors in computing systems, Atlanta, Georgia.

Hazlewood, W. R., Stolterman, E., & Connelly, K. (2011). *Issues in evaluating ambient displays in the wild: Two case studies.* Paper presented at the proceedings of the SIGCHI conference on human factors in computing systems, Vancouver, BC, Canada.

Holtzblatt, K., Wendell, J., & Wood, S. (2004). *Rapid contextual design: A how-to guide to key techniques for user-centered design (interactive technologies).* San Francisco: Morgan Kaufmann.

Jin, Z. X., Plocher, T., & Kiff, L. (2007). *Touch screen user interfaces for older adults: Button size and spacing.* Paper presented at the proceedings of the 4th international conference on Universal access in human computer interaction: Coping with diversity, Beijing, China.

Kharrazi, H., Chisholm, R., VanNasdale, D., & Thompson, B. (2012). Mobile personal health records: An evaluation of features and functionality. *International Journal of Medical Informatics, 81*(9), 579–593. doi:10.1016/j.ijmedinf.2012.04.007.

Klasnja, P., Consolvo, S., & Pratt, W. (2011). *How to evaluate technologies for health behavior change in HCI research.* Paper presented at the proceedings of the SIGCHI conference on human factors in computing systems, Vancouver, BC, Canada.

Kobayashi, M., Hiyama, A., Miura, T., Asakawa, C., Hirose, M., & Ifukube, T. (2011). *Elderly user evaluation of mobile touchscreen interactions.* Paper presented at the proceedings of the 13th IFIP TC 13 international conference on Human-computer interaction – Volume Part I, Lisbon, Portugal.

Lopetegui, M., Yen, P. Y., Lai, A. M., Embi, P. J., & Payne, P. R. (2012). Time capture tool (TimeCaT): Development of a comprehensive application to support data capture for time motion studies. *AMIA Annual Symposium Proceedings, 2012*, 596–605.

Lopetegui, M., Yen, P. Y., Lai, A., Jeffries, J., Embi, P., & Payne, P. (2014). Time motion studies in healthcare: What are we talking about? *Journal of Biomedical Informatics.* doi:10.1016/j.jbi.2014.02.017.

MacLean, D., Roseway, A., & Czerwinski, M. (2013). *MoodWings: A wearable biofeedback device for real-time stress intervention.* Paper presented at the 6th international conference on PErvasive technologies related to assistive environments, Rhodes, Greece.

Mauriello, M., Gubbels, M., & Froehlich, J. E. (2014). *Social fabric fitness: The design and evaluation of wearable E-textile displays to support group running.* Paper presented at the proceedings of the SIGCHI conference on human factors in computing systems, Toronto, ON, Canada.

Motti, L. G., Vigouroux, N., & Gorce, P. (2013). *Interaction techniques for older adults using touchscreen devices: A literature review.* Paper presented at the 25ème conférence francophone sur l'Interaction Homme-Machine, IHM'13.

Nischelwitzer, A., Pintoffl, K., Loss, C., & Holzinger, A. (2007). *Design and development of a mobile medical application for the management of chronic diseases: Methods of improved data input for older people.* Paper presented at the proceedings of the 3rd Human-computer interaction and usability engineering of the Austrian computer society conference on HCI and usability for medicine and health care, Graz, Austria.

Sarcevic, A., Weibel, N., Hollan, J. D., & Burd, R. S. (2012, May 21–24). *A paper-digital interface for information capture and display in time-critical medical work.* Paper presented at the pervasive computing technologies for healthcare (PervasiveHealth), 2012 6th international conference on.

Siek, K. A., Connelly, K. H., & Rogers, Y. (2006). *Pride and prejudice: Learning how chronically ill people think about food.* Paper presented at the proceedings of the SIGCHI conference on human factors in computing systems, Montréal, QC, Canada.

Stone, A., Shiffman, S., Schwartz, J., Broderick, J., & Hufford, M. (2003). Patient compliance with paper and electronic diaries. *Controlled Clinical Trials, 24*(2), 182–199.

Suh, H., Porter, J. R., Hiniker, A., & Kientz, J. A. (2014). *@BabySteps: Design and evaluation of a system for using twitter for tracking children's developmental milestones.* Paper presented at the CHI'14 proceedings of the SIGCHI conference on human factors in computing systems, Toronto, Canada.

Toscos, T., Faber, A., An, S., & Gandhi, M. P. (2006). *Chick clique: Persuasive technology to motivate teenage girls to exercise.* Paper presented at the CHI'06 extended abstracts on human factors in computing systems, Montréal, QC, Canada.

Chapter 14
Visual Analytics: Leveraging Cognitive Principles to Accelerate Biomedical Discoveries

Suresh K. Bhavnani

14.1 Introduction

The *Open Science* movement (e.g., data from NIH-funded studies being made publicly available), combined with digital access to patient clinical records, in addition to rapid advances in the development of inexpensive high throughput technologies (e.g., multiplex assays for measuring whole genome data across many patients) has resulted in vast digital resources accessible by both scientists and the lay public (Molloy 2011). However, the sheer magnitude of such resources far exceeds our cognitive abilities to exploit them for the prevention, diagnosis, and treatment of diseases. For example, translational teams consisting of biologists, clinicians, and epidemiologists increasingly need to integrate and comprehend the relationships among large and disparate types of information including molecular, biochemical, and environmental variables, with the goal of comprehending complex phenomena such as heterogeneities and corresponding pathways underlying different diseases.

Portions of this chapter in sections "VISUAL ANALYTICS: THEORETICAL FOUNDATIONS", and "STRENGTHS AND LIMITATIONS OF NETWORK ANALYSIS" appeared in Bhavnani, Drake, and Divekar, 2014. With kind permission from Springer Science + Business Media: Bhavnani et al. (2014b). Portions of this chapter in the section "NETWORK ANALYSIS: MAKING DISCOVERIES IN COMPLEX BIOMEDICAL DATA", appeared in an article in the *Proceedings of the AMIA Summit on Translational Bioinformatics* (2014), Bhavnani, S.K., Dang, B, Caro, M., Bellala, G., Visweswaran, S., Heterogeneity within and across Pediatric Pulmonary Infections: From Bipartite Networks to At-Risk Subphenotypes".

S.K. Bhavnani, Ph.D. (✉)
Institute for Translational Sciences, University of Texas Medical Branch, 301 University Blvd, Galveston, TX 77555, USA
e-mail: skbhavnani@gmail.com

© Springer International Publishing Switzerland 2015
V.L. Patel et al. (eds.), *Cognitive Informatics for Biomedicine*, Health Informatics,
DOI 10.1007/978-3-319-17272-9_14

One approach to integrate and comprehend such vast and disparate information is through methods being developed in the new field of visual analytics. This chapter begins by presenting an overview of the evolving theoretical foundations for visual analytics, and the cognitive and task-based motivations to use methods from this field to help comprehend complex biomedical data. Next, the chapter provides a brief overview of visual analytical applications in the biomedical domain, with a demonstration of how to use one of the most advanced forms of visual analytics called networks, which are particularly useful for analyzing complex molecular and clinical data. These analyses reveal the strengths and limitations of network analysis, which are critical for its practical use to analyze ever increasing and complex biomedical data. The chapter concludes with theoretical, applied, and pedagogical hurdles that need to be addressed through future, research which will enable visual analytics to fully realize its potential in accelerating biomedical discoveries.

14.2 Visual Analytics: Theoretical Foundations

Visual analytics is defined as the science of analytical reasoning, facilitated by interactive visual interfaces (Thomas and Cook 2005). The primary goal of visual analytics is to augment cognitive reasoning by translating symbolic data (e.g., numbers in a spreadsheet) into *visualizations* (e.g., a scatter plot) which can be manipulated through *interaction* (e.g., highlight only some data points in the scatter plot). As discussed below, visualizations, and interaction with those visualizations, are powerful for helping analysts comprehend complex relationships in biomedical data because of the nature of human cognition, and the nature of tasks performed by analysts.

14.2.1 Why Do Visualizations Matter?

Visualizations of data are often powerful because they leverage the massively parallel architecture of the human visual system consisting of the eye and the visual cortex of the brain (Card et al. 1999). This parallel cognitive architecture enables the rapid comprehension of multiple graphical relationships simultaneously, which often leads to insights about relationships in complex data such as similarities, trends, and anomalies (Thomas and Cook 2005). For example, Fig. 14.1a shows a spreadsheet representing the systolic blood pressure of patients before and after taking a drug. The task of determining which of the two conditions have more patients with systolic >140 is time consuming and error prone because the analyst has to compare the number in each cell with 140, remember the result of each comparison, and then make a final count to determine which column has a higher number of patients with systolic >140. Such symbolic processing is serial in nature,

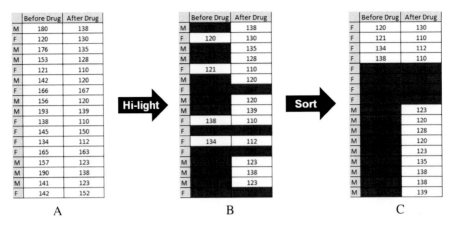

Fig. 14.1 An example of how symbolic data in a spreadsheet (**a**) when converted into a visual representation (**b**) leverages the parallel processing abilities of the visual cortex which enables faster comprehension of patterns in the data. Because visual processing is parallel in nature, it scales to handle large amounts of data. When the same data is sorted by gender (**c**), the visual representation reveals yet another pattern demonstrating how interaction with the data is a critical aspect of visual analytics, and can guide the verification of the patterns using the appropriate quantitative measures

and therefore highly dependent on the number of data points, which when large can quickly overwhelm an analyst.

In contrast, as shown in Fig. 14.1b, if all cells in the spreadsheet with values >140 are colored red, the resulting visual representation enables processing of red cells in each column to be conducted in parallel, resulting in a more rapid determination that the left column has more red cells compared to the right column. Such parallel processing is independent of the number of cells, and therefore scales up well to large amounts of data. Data visualizations therefore help to shift processing from the slower symbolic processing areas of the human brain, to the faster graphical parallel processing of the visual cortex enabling detection of patterns in large and complex biomedical data sets. Furthermore, by externalizing key aspects of the task, the representation in Fig. 14.1b shifts information from an internal to an external representation, making other tasks such as counting the number of patients with systolic >140 in each column much easier (Zhang and Norman 1994).

Unfortunately, not all data visualizations are effective in augmenting cognition. For example, a road map pointing south is not effective for a driver who is facing north because it requires a mental rotation of the map before it can be useful for navigation. Similarly, an organizational chart of employee names and their locations laid out in a hierarchy based on seniority is not very useful if the task is to determine patterns related to the geographical distribution of the employees. Finally, if a chart has an incorrect or missing legend and axes labels, the visualization is difficult to comprehend because it cannot be mapped to concepts in the data. Therefore visualizations need to be aligned with mental representations of the user (Tversky et al. 2002), tasks (Norman 1993), and data, before those visualizations can be effective in augmenting cognition.

14.2.2 Why Does Interactivity Matter?

While static visualizations of data can be powerful if they are aligned with mental representations, tasks, and data, they are often insufficient for comprehending complex data. This is because data analysis typically requires many different tasks performed on the same data such as discovery, inspection, confirmation, and explanation (Bhavnani et al. 2012), each requiring different transformations of the data. For example, if the task in Fig. 14.1b is to understand the relationship of the drug to gender, then the data can be sorted based on gender. As shown, interaction with the data through such sorting reveals that the drug has no effect on females (low values remain low, and high values remain high), whereas it has a dramatic effect on lowering systolic values in males (all high values become low). Therefore, while it is well accepted that interactivity is crucial for the use of most computer systems, interaction with data visualizations can help to reveal relationships that are otherwise hidden when using a single representation of the data.

Interactivity is also critical when analysis is done in teams consisting of different disciplines, where each member often requires a different representation of the same data. For example, a molecular biologist might be interested in which genes are co-expressed across patients, whereas a clinician might be interested in the clinical characteristics of patients with similar gene profiles, and later how they integrate with the molecular information. To address these changes in task and mental representation, visualizations require interactivity or the ability to transform parts, or the entire visual representation.

14.2.3 Theories Related to Visual Analytics

Although the field of visual analytics has drawn on theories and heuristics from different disciplines such as cognitive psychology, computer science, and graphic design, the development of theories and taxonomies for visual analytics are still in early stages of development (Thomas and Cook 2005). For example, there are a number of attempts to classify visual analytical representations (Heer et al. 2010; Shneiderman 1996), and interaction intents at different levels of granularities (Yi et al. 2007; Amar et al. 2005).

One attempt to classify visual analytical representations groups them into (1) time series (e.g., line graphs showing how the expression of different genes change over time), (2) statistical distributions (e.g., box-and-whisker plots), (3) maps (e.g., pie charts showing percentages of different races at different city locations on the US map), (4) hierarchies (e.g., top-down tree showing the management structure of an organization), and networks (e.g., a social network of how friends connect to other friends such as on Facebook). Once these visualizations are generated, they are considered visual analytical if they enable interaction directly or indirectly with part, or all of the information being represented. Examples for such interactivity include transforming a top-down tree into a circular tree, coloring nodes in the tree based on specific properties such as gender, or dragging a node in the tree to swap its location with another sibling node.

Similarly, there have been several attempts to classify interactions with visualizations at different levels of granularity. For example, Amar et al. (2005) proposed 8 low-level interaction intents: retrieve value, filter, compute derived value, find extremum, sort, determine range, characterize distribution, find anomalies, and cluster and correlate. In contrast, Yi et al. (2007) proposed 6 higher level interaction intents typically used: select, explore, reconfigure, encode, abstract/elaborate, filter and connect.

While the above classifications of visual analytical representations and interaction with them are useful as check lists for building effective visual analytical systems, they do not provide an integrated understanding of how they work together to enable analytical reasoning, a primary goal of visual analytics. To address this gap, Liu and Stasko (2010) proposed a framework which integrates visual representation, interaction, and analytical reasoning. The framework specifies that central to reasoning with an external visual analytical representation (e.g., the table in Fig. 14.1b) is a *mental model* which is an analog of the external representation stored in working memory, and which is "runnable" to enable reasoning of the data and relationships. This is achieved by creating a mental model in working memory which is a "collage" of some or all of the structural, semantic, and elemental details present in the visual representation, in addition to other information from long term memory relevant to the task. For example as shown in Fig. 14.1b, an analyst conducting the task of determining which of the two columns have more patients with systolic >140 might construct a mental model in working memory consisting of two columns with cells colored red and white, but excluding elements such as the numbers in the cells. Similar to the speed of accessing information stored in the memory of a computer versus from disk, a mental model stored in the brain's working memory can be used to rapidly achieve tasks such as determining which of the two columns have more red cells, or even determining that the first column has approximately three times more red cells compared to the second column.

The framework further specifies that because working memory has size constraints, a mental model can typically contain only some of the information present in the external visualization at any given time. Therefore, when the task changes, it motivates a tight interactive coupling between the internal mental model and the external visual representation, through which new information is extracted from the existing state of the visualization or from long term memory, irrelevant information in the mental model is discarded to make room for new information, the external visual representation itself is transformed to reveal new relationships, or the conceptual information is externalized onto the visual representation to enable future tasks. For example, when the task described in Fig. 14.1 involves exploring or determining the relationship of systolic blood pressure to gender, then a tight coupling between the internal and external representations is triggered enabling the extraction of gender-related information and its relationship to systolic blood pressure. This can be done either by extracting the information from the current representation (requiring often costly mental manipulations) to identify patterns, or by transforming the external representation through manipulations such as sorting (requiring relatively cheaper physical actions) to reveal new relationships, which are then immediately available for internal reasoning tasks such as determining inequalities between the columns. Furthermore, information about the current or previous task such as a discovered pattern can be externalized onto the visual representation through annotations, and therefore freeing up working memory for subsequent tasks.

The framework proposes that the coupling of internal and external representations can be characterized by three interacting goals: (1) *External anchoring* or the process of connecting conceptual structures (e.g., systolic blood pressure >140) to material elements of the visualization (red colored cells), (2) *Information foraging* or the process of exploring the external visual representation through extraction (e.g., counting the red cells related to female patients) or through transformation (e.g., sorting) of the representation, and (3) *Cognitive offloading* or the process of transferring a conceptual structure onto the visual representation to reduce working memory demands (e.g., encircling or annotating in Fig. 14.1c all female patients who have systolic >140 before and after taking the drug).

While the above integrated framework of visual representation, interaction, and analytical reasoning still needs to be elaborated into a theory and tested through predictive models, it provides a first step into how the critical concepts of visual analytics could be working together to enable analytical reasoning, leading to implications for the design and evaluation of effective visual analytical systems.

Finally, it is important to note that visual analytics has considerable overlap with the fields of scientific visualization (focused on modeling real-world geometric structures such as earthquakes), and information visualization (focused on modeling abstract data structures such as relationships). However, as described above, visual analytics places a large emphasis on approaches that facilitate reasoning and making sense of complex information individually and in groups (Thomas and Cook 2005).

14.3 Visual Analytics: Biomedical Applications

The use of visual analytical representations is increasingly becoming pervasive in the biomedical domain. The selection of visual analytical representations is highly dependent on the users of the information and their goals, which can be classified in the following two broad categories:

14.3.1 Information Consumers

The primary goal of information consumers is to make biomedical information actionable in terms of directly affecting change in health-related behaviors. An important class of information consumers is patients and care providers whose primary goal is to track and modify personal health and life style behaviors through the use of biomedical and social data. For example, the website *PatientsLikeMe* (2014) enables users to input health and lifestyle variables of specific individuals. As shown in Fig. 14.2, this information is displayed using visual analytical representations such as longitudinal charts and graphs which can be modified to display

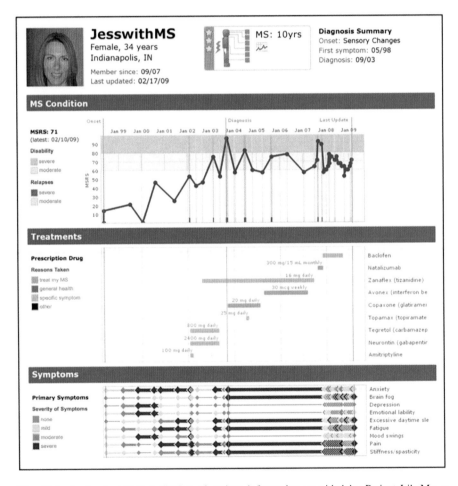

Fig. 14.2 A visual analytical display of patient information provided by PatientsLikeMe, a website that enables patients and caregivers to upload information about individuals, and search for other patients with a similar condition (Reprinted by permission from Macmillan Publishers Ltd: Nature Biotechnology (Brownstein et al. 2009), copyright 2009)

different granularities of data. Users can also find patients who are similar to their profile, and learn about their real-world experiences of dealing with their diseases, with the goal of improving the quality of life for themselves or for those they provide care. Similarly, personal and wearable activity monitors (e.g., fitbit) have been developed to motivate behavior change such as weight loss by monitoring how many steps a user has taken on a particular day, and displaying that information on a smart phone using visualizations such as a progress bar and the recommended target. Such information can be shared with other users in a social network to provide additional motivation through competition.

Another important class of information consumers consists of healthcare providers such as physicians and first-responders whose primary goal is to make healthcare decisions relevant to specific patients and situations by extracting relevant information from databases such as electronic health records. For example, the Twinlist system (Plaisant et al. 2013) was developed to reconcile multiple lists of drugs (e.g., from the hospital records versus what the patient reports taking) associated with a patient by graphically displaying what is similar and different among the different lists. The goal of this prototype was to enable caregivers to rapidly reconcile contradictory information with the goal of reducing errors in treatment.

A third class of information consumers consists of policy makers from federal and state agencies whose primary goal is to make policy decisions based on public health information. For example, the Centers of Disease Control provides interactive maps showing the incidence of different disease outbreaks across the US (CDC 2014), with the goal of enabling faster response.

Given that the primary goal of information consumers is to make specific forms of biomedical information actionable, an active area of research is to determine which visual analytical representations are appropriate for which classes of users and goals, and to design and evaluate systems which are easy to learn, and intuitive to use (Shneiderman et al. 2013). For example, while interactive time series, maps, and hierarchies when designed carefully are considered easy to comprehend and to interact with, other representations such as networks with more than a few dozen nodes are considered more difficult to comprehend and tend to be avoided as representations for information consumers.

14.3.2   Information Analysts

In contrast to information consumers, the primary goal of information analysts in academic and industrial settings is to make contributions to biomedical scientific knowledge. While the goal of all biomedical information users is to ultimately improve health outcomes, the process of reaching that long-term goal is achieved by information analysts through progressive contributions to scientific knowledge. An important class of information analysts consists of biologists and bioinformaticians whose primary goal is to decipher the biological mechanisms involved

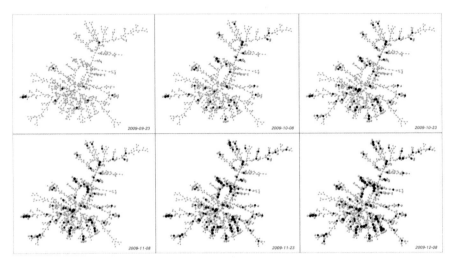

Fig. 14.3 Progression of the flu infection through a social network of students from Harvard University (Christakis and Fowler 2010). The *red nodes* represent infected students, the *yellow nodes* represent friends of infected students, and the edges connecting the nodes represent self-reported friendship links (Reprinted under the Creative Commons Attribution license)

in different diseases. For example, biologists often use network visualization and analysis tools like Cytoscape (2014) to comprehend complex disease-protein associations (Ideker and Sharan 2008) with the goal of deciphering the functions and pathways related to proteins of interest.

A second class of information analysts consists of clinical researchers and medical informaticians whose primary goal is to develop new methods to improve patient treatment by analyzing the relationship between clinical variables and outcomes. For example, networks visualizations have been used to analyze Medicare claims from more than 30 million patients, which enabled researchers to infer patterns in the progression of different diseases (Hidalgo et al. 2009). One of the their observations was that that highly connected nodes in the network had high lethality implying that patients with such diseases are more likely to have an advanced stage of disease.

A third class of information analysis consists of epidemiologists whose primary goal is to analyze public health information. For example as shown in Fig. 14.3, Christakis and Fowler (2010) found that the flu infection in a social network consisting of Harvard students peaked two weeks earlier compared to a random set of students from the same population. Such advanced warning could be effective for planning immunizations during outbreaks of infectious diseases.

An active area of visual analytics research is to develop new approaches that integrate molecular, clinical, and epidemiological information, in a single representation. For example, translational scientists working in teams have used network visualization and analyses to integrate molecular and clinical information with the goal of inferring heterogeneity in asthma, and the respective biological mechanisms (e.g., Bhavnani et al. 2014a, b).

Given the importance of networks for the analysis and presentation of complex relationships in a wide range of data types, and because it is one of the most advanced form of visual analytics, the rest of this chapter focuses on providing a concrete understanding of this approach as applied to the integrative analysis of molecular and clinical information.

14.4 Network Analysis: Making Discoveries in Complex Biomedical Data

Networks (Newman 2010) are an effective representation for analyzing biomedical data because they enable an interactive visualization of complex associations. Furthermore, because they are based on a graph representation, they also enable the quantitative analysis and validation of the patterns that become salient through the visualization. Networks are increasingly being used to analyze a wide range of molecular measurements related to gene regulation (Albert 2004), disease-gene associations (Goh et al. 2007), and disease-protein associations (Ideker and Sharan 2008). A network (also called a graph) consists of a set of nodes, connected in pairs by edges; nodes represent one or more types of entities (e.g., patients or genes). Edges between nodes represent a specific relationship between the entities (e.g., a patient has a particular gene expression[1] value). Figure 14.4 shows a sample bipartite network where edges exist only between different types of entities (Newman 2010), in this case between patients and genes.[2]

Network analysis of biomedical data typically consists of three steps: (1) **exploratory visual analysis** to identify emergent bipartite relationships such as between patients and genes; (2) **quantitative analysis** through the use of methods suggested by the emergent visual patterns; (3) **inference** of the biological mechanisms involved across different emergent phenotypes. This three-step method used across several studies (Bhavnani et al. 2010, 2011b, 2012) have revealed complex but comprehensible visual patterns, each prompting the use of quantitative methods that make the appropriate assumptions about the underlying data, which in turn led to inferences about the biomarkers and underlying mechanisms involved. Each of the three steps of this method is described below, followed by its application to analyze a data set of subjects and gene expressions.

---

[1] Gene expression is the process by which the information in a gene is translated into a gene product such as a protein which can be involved in biological processes like inflammation during an infection.

[2] Researchers have explored a wide range of network types including unipartite, directed, dynamic, and networks laid out in three dimensions to analyze complex data. As this wide range is beyond the scope of this chapter, we suggest other excellent sources (Newman 2010) for such information.

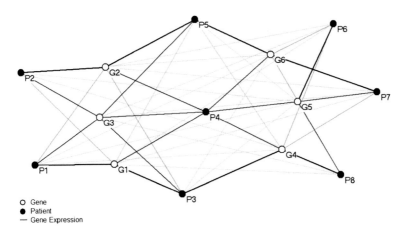

Fig. 14.4 A sample bipartite network where edges exist only between two different types of nodes. In this case, nodes represent either patients (*black*) or genes (*white*), and edges connecting the two represent gene expression

14.4.1   Exploratory Visual Analysis

Network analysis typically begins by transforming symbolic data into graphical elements in a network. To achieve this, the analyst needs to decide which *entities* in the data represent the nodes in the network, in addition to how other useful information can be mapped onto the node's shape, color, and size. Similarly, the analyst needs to decide which *relationships* between the entities in the data are represented by the edges in the network, in addition to how to map other useful information to the edge's thickness, color, and style. These selections are made based on an understanding of the kinds of relationships that need to be explored, and is often an iterative process based on an understanding of the domain and the nature of the data being processed.

Once the symbolic data has been mapped to graphical elements, the resulting network is laid out so the nodes and edges can be visualized. The layout of nodes in a network can be done where either the distances between nodes has no meaning (e.g., nodes laid out randomly or along a geometric shape such as a line or circle), or where the distance between nodes represents a relationship such as similarity (e.g., similar cytokine expression profiles). Layouts where distance has meaning are typically generated through force-directed layout algorithms. For example, the application of the *Kamada-Kawai* (1989) layout algorithm to a network results in nodes with a similar pattern of connecting edge weights to be pulled together, and those with different patterns to be pushed apart.

Figures 14.5, 14.6, 14.7 and 14.8 show the steps that were used to generate a bipartite network of 101 subjects and 18 genes, data which is described in more detail in the original study (Ioannidis et al. 2012). The 101 subjects consisted of 28 influenza (flu), and 51 respiratory syncytial virus (RSV) cases, and 22 age,

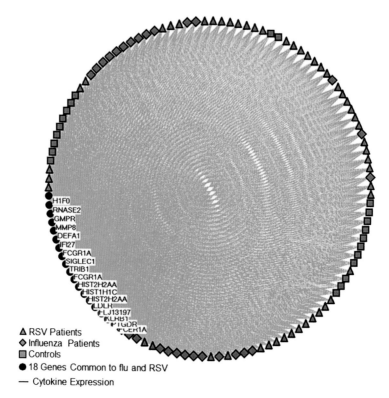

H1F0
RNASE2
GMPR
MMP8
DEFA1
IFI27
FCGR1A
SIGLEC1
TRIB1
FCGR1A
HIST2H2AA
HIST1H1C
HIST2H2AA
LDLR
LJ13197
KLRB1
PTGDR
CCR1A

△ RSV Patients
◇ Influenza Patients
▢ Controls
● 18 Genes Common to flu and RSV
— Cytokine Expression

Fig. 14.5 A bipartite network showing subject nodes (RSV patients = *triangles*, flu patients = *diamonds*, and controls = *squares*) and gene nodes (*black circles*) connected in pairs by edges, which represent normalized gene expression. Patient and gene nodes were separately grouped and randomly laid out equidistantly around a circle

gender, and race matched healthy controls. The 18 genes were highly significant, differentially-expressed genes that were common to both infections. The goal of this analysis was to identify subgroups of cases that had different molecular profiles and therefore could suggest sub-phenotypes that require different treatments. Figure 14.5 shows how the three types of subjects were represented as RSV (gray triangles), flu (gray diamonds), and controls (gray squares), and the genes were represented as circular black nodes. Furthermore, normalized gene expression values were represented as edges connecting each subject to each gene. These nodes were laid out equidistantly around a circle. Figure 14.6 shows the same network but where the edge thicknesses are proportional to the normalized gene expression values. Therefore, thicker edges represent higher gene expression values as compared to the thinner edges. Furthermore, the size of the node was made proportional to the total expression value of the connecting edges. Therefore, larger patient nodes have overall higher aggregate gene expression values compared to smaller patient nodes.

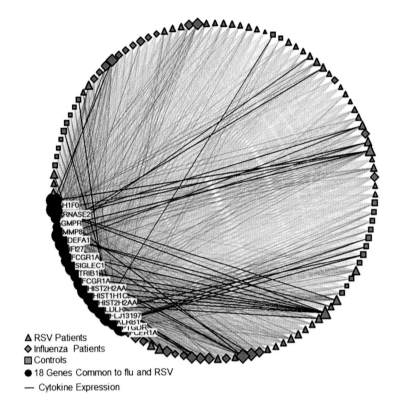

Fig. 14.6 The same network as in Fig. 14.5 but where edge thickness is proportional to the normalized gene expression value and the size of each node is proportional to the total expression values of the connecting edges. Thick edges represent higher gene expression values compared to thin edges. Similarly, larger subject nodes have higher aggregate gene expression values compared to smaller patient nodes

Although the patients, genes, and the gene expression have been visually represented, the distances between the nodes have no meaning. To better comprehend the data, the subjects that have higher expression value for a particular gene should be spatially closer to that gene compared to those that have lower gene expressions. This approach of using short distances between entities to show similarity, and long distances between entities to show dissimilarity is typical across clustering algorithms. As shown in Fig. 14.7 and previously reported (Bhavnani et al. 2014a, b), application of the forced-directed algorithm Kamada-Kawai to the circular layout results in nodes that have a similar pattern of gene expression to be pulled together, and those that are not similar to be pushed apart.

The resulting layout suggests that there exist distinct clusters of subjects and genes. As shown in Fig. 14.7, the subjects had a complex but understandable topology consisting of a majority of the cases (triangles and diamonds) on the top cluster which had a preferential expression of the top 14 genes, and a majority of the

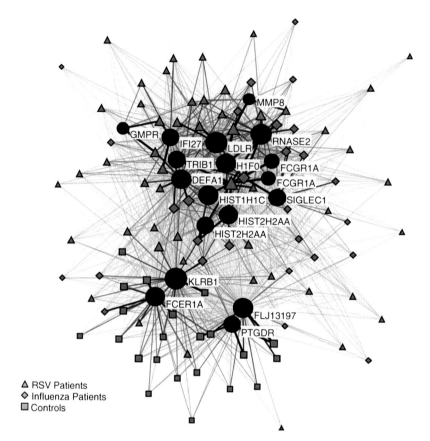

Fig. 14.7 Application of *Kamada-Kawai*, a force-directed algorithm, to the circular layout. The algorithm pulls nodes with similar gene expression patterns closer together while pushing apart those with dissimilar expression patterns. The layout of the network suggested the existence of distinct subject and gene clusters, and revealed inter-cluster relationships such as how the subject clusters express particular gene clusters. However, quantitative methods must be used to identify cluster boundaries

controls (squares) at the bottom of the network which had preferential expression of the bottom 4 genes. In addition, the cases on the top had a core-periphery topology, where there were some cases with high overall gene expression in the center, and many patients with low overall gene expression in the periphery. Finally, there were four cases (triangles and diamonds) that were clustered with the controls at the bottom of the network.

While the network layout suggests the existence of distinct clusters, it is not designed to reveal the members of each cluster. We therefore need to use quantitative methods that are explicitly designed to identify the boundaries of clusters based on a multivariate analysis of the data.

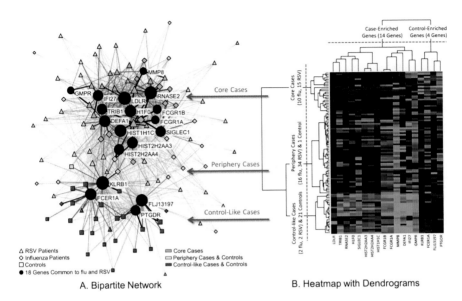

A. Bipartite Network   B. Heatmap with Dendrograms

Fig. 14.8 A heatmap with dendrogram generated through hierarchical clustering helped to identify the boundaries of three subject clusters, which were superimposed onto the network shown in Fig. 14.4 using colored nodes to denote cluster membership. The network also shows the relationship of the subject clusters to the top gene cluster consisting of 11 genes, and bottom gene cluster consisting of 4 genes (Bhavnani et al. 2014a)

14.4.2 Quantitative Verification and Validation

There exist a wide range of quantitative methods to verify and validate patterns discovered through network visualization methods. While in principle any statistical method can be used to quantitatively analyze a pattern observed in a network, many patterns are often analyzed using graph-based methods (Newman 2010) that specialize in analyzing complex relationships. For example, *degree assortativity* measures whether one type of nodes in a network which have high weighted degree (e.g., subjects that have large nodes in Fig. 14.7), are preferentially connected to another type of nodes that have high degree (e.g., genes that have large nodes in Fig. 14.7), or vice versa.

Another approach that can be used to verify patterns in a network is hierarchical clustering (Johnson and Wichern 1998). This unsupervised learning method attempts to identify the number and boundary of clusters in the data. For example, hierarchical clustering can be used to identify clusters of patients based on their relationship to genes, or clusters of genes based on their relationship to patients. The method begins by putting each node in a separate cluster, and then progressively joins nodes that are most similar based on their relationship to connected nodes. This progressive grouping generates a tree structure called a *dendrogram*, where distances between subsequent layers of the tree represent the strength of dissimilarity between the respective clusters; the larger the distance between two subsequent layers, the stronger the clustering. Analysts therefore determine the number and membership of the clusters by identifying relatively large breaks between the layers in the dendrogram.

Given the wide range of quantitative methods available, the patterns in the network are used to guide the selection of the appropriate method. For example, if distinct clusters do not exist in a network, then it is not appropriate to apply a clustering algorithm to the network. This approach of selecting methods based on the inspection of the data is similar to how statisticians determine whether to use parametric or non-parametric inferential methods based on the underlying distribution of the data.

Because the network in Fig. 14.7 suggested the existence of distinct clusters, hierarchical clustering was used to identify the boundary and members of the clusters. As shown in Fig. 14.8b, the horizontal dendrogram represents the gene clusters, the vertical dendrogram represents the patient clusters, and the colored cells represent normalized gene expression ranging from green (0) to red (1). The dendrograms shows a clear break at two clusters for the genes, and three clusters for subjects (as shown by the corresponding blue dotted lines across each dendrogram).

While there may be clear breaks in the dendrograms, the overall pattern could have occurred by random chance. Patterns discovered in networks, and subsequently the dendrograms, are therefore, validated by determining their significance. One approach to do this is to compare the patterns in the data to random permutations of the network.

To test whether there were significant breaks in the dendrogram (denoting the existence of distinct clusters), the variance, skewness, and kurtosis of the dissimilarities (generated by the hierarchical clustering algorithm) in the flu/RSV network were compared to 1,000 random permutations of the data. For each network permutation, the number of nodes and the number of edges connected to each node, in addition to the edge weight distribution of subjects were preserved when analyzing the gene dendrogram, and vice versa. Significant breaks in the subject or gene dendrograms would result in a significantly larger variance, skewness, and kurtosis of the dissimilarity measures, compared to the same measures generated from the random networks. As previously reported (Bhavnani et al. 2014a, b) the results showed the clusteredness of the subjects in the network was significant as measured by the variance of the dissimilarities (flu/RSV $= 2.75$, Random-Mean $= 0.88$, $p < .001$ two-tailed test), skewness of the distribution of dissimilarities (flu/RSV $= 5.55$, Random-Mean $= 3.94$, $p < .001$ two-tailed test), and kurtosis of the distribution of dissimilarities (flu/RSV $= 38.69$, Random-Mean $= 25.03$, $p < .001$ two-tailed test).

The same approach was used to test the clusteredness of the gene clusters. The results showed that the gene clustering was also significant when compared to 1,000 random networks based on variance of the dissimilarities (flu/RSV $= 2.91$, Random-Mean $= 0.24$, $p < .001$ two-tailed test), skewness of the distribution of dissimilarities (flu/RSV $= 2.01$, Random-Mean $= 0.80$, $p < .001$ two-tailed test), and kurtosis of the distribution of dissimilarities (flu/RSV $= 7.81$, Random-Mean $= 3.16$, $p < .001$ two-tailed test).

To understand why the subjects and genes were clustered, and how they related to each other, the cluster memberships were superimposed onto the network. As shown in Fig. 14.8a, the subject nodes were colored (blue, yellow, and pink) to denote their membership in three separate clusters referred to as core cases, periphery cases, and control-like cases. Furthermore, the 14 genes on the top, and the 4 genes at the bottom also formed distinct clusters, but because they were easy to distinguish by their spatial separation, they were kept black to reduce visual complexity.

As shown in Fig. 14.7, in addition to the above clustering, the core cases appeared to have higher overall gene expression (based on their size which is proportional to the sum of their edge weights) compared to the periphery cases. This pattern was quantitatively verified by comparing the weighted degree centrality (sum of edge weights) of the core cases to those of the periphery cases. This can be done with well-known statistical tests such as the Mann Whitney U test, a non-parametric test, which can be used to determine if the median of a variable is significantly different across two groups.

The results showed that the core cases (Median $= 4.55$) was significantly different ($U = 49.00$, $p < .001$, two-tailed test) compared to the periphery cases (Median $= 2.52$) verifying that the overall gene expression of the patients in the core was higher compared to those in the periphery. Furthermore, the median gene expression of the 14 genes across the 25 core cases (Median $= 4.22$) was significantly higher ($U = 16$, $p < .001$, two-tailed test) compared to the 50 periphery cases (Median $= 1.95$). This pattern can also be seen in the high expression values (shown in mostly red cells) in the upper left-hand corner of the heatmap in Fig. 14.8b. Finally, there was no significant difference ($\chi^2(2, N = 79) = 0.86$, $p = 0.652$) in the proportion of flu vs. RSV patients across the three case clusters, suggesting that the gene-based clustering was common across both types of infection.

The above results of the cluster analysis superimposed over the network, in addition to quantitative analysis of gene expression across the clusters enabled the identification of three potential sub-phenotypes: (1) **core-cases** who had a significantly higher gene expression of the top cluster of 14 genes, (2) **periphery cases** who had a medium expression of the top 14 genes, and (3) **control-like cases** whose profiles were similar to the controls with high expression of the bottom cluster 4 genes. These three sub-phenotypes were common across both infections.

14.4.3   Inference of Sub-phenotypes and Biological Mechanisms

While the visual and quantitative analysis helped to reveal patterns in the data, the ultimate goal of the network analysis is to infer the biological mechanisms involved, and the emergent sub-phenotypes in the data. This inferential step requires an integrated understanding of the molecular and clinical variables.

One approach to conduct such an integrated analysis, is to analyze how the patients in each emergent cluster (based on molecular profiles), differ in their clinical variables. As the primary data included disease severity of each patient (Ioannidis et al. 2012), we used the Mann Whitney U test to analyze if the core and periphery cases were significantly different in their disease severity. The test revealed that the disease severity of core cases (Median $= 7$) was significantly higher ($U = 261.50$, $p < .001$, two-tailed test) compared to periphery cases (Median $= 2$). This result suggested a significant association between the high gene expression of the 14 top genes in the core-cases, and higher disease severity.

The bipartite visualization and quantitative verifications therefore revealed not only sub-phenotypes based on the molecular profiles, but also how they related to clinical variables, which enabled the domain experts to infer three possible sub-phenotypes and their potential pathways (Bhavnani et al. 2014a, b).

1. The **core cases** have significantly higher expression of 14 up-regulated genes, which included 4 histone genes, 4 genes with to date have unknown function in antiviral response, and 6 immune-related genes each of which has a well-known non-overlapping antiviral function. An Ingenuity Pathway Analysis (Ingenuity 2014) of the 14 genes suggested an indirect but strong interferon signature including TNFα and IL-6 cytokines involved in antiviral and innate inflammatory responses. Because the core cases also had a significantly higher disease severity score, they represent a distinct at-risk sub-phenotype that are hyper responsive to pathways targeted to viral clearance, and possibly carry a risk for long-term epithelial cell damage.
2. The **periphery cases** have a medium expression of all 18 genes and therefore suggest a second subphenotype with a subdued anti-viral response relative to the above hyperresponders.
3. The **control-like cases** have a high expression of 4 down-regulated genes, and low expression of the 14 up-regulated genes, and therefore mirror the expression patterns in uninfected controls. The results therefore suggest that the down-regulation of these 4 genes indicates a "protective" phenotype making them similar to the uninfected controls. Existing literature on these genes provide some confirmatory evidence. While the exact role of the high-affinity receptor which binds to the constant portion of IgE (FcER1) is unknown in viral pathogenesis, SNPs included on this gene have been shown to be associated with severe RSV disease (Janssen et al. 2007). Additionally, KLRB1, which has been shown to have inhibitory functions on natural killer (NK) cells (Pozo et al. 2006) was downregulated, suggesting an enhanced antiviral response in patients resembling the immune response of controls. Finally, PTGDR a receptor important in mast cell function was downregulated, but the exact role of this receptor in viral infection is still unknown. Overall, control-like cases suggests a third subphenotype which have a "just enough" response to the virus, without overt

stimulation of virally induced genes, and therefore potentially with reduced bystander damage.

One might argue that the above result could also be the result of the progression of infection over time. For example, the core cases could be at the peak of infection, the periphery cases could be later in the infection, and the control-like cases could be recovering from the infection. However, an additional analysis revealed that the 3 case clusters were not significantly different ($H(2, N = 79) = 2.56$, $p = 0.278$) in time of sample collection after hospitalization. There is of course the possibility that the children were infected at very different times before hospitalization, but controlling such a variable is practically impossible in the analysis of naturally infected humans. Therefore, we provide two explanations for why sample collection time is probably not an adequate explanation for the results: (1) Because all case samples were collected from patients that were hospitalized indicating severe illness, a resolution of such severity in the short time window of 42–72 h is unlikely to occur. (2) The gene expression changes in the PBMCs of the patients suggest a specific induced innate immune response (e.g., Toll-like receptor) to viruses. Such signaling pathways (which induce interferon secretion and contribute to anti-viral immunity) last several days which exceeds the sample collection time window in this study. We therefore propose that the three case clusters are more likely the result of inherent host differences in anti-viral responses, and therefore represent distinct sub-phenotypes.

Informed by these underlying molecular processes, the network analysis of subjects and genes therefore helped to infer not only the sub-phenotypes, but also the possible mechanisms involved, and which sub-phenotypes had a high risk of developing severe complications. The results therefore provided data-driven hypotheses of sub-phenotypes and their mechanisms which can be validated in future research with other datasets. Such analysis therefore could lead to future treatments that are targeted to specific sub-phenotypes, and is therefore an important step towards precision medicine.

14.5   Strengths and Limitations of Network Analysis

Network analysis has several strengths and limitations, whose understanding can lead to informed uses of the method, appropriate interpretation of the results, and insights for future enhancements and complementary methods.

14.5.1   Strengths

Network visualization and analysis provide four distinct strengths for enabling rapid discovery of patterns in complex biomedical data.

1. **Provides Integrative Visualizations.** Because networks are based on graph theory, they provide a tight integration between visual and quantitative analysis. For example as shown in the Fig. 14.8a, networks enable the integrative visualization of multiple raw values (e.g., subject-gene associations, gene expression values, subject phenotype), aggregated values (e.g., sum of gene values), and emergent global patterns (e.g., clusters) in a single representation. This uniform visual representation leverages the parallel processing power of the visual cortex enabling the comprehension of complex multivariate, quantitative relationships.

2. **Guides Quantitative Analysis.** Networks do not require *a priori* assumptions about the relationship of nodes within the data, in contrast to hierarchical clustering or k-means which assume the data is hierarchically organized or contain disjoint clusters, respectively. Instead, by using a simple pairwise representation of nodes and edges, network layouts enable the identification of multiple structures (e.g., hierarchical, disjoint, overlapping, nested) in a single representation (Nooy et al. 2005). Therefore, while layout algorithms such as Kamada-Kawai depend on the force-directed assumption and its implementation, such algorithms are viewed as less biased for data exploration because they do not impose a particular cluster structure on the data, often leading to the identification of more complex structures in the data (Bhavnani et al. 2010). The overall approach therefore enables a more informed selection of quantitative methods to verify the patterns in the data.

3. **Enables Pathway Inference through Co-occurrence.** Network layouts such as the one shown in Fig. 14.8a, preserve highly-correlated variables (such as genes) and display them through clustering. Furthermore, the bipartite network representation enables the comprehension of inter-cluster relationships such as between variable (e.g., genes) clusters and subject clusters. These features provide important clues to domain experts about the pathways that involve those variables. This is in contrast to many supervised learning methods which drop highly correlated variables in an attempt to identify a small number of variables that together can explain the maximum amount of variance in the data. While this approach is powerful for developing predictive models, the reduction in variables could limit the inference of biological pathways involved in the disease.

4. **Accelerates Discovery through Interactivity.** Networks enable high interactivity enabling the rapid modification of the visual representation to match the changing task and representation needs of analysts during the analysis process. For example, nodes that represent patients in a network can be interactively colored or reshaped to represent different variables such as gender and race, enabling the discovery of how they relate to the rest of the network.

14.5.2 Limitations

Networks have three important limitations that are important to understand for their current use, and need to be addressed in future research.

1. **Constrains Number of Node Properties.** While node shape, color and size can represent different variables, there is a limit on the number of variables that can be simultaneously represented. Furthermore, a visual representation can get overloaded with too many colors and shapes, which can mask rather than reveal important patterns in the data. Therefore, while networks can reveal complex multivariate patterns in the data based on a few variables, they often require complimentary visual analytical representations such as Circos ideograms (Krzywinski et al. 2009; Bhavnani et al. 2011a) to explore data that is high-dimensional (e.g., large number of attributes related to entities such as subjects in the network).

2. **Requires Advanced Computational Skills.** While networks provide a rich vocabulary of graphical elements to represent data, their design and use requires iterative refinement based on an understanding of the domain, knowledge of graphic design and cognitive heuristics, and the use of complex interfaces that are designed for those facile in computation. This combination of knowledge required to conduct network analyses makes domain experts dependent on network analysts to generate and refine the representations, which can limit the rapid exploration and interpretation of complex data.

3. **Lacks Systematic Approaches for Finding Structure in Hairballs.** While network layout algorithms are designed to reveal complex and unbiased patterns in multivariate data, they often fail to show any patterns in the data resulting in what is colloquially called a "hairball". In such cases, the nodes appear to be randomly laid out providing little guidance for how to proceed with the analysis. While network applications offer many interactive methods to filter data such as by dropping edges and nodes based on different thresholds, many of these methods are arbitrary and therefore unjustifiable to use when searching for patterns especially in important domains such as biomedicine. There is therefore a need to develop more systematic and defensible methods to find hidden patterns in network hairballs.

14.6 Future Directions in Network Analysis of Biomedical Data

The limitations of networks discussed above motivate future research with the goal of overcoming theoretical, practical, and pedagogical hurdles. **Theoretically**, we need better frameworks that tightly integrate existing theories from cognition, mathematics, and graphic design. Such theories can help predict for example which combination of visual representations can together help researchers to best comprehend patterns in different types of data such as genes versus cytokines. Furthermore, given that many network layouts show no structure, future algorithms should attempt to integrate different methods from machine learning to enable the discovery of hidden patterns. These research directions could enable the rapid discovery of patterns in the age of big data and translational medicine. **Practically**, visual analytical tools tend to be designed for analysts, often requiring substantial programming to make a dataset ready for visualization, and therefore limiting the use of the methods to only a few biologists and physicians. This hurdle motivates the need for tools that enable biologists and physicians to explore data on their own so that they can better leverage their domain knowledge in interpreting the patterns in the data. Of course such patterns need to be statistically validated by subsequent analyses, but currently the exploration and validation is done mostly by analysts, who could miss important associations due to the lack of domain knowledge. **Pedagogically** there needs to be a concerted effort to train the next generation of biomedical informaticians for developing and using novel visual analytical approaches, and to train biologists and physicians on how to make important biomedical discoveries in visual analytical representations of their data. Such advances should enable visual analytics to fully realize its potential to accelerate discoveries in increasingly complex and big biomedical data.

Discussion Questions

1. Why are visualizations and interactivity critical in making discoveries in complex biomedical data?
2. What are the strengths and limitations of networks, and how can future research fully exploit the strengths, and overcome the limitations?

Acknowledgements I thank Shyam Visweswaran, Rohit Divekar, and Bryant Dang for their contributions to this chapter. This research was supported in part by NIH CTSA #UL1TR000071, the Institute for Human Infections and Immunity at UTMB, the Rising Star Award from University of Texas Systems, and CDC/NIOSH #R21OH009441-01A2.

Additional Readings

Card, S., Mackinlay, J. D., & Shneiderman, B. (1999). *Readings in information visualization: Using vision to think*. San Francisco: Morgan Kaufmann Publishers.

Newman, M. E. J. (2010). *Networks: An introduction*. Oxford: Oxford University Press.

Thomas, J. J., & Cook, K. A. (2005). *Illuminating the Path: The R&D agenda for visual analytics national visualization and analytics center*.

Tufte, E. R. (1983). *The visual display of quantitative information*. Chesire: Graphics Press.

References

Albert, R. K. (2004). Boolean modeling of genetic regulatory networks. *Complex Networks, 21*, 459–481.

Amar, R., Eagan, J., & Stasko, J. (2005, October). Low-level components of analytic activity in information visualizations. In *Proceedings of IEEE InfoVis'05*, Minneapolis, MN, USA (pp. 111–117).

Bhavnani, S. K., Bellala, G., Ganesan, A., et al. (2010). The nested structure of cancer symptoms: Implications for analyzing co-occurrence and managing symptoms. *Methods of Information in Medicine, 49*, 581–591.

Bhavnani, S. K., Pillai, R., Calhoun, W. J., et al. (2011a). How circos ideograms complement networks: A case study in asthma. In *Proceedings of AMIA summit on translational bioinformatics*, Bethesda, MD.

Bhavnani, S. K., Victor, S., Calhoun, W. J., et al. (2011b). How cytokines co-occur across asthma patients: From bipartite network analysis to a molecular-based classification. *Journal of Biomedical Informatics, 44*, S24–S30.

Bhavnani, S. K., Bellala, G., Victor, S., et al. (2012). The role of complementary bipartite visual analytical representations in the analysis of SNPs: A case study in ancestral informative markers. *Journal of the American Medical Informatics Association, 19*, e5–e12.

Bhavnani, S. K., Dang, B., Caro, M., Bellala, G., & Visweswaran, S. (2014a). Heterogeneity within and across pediatric pulmonary infections: From bipartite networks to at-risk subphenotypes. In *Proceedings of AMIA summit on translational bioinformatics*, Bethesda, MD.

Bhavnani, S. K., Drake, J. A., & Divekar, R. (2014b). The role of visual analytics in asthma phenotyping and biomarker discovery. In A. Brasier (Ed.), *Heterogeneity in asthma* (pp. 289–305). New York: Springer.

Brownstein, C. A., Brownstein, J. S., Williams, D. S., III, Wicks, P., & Heywood, J. A. (2009). The power of social networking in medicine. *Nature Biotechnology, 27*, 888–890.

Card, S., Mackinlay, J. D., & Shneiderman, B. (1999). *Readings in information visualization: Using vision to think*. San Francisco: Morgan Kaufmann Publishers.

Centers for Disease Control and Prevention. (2014, April 28). Retrieved from the website http://nccd.cdc.gov/DHDSPAtlas/#

Christakis, N. A., & Fowler, J. H. (2010). Social network sensors for early detection of contagious outbreaks. *PLoS ONE, 5*(9), e12948.

Cytoscape. (2014, April 28). Retrieved from the website http://www.cytoscape.org/

Goh, K., Cusick, M., Valle, D., et al. (2007). The human disease network. *Proceedings of the National Academy of Sciences of the United States of America, 104*, 8685.

Heer, J., Bostock, M., & Ogievetsky, V. (2010). A tour through the visualization zoo. *Communications of the ACM, 53*, 59–67.

Hidalgo, C. A., Blumm, N., Barabási, A.-L., & Christakis, N. A. (2009). A dynamic network approach for the study of human phenotypes. *PLoS Computational Biology, 5*(4), e1000353.

Ideker, T., & Sharan, R. (2008). Protein networks in disease. *Genome Research, 18*, 644.

Ingenuity. (2014, April 28). Retrieved from the website http://www.ingenuity.com/products/ipa

Ioannidis, I., McNally, B., Willette, M., et al. (2012). Plasticity and virus specificity of the airway epithelial cell immune response during respiratory virus infection. *Journal of Virology, 86*(10), 5422–5436.

Janssen, R., Bont, L., Siezen, C. L., et al. (2007). Genetic susceptibility to respiratory syncytial virus bronchiolitis is predominantly associated with innate immune genes. *Journal of Infectious Diseases, 196*(6), 826–834.

Johnson, R. A., & Wichern, D. W. (1998). *Applied multivariate statistical analysis*. Upper Saddle River: Prentice-Hall.

Kamada, T., & Kawai, S. (1989). An algorithm for drawing general undirected graphs. *Information Processing Letters, 31*, 7–15.

Krzywinski, M., Schein, J., Birol, I., et al. (2009). Circos: An information aesthetic for comparative genomics. *Genome Research, 19*, 1639–1645.

Liu, Z., & Stasko, J. T. (2010). Mental models, visual reasoning and interaction in information visualization: A top-down perspective. *IEEE Transactions on Visualization and Computer Graphics, 16*(6), 999–1008.

Molloy, J. C. (2011). The open knowledge foundation: Open data means better science. *PLoS Biology, 9*, e1001195.

Newman, M. E. J. (2010). *Networks: An introduction*. Oxford: Oxford University Press.

Nooy, W., Mrvar, A., & Batagelj, V. (2005). *Exploratory social network analysis with Pajek*. Cambridge: Cambridge University Press.

Norman, D. (1993). *Things that make us smart*. New York: Doubleday/Currency.

PatientsLikeMe. (2014, April 28). *PatientsLikeMe*. Retrieved from the website http://www.patientslikeme.com/

Plaisant, C., Chao, T., Wu, J., Hettinger, A. Z., Herskovic, J. R., Johnson, T. R., Bernstam, E. V., Markowitz, E., Powsner, S., & Shneiderman, B. (2013, November 16). Twinlist: Novel user interface designs for medication reconciliation. In *Proceedings of AMIA annual symposium* (pp. 1150–1159).

Pozo, D., Valés-Gómez, M., Mavaddat, N., Williamson, S. C., Chisholm, S. E., & Reyburn, H. (2006). CD161 (human NKR-P1A) signaling in NK cells involves the activation of acid sphingomyelinase. *Journal of Immunology, 176*(4), 2397–2406.

Shneiderman, B. (1996). The eyes have it: A task by data type taxonomy for information visualization. *Visual Languages, 93*, 336–343.

Shneiderman, B., Plaisant, C., & Hesse, B. (2013). Improving health and healthcare with interactive visualization tools. *IEEE Computer, 46*(5), 58–66.

Thomas, J. J., & Cook, K. A. (2005). *Illuminating the path: The R&D agenda for visual analytics national visualization and analytics center*.

Tversky, B., Morrison, J. B., & Betrancourt, M. (2002). Animation: Can it facilitate? *International Journal of Human-Computer Studies, 57*, 247–262.

Yi, J. S., Kang, Y. A., Stasko, J., et al. (2007). Toward a deeper understanding of the role of interaction in information visualization. *IEEE Transactions on Visualization and Computer Graphics, 13*, 357–369.

Zhang, J., & Norman, D. A. (1994). Representations in distributed cognitive tasks. *Cognitive Science, 18*, 87–122.

Index

© Springer International Publishing Switzerland 2015
V.L. Patel et al. (eds.), *Cognitive Informatics for Biomedicine*, Health Informatics,
DOI 10.1007/978-3-319-17272-9

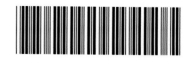